EMQs in Ophthalmology, Dermatology and ENT

An essential revision guide with
comprehensive answers

MUKHTAR BIZRAH
MBBS, BSc
ST1 Ophthalmology Trainee
London Deanery

and

MANAF KHATIB
MBBS
CT1 Core Surgical Trainee
East of England Deanery

Foreword by
JANICE RYMER
Dean of Undergraduate Medicine
King's College London School of Medicine

Radcliffe Publishing
London • New York

Radcliffe Publishing Ltd
33–41 Dallington Street
London
EC1V 0BB
United Kingdom

www.radcliffehealth.com

British Library Cataloguing in Publication Data

A catalogue record for this book is available from the British Library.

ISBN-13: 978 184619 552 5

The paper used for the text pages of this book
is FSC® certified. FSC (The Forest Stewardship
Council®) is an international network to promote
responsible management of the world's forests.

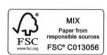

Typeset by Darkriver Design, Auckland, New Zealand
Printed and bound by TJI Digital, Padstow, Cornwall, UK

Contents

Foreword

The General Medical Council has determined that medical school curricula must focus on the 'core' curriculum and, as a result of this, a number of specialty areas have been squeezed out and, because of heavy demands on teaching time, are often completely neglected. Not only does this limit the knowledge that the students graduate with but it restricts the opportunities for the students to be exposed to these specialties and perhaps choose them as their career pathways. These specialties often appear in exam questions but as students have not had adequate preparation for them they often find them challenging.

In their training Drs Mukhtar Bizrah and Manaf Khatib appreciated this and have produced this book to help increase students' and junior doctors' knowledge of three important specialty areas, namely ophthalmology, ENT and dermatology, which is helpful for not only those wishing to consider these areas as career pathways but also for those destined for general practice where knowledge of these areas is pivotal.

Extended Matching Questions are difficult to design and Drs Bizrah and Khatib have done a great job of covering the very wide syllabuses for these subjects while at the same time making reading the book such a pleasurable learning experience. Each junior doctor and medical student could use this book to give them a comprehensive, yet adequately detailed, insight into these specialties. Having all three together makes it a much less daunting prospect than having to go through three textbooks.

It is a delight to read a book written by recently qualified enthusiasts who are now at the coal face of their surgical specialties and so are ideally placed to define what is crucial for treating patients and ensuring patient safety.

Professor Janice Rymer
Dean of Undergraduate Medicine
King's College London School of Medicine
February 2013

Preface

This book presents challenging questions in commonly asked-about topics in the fields of Ophthalmology, Dermatology and ENT. The rationale behind the comprehensive answers provided here is to make this book an all-in-one study and revision tool for these clinical specialties.

Ophthalmology, Dermatology and ENT are known to be areas in which both medical students and clinical trainees lose valuable marks in medical school and college membership examinations. The aim of this book is to help students and clinical trainees overcome barriers to achieving merits and distinctions.

More importantly, signs and symptoms relating to clinical specialties may be the presentation of a sinister disorder, or a disorder significantly affecting a patient's quality of life. This book aims to enable clinicians to have a thorough understanding of the clinical presentation and management of common and important Ophthalmological, Dermatological and ENT disorders.

Mukhtar Bizrah
Manaf Khatib
February 2013

About the authors

Mukhtar Bizrah graduated from St George's University of London in 2010. He received merits in medical and clinical sciences, and he was awarded the London Student of the Year Award. He then completed the 2-year Academic Foundation Programme at Guy's and St Thomas' Hospitals NHS Foundation Trust in London, during which he carried out research in medical education and was awarded a South Thames Foundation School Teaching Merit. He commenced full-time run-through training in Ophthalmology at the London Deanery in 2012.

Manaf Khatib graduated from St George's University of London in 2010. He received distinction in medical science and merit in clinical practice, and he received the Gold-Level Community Education Award. He then completed the 2-year Academic Surgery Foundation Programme at the North West Thames Foundation School and received the Imperial College Teaching Hero Award. He is currently a core surgical trainee at St Andrews Centre for Plastic Surgery and Burns in the East of England Deanery. He is also completing a part-time Master of Science degree in Surgical Sciences at the University of Edinburgh.

List of contributors

Mohamad Fahed Barakat, MBBS, BSc
MSc Medical Statistics Programme
London School of Hygiene and Tropical Medicine

Nana Seiwaa Opare, MBBS, BSc
MSc Clinical Embryology Programme
University of Oxford

Laura-Reim Ismail, MBBS, BSc
ST1 Obstetrics and Gynaecology
St Mary's Hospital
Imperial College Healthcare NHS Trust
London Deanery

Dedication

*In memory of the peaceful demonstrators who bravely
sacrificed for justice, equality, and human rights.*

MB

To my father and grandfather, for being inspirational role models,
for the great gift of education and for their relentless motivation.

To my mother, for her overwhelming love and warmth.
To my wife, for her support and beautiful patience.

To Bahlubi, for driving me to school every day.

MK

To my beloved parents whom I owe everything to. I can't express
enough thanks and gratitude to be able to repay you. Your
unconditional love, selflessness, sacrifices and unwavering support
is something I aspire to be able to provide to my future family.

To my dear friend Mukhtar, your drive and spirit is contagious.
The book will not exist without you! You are a role model
for any clinician. I am blessed to have met you.

To my brothers Karim and Faisal for their
continuous support and encouragement.

Section A

Ophthalmology EMQs

Q **Ophthalmology Q1 – Sudden painless visual loss**
A. Acute anterior uveitis
B. Anterior ischaemic optic neuropathy
C. Central retinal artery occlusion
D. Central retinal vein occlusion
E. Diabetic maculopathy
F. Meningitis
G. Migraine
H. Optic neuritis
I. Retinal detachment
J. Vitreous haemorrhage

From the list above, choose the most likely diagnosis for each of the following examples.

1. A 70-year-old woman presents to A&E complaining of a 1-day history of sudden loss of vision in her left eye. She denies any redness or pain in her eye, but she does complain of a severe left-sided headache. She has been feeling generally unwell over the past few weeks and has unintentionally lost about 4 kg in weight. Funduscopy reveals left-sided optic disc swelling, flame haemorrhages and cotton wool spots.

2. A 70-year-old man presents to A&E complaining of a 2-hour history of sudden loss of vision in his left eye. He denies any other ocular symptoms. He reports experiencing temporary visual loss in his other eye a few months ago. His eye is not red or painful, and can move normally without pain. He has a past medical history of type 2 diabetes, hypertension, angina and ankylosing spondylitis. His visual acuity is 6/9 on the right, but he can only see light with his left eye. Funduscopy reveals an unremarkable right fundus, while on the left side the retina is generally pale with a dense red spot at the fovea.

3. A 70-year-old man presents to A&E complaining of sudden loss of vision in his left eye that occurred 2 hours ago. He does not complain of any other ocular symptoms. His eye is not red or painful, and can move normally without pain. He has a past medical history of type 2 diabetes, hypertension and angina. His visual acuity is 6/12 on the left and 6/60 on the right. Red eye reflex is present on the right but absent on the left. Funduscopy reveals proliferative diabetic retinopathy in the right eye, but nothing can be visualised in the left eye.

4. A 70-year-old man presents to A&E complaining of a 2-hour history of sudden loss of vision in his left eye. He does not complain of any other ocular symptoms. His eye is not red or painful, with normal painless ocular movement. He has a past medical history of type 2 diabetes, hypertension and angina. He has a 22-pack-year history of smoking. His visual acuity is 6/12 on the right and 6/60 on the left. Funduscopy reveals optic disc swelling, venous dilation and tortuosity and retinal flame-shaped haemorrhages in the left fundus. There are a few microaneurysms in the right fundus.

5. A 70-year-old male presents to A&E complaining of sudden loss of vision in his left eye. He says he has been seeing black spots and flashing lights with his left eye for the past few days. This morning he saw a black shadow coming down his left eye, and his vision is very blurry now. On examination, his visual acuity is 6/9 in the right eye but he can only see hand movements with the left eye.

Ophthalmology Q2 – Painful eye

A. Acute primary angle-closure glaucoma
B. Anterior uveitis
C. Bacterial conjunctivitis
D. Bacterial keratitis
E. Endophthalmitis
F. Episcleritis
G. Optic neuritis
H. Orbital cellulitis
I. Scleritis
J. Viral keratitis

From the list above, choose the most likely diagnosis for each of the following examples.

1. A 41-year-old woman presents to A&E with a 1-day history of nausea, vomiting and abdominal pain. She also complains of a severe frontal headache and a right eye pain that she describes as worse than labour. She has a past medical history of hypertension and type 1 diabetes mellitus. On examination, her right eye is red and her cornea is cloudy. She only lets you shine light into her right eye for a few seconds, but unlike her left pupil, her right pupil is clearly unreactive to light. Vision is 6/60 in the right eye and 6/9 in the left.

2. A 38-year-old woman presents to A&E with a 2-day history of a red and painful right eye. The pain is described as 8 out of 10 in severity. She has a past medical history of hypertension and a chronic cough. She is wearing sunglasses and refuses to let you shine any direct light into her eyes. On taking off her glasses, you note that her right pupil is constricted. Visual acuity is 6/90 in the right eye and 6/6 in the left. You also notice raised red lesions on her shins.

3. A 68-year-old woman presents to A&E with a 1-day history of a red and painful right eye. She complains that her ocular pain and vision are worsening by the hour. Her right and left cataracts were operated on 4 days ago and 5 months ago, respectively. On examination, her right conjunctiva is inflamed, cornea is opaque, and there is a profuse green discharge. She also has a white fluid level in the anterior chamber. She can only count fingers with her right eye, while her visual acuity is 6/9 on the left. She has a relative afferent pupillary defect in the right eye.

4. A 71-year-old woman presents to A&E with a red, irritable right eye. She is very scared as her right eye is producing a sticky green discharge. She does not have photophobia and has not noticed any change to her vision. She has a past medical history of hypertension and type 2 diabetes mellitus. Her pupils are equal and reactive to light. Visual acuity is unchanged from her previous tests.

5. A 42-year-old woman presents to A&E complaining of loss of vision in her left eye. She says that she noticed her vision was blurred when she woke up this morning. She has also had pain behind her left eye for the past 2 days. There is no eye redness or discharge. On examination, her visual acuity is 6/9 in her right eye and 6/36 in her left eye. She has a full range of eye movements bilaterally, and a left relative afferent pupillary defect. Visual field testing reveals a central scotoma in the left eye. She has a past medical history of rheumatoid arthritis, asthma and hay fever. Funduscopy is unremarkable in both eyes.

Ophthalmology Q3 – Red eye

A. Anterior uveitis
B. Bacterial conjunctivitis
C. Bacterial keratitis
D. Corneal laceration
E. Herpes simplex virus keratitis
F. Herpes zoster ophthalmicus
G. Marginal keratitis
H. Orbital cellulitis
I. Sjögren's syndrome
J. Viral conjunctivitis

From the list above, choose the most appropriate diagnosis for each of the following examples.

1. A 56-year-old woman presents to A&E with a painful red right eye. She says that her eye is very painful, sensitive to light and watery. She feels like there is something in her eyelid, although she has removed her contact lenses. Blinking worsens her pain. Her visual acuity is 6/36 in the right eye, and 6/6 in the left. She has multiple small, white opacities in the right corneal stroma. After administering anaesthetic and fluorescein eye drops, a small irregular lesion stains green on her right cornea.

2. A 45-year-old woman presents to A&E with a red and painful left eye. She has had a kidney transplant 3 weeks ago but has been fine otherwise. On examination, there is conjunctival injection in the left eye, and fluorescein staining reveals a dendritic defect with terminal bulbs on the left cornea. Visual acuity is 6/6 on the right and 6/9 on the left.

3. An 81-year-old man presents to A&E with a vesicular rash over his right forehead. The rash extends to the midline, involving the upper eyelid. The patient complains of visual loss, pain and photophobia in the right eye. Visual acuity is 6/60 in the right eye, and 6/9 in the left. On examination, the patient has signs of right eye conjunctivitis and anterior uveitis.

4. A 79-year-old man presents to A&E with an extremely painful and photophobic red right eye that has been this way for the past 24 hours. Although his eyes are normally very dry, his right eye has been very tearful. He has also noticed blurring of his vision. He is known to have chronic blepharitis, asthma and hypertension. On slit-lamp examination, there are multiple

superficial infiltrates in the peripheral cornea, but the corneal epithelium is intact. Visual acuity is 6/36 in the right eye and 6/9 in the left.

5. A 16-year-old girl presents with painful and reduced right eye movements. Her right eye vision is blurry, and she also complains of double vision. She has no significant past medical history. On examination, her right eyelid is red and swollen, and her right eye is slightly proptosed. Her body temperature is 38.2°C.

Q **Ophthalmology Q4 – Management of red eye**
A. Advice on infection control
B. Conjunctival swab and topical antibiotics
C. Lid hygiene and topical antibiotics
D. Lid hygiene and artificial tears
E. Lid hygiene, artificial tears and topical antibiotics
F. Oral non-steroidal anti-inflammatory drugs (NSAIDs)
G. Topical and systemic steroids
H. Topical antibiotics
I. Topical antihistamines
J. Topical antihistamines and mast cell stabilisers

From the list above, choose the most appropriate mainstay of treatment for each of the following examples.

1. A 67-year-old woman presents to the GP with irritable red eyes. Her eyes have been red and sticky for the past 3 days, and there is now a green discharge in both eyes. She has been having intermittent redness and grittiness of both eyes over the past 3 years, and her eyes are always dry. On examination, some of her eyelashes are clumped together, with crusts at the base of the eyelashes. Her eyelids look inflamed. Her vision is unaffected bilaterally.

2. A 36-year-old woman presents to her GP with redness and a severe pain in her left eye that has been worsening over the past 3 days. There is no discharge from the eyes, and she has not noticed a difference in her vision. She has not been in contact with anyone with similar symptoms. She has a past medical history of Crohn's disease and rheumatoid arthritis. On examination her vision is unaffected, and there is a diffuse redness in the sclera. She requests painkillers, as the eye pain is terrible and has kept her up all night.

3. A 33-year-old woman presents to the GP with irritable red eyes. Her eyes have been red and watery for the past 3 days, and she describes a sensation of 'discomfort' in her eyes, but denies any pain. She has never had this before, although her husband had similar symptoms a week ago. She has a past medical history of asthma and hay fever. She says her vision is blurry first thing in the morning, but on examination her visual acuity is unaffected.

4. A 33-year-old woman presents to the GP with irritable red eyes. Her eyes have been red and watery for the past 3 days, and she

describes a sensation of itchiness in both eyes. She gets similar symptoms at the same time every year. She has a past medical history of asthma and hay fever. Her vision is unaffected.

5. A 3-day-old baby develops redness in her left eye with a greenish discharge. She was born at term via a vaginal delivery. There were no complications during delivery, although labour took about 20 hours. Both the baby and her 22-year-old mother are otherwise well.

Q Ophthalmology Q5 – Diplopia

A. Carotid artery dissection
B. Carotid cavernous sinus fistula
C. Fourth cranial nerve palsy
D. Graves' ophthalmopathy
E. Lung cancer
F. Myasthenia gravis
G. Ocular myositis
H. Orbital blowout fracture
I. Orbital cellulitis
J. Posterior communicating artery aneurysm

From the list above, choose the most appropriate diagnosis for each of the following examples.

1. A 56-year-old lady presents with double vision and increased lacrimation. Double vision is worse on upgaze. Her eyes are red and gritty. There is bilateral conjunctival oedema and proptosis. She has lost 5 kg in the past 2 months, despite having a good appetite. She has a past medical history of diabetes insipidus and antiphospholipid syndrome. Her visual acuity is 6/9 in both eyes. No abnormalities are seen on ophthalmoscopy. A CT scan shows ocular muscle thickening.

2. An 86-year-old lady presents following a fall with right eye redness and double vision. She has a past medical history of hypertension, osteoporosis and Alzheimer's disease. On examination, her right conjunctiva is injected and swollen. You can hear a right ocular bruit on auscultation. Visual acuity is 6/18 in the right eye and 6/9 in the left eye. No abnormalities are seen on ophthalmoscopy.

3. An 86-year-old lady presents with a headache and a left eye ptosis. She has a past medical history of hypertension, osteoporosis and Alzheimer's disease. On lifting her eyelid, her left pupil is dilated and unreactive to light, and she complains of double vision. Her right pupil is normal. Her visual acuity is 6/9 in both eyes. No abnormalities are seen on ophthalmoscopy.

4. A 48-year-old lady presents with neck pain. She also has a slight right eye ptosis with a constricted right pupil. She has a past medical history of hypertension and type 2 diabetes mellitus. Her visual acuity is 6/9 in both eyes. No abnormalities are seen on ophthalmoscopy.

5. A 54-year-old lady presents to her GP complaining of double vision that comes on and off during the day. She has also noticed that her eyelids become droopy towards the end of the day. She has a past medical history of hypertension, type 2 diabetes mellitus and rheumatoid arthritis. On examination, her pupils are equal and reactive to light, and there is slight bilateral ptosis. Visual acuity is 6/6 in both eyes. No abnormalities are seen on ophthalmoscopy. After placing an ice pack over her right, closed eyelid, her ptosis resolves.

Q Ophthalmology Q6 – Management of ocular conditions

A. Acetazolamide
B. Aciclovir
C. Aciclovir and prednisolone
D. Cyclopentolate
E. Iridotomy
F. Latanoprost
G. Pilocarpine
H. Prednisolone
I. Timolol
J. Trabeculectomy

From the list above, choose the most appropriate option for each of the following examples.

1. Topical agent used to reduce formation of aqueous humour in acute angle-closure glaucoma.
2. Definitive management of acute angle-closure glaucoma.
3. Used to relieve pain and photophobia in anterior uveitis.
4. Used to treat a dendritic corneal ulcer caused by herpes simplex keratitis.
5. Used to treat herpes zoster ophthalmicus.

Q Ophthalmology Q7 – Ophthalmological terms

A. Amblyopia
B. Anisocoria
C. Astigmatism
D. Diplopia
E. Emmetropia
F. Flare
G. Floaters
H. Hypermetropia
I. Hyphaema
J. Hypopyon
K. Myopia
L. Photopsia
M. Scotoma
N. Stereoscopic vision
O. Strabismus

From the list above, choose the most appropriate option for each of the following examples.

1. An ophthalmological term for long-sighted vision.
2. Refers to unilateral or bilateral reduced visual acuity for which no organic cause can be found.
3. Refers to visualisation of the slit-lamp beam due to increased protein in the anterior chamber fluid.
4. Is when light rays from different angles do not meet at a single focal point in the retina because of a non-spherical cornea.
5. Refers to a white fluid level in the anterior chamber.

Q **Ophthalmology Q8 – Eye structure and function**

A. Ciliary body
B. Cornea
C. Iris
D. Lens
E. Levator palpebrae superioris
F. Müller's muscle
G. Orbicularis oculi
H. Retina
I. Trabecular meshwork
J. Zonules

From the list above, choose the most appropriate option for each of the following examples.

1. Major refractive structure of the eye.
2. Is innervated by the seventh cranial nerve.
3. Is innervated by sympathetic fibres.
4. Responsible for aqueous humour formation.
5. Contraction of this structure increased the refractive power of the eye.

Q Ophthalmology Q9 – Features of chronic ocular disorders

A. Annular mid-peripheral scotoma
B. Arcuate scotoma
C. Central scotoma
D. Cherry-red spot at the fovea
E. Choroidal neovascular membrane
F. Roth's spots
G. Loss of red reflex
H. Optic disc:cup ratio of 0.3
I. Pigmented fundus lesion
J. Proliferative retinopathy

From the list above, choose the most appropriate clinical finding for each of the following examples.

1. A 71-year-old patient presents to his GP with blurry vision. He says this started a few days ago. He has a past medical history of hypertension and chronic renal failure. Visual acuity is 6/9 in the right eye and 6/18 in the left. Visual acuity was 6/9 in both eyes last year. Visual fields are normal. Amsler grid testing reveals left eye metamorphopsia. What is the characteristic visual field defect in this disease?

2. A 62-year-old patient presents to his GP for review of his blood pressure control. He has a past medical history of hypertension and rheumatic fever. His blood pressure is 170/97. His blood glucose level is normal. Visual acuity is 6/9 bilaterally. Funduscopy reveals bilateral optic disc cupping. What is a characteristic visual field defect in this disease?

3. An 18-year-old woman presents to her GP. She has just acquired a full driving licence, but she is complaining of difficulty driving at night because she cannot see clearly. She has no significant past medical history. Her visual acuity is 6/5 in both eyes. Her visual field is slightly constricted. Funduscopy reveals arteriolar narrowing and bone-spicule pigmentation. An electroretinogram shows reduced signals. What is the most characteristic finding in this disease?

4. A 78-year-old patient presents to his GP with blurry vision that he says has been getting worse over the past few months. Visual acuity is 6/9 in the right eye and 6/18 in the left. Visual fields are normal. Funduscopy reveals bilateral drusen deposits. What is the characteristic visual field defect in this disease?

5. A 68-year-old patient presents to his GP complaining of blurred vision. He is finding it increasingly difficult to drive at night because of the dazzling rays of light from oncoming car headlights. He has a past medical history of type 2 diabetes mellitus and hypertension. Visual acuity is 6/9 in the right eye and 6/12 in the left. What is a characteristic finding in this disease?

Q **Ophthalmology Q10 – Management of chronic ocular disorders**
A. 5-Fluorouracil
B. Dorzolamide
C. Focal laser photocoagulation
D. Laser trabeculoplasty
E. Panretinal laser photocoagulation
F. Photodynamic therapy
G. Prednisolone
H. Ranibizumab
I. Timolol
J. Trabeculectomy

From the list above, choose the most appropriate first-line management option for each of the following examples.

1. A 60-year-old patient is referred to an ophthalmologist, after having been found to have a raised intraocular pressure by the optometrist. He does not complain of any visual symptoms. He has a past medical history of hypertension, ischaemic heart disease, congestive heart failure and psoriasis. On examination, his visual acuity is 6/9 in both eyes. Automated perimetry reveals bilateral superior visual field defects. Funduscopy reveals bilateral optic disc cupping as well as inferior optic disc rim notching.

2. A 64-year-old patient is referred to an ophthalmologist after having been found to have retinal neovascularisation. He does not complain of any visual symptoms. He has a past medical history of hypertension, ischaemic heart disease and type 2 diabetes mellitus. On examination, his visual acuity is 6/6 in the right eye and 6/9 in the left eye. He does not have visual field loss. Funduscopy reveals bilateral flame shaped haemorrhages, cotton wool spots and retinal neovascularisation.

3. A 64-year-old patient is referred to an ophthalmologist after having been found to have diabetic retinopathy. He says that his vision has been deteriorating for months. He has a past medical history of hypertension, ischaemic heart disease, congestive heart failure and type 2 diabetes mellitus. On examination, his visual acuity is 6/12 in the right eye and 6/18 in the left eye. He does not have visual field loss. Funduscopy reveals hard exudates and an oedematous looking retina. An ocular coherence tomography scan confirms the presence of bilateral macular oedema.

4. A 73-year-old patient is referred to an ophthalmologist with visual blurring. He says that straight lines look distorted, and this is confirmed with an Amsler grid. He has a past medical history of hypertension, asthma and cataracts removal. Investigations reveal that he has wet age-related macular degeneration. He is very distressed by this and asks if there is a treatment that can improve his vision.

5. A 60-year-old patient has tried several medications to control his glaucoma, all of which have failed. He does not mind trying non-medical treatment options, and wants the most effective and reliable treatment available for his glaucoma.

Q Ophthalmology Q11 – Ophthalmic tests

A. Amsler grid
B. Biometry
C. Fundus fluorescein angiography
D. Gonioscopy
E. Ishihara test
F. Keratometry
G. LogMAR charts
H. Perimetry
I. Seidel test
J. Tonometry

From the list above, choose the most appropriate answer for each of the following examples.

1. Used to measure visual acuity.
2. Used to plot visual fields.
3. Used to calculate the power of the intraocular lens to be implanted after cataract removal.
4. Used to view the anterior chamber angle.
5. Used to detect a corneal leak.

Ophthalmology Q12 – Ocular manifestations of vascular diseases
A. Central retinal artery occlusion
B. Diabetic maculopathy
C. Grade 1 hypertensive retinopathy
D. Grade 2 hypertensive retinopathy
E. Grade 3 hypertensive retinopathy
F. Grade 4 hypertensive retinopathy
G. Mild non-proliferative diabetic retinopathy
H. Moderate non-proliferative diabetic retinopathy
I. Severe non-proliferative diabetic retinopathy
J. Sickle cell retinopathy

From the list above, choose the most likely diagnosis for each of the following examples.

1. A 68-year-old patient presents to his GP feeling generally unwell. He has recently registered at the GP practice and has not seen a doctor in years. His blood pressure is 170/95, and his blood glucose level is 10. Funduscopy reveals prominent intraretinal microvascular abnormalities, intraretinal haemorrhages and fluffy white lesions.

2. A 68-year-old patient presents to his GP feeling generally unwell. He has recently registered at the GP practice and has not seen a doctor in years. His blood pressure is 170/95, and his blood glucose level is 10. Funduscopy reveals arterioles with a broad light reflex, as well as narrowing of the veins at their crossing with arteries.

3. A 68-year-old patient presents to his GP with a blurry vision in the right eye that has been gradually worsening for the past 3 months. He has recently registered at the GP practice and has not seen a doctor in years. His blood pressure is 170/95, and his blood glucose level is 10. Funduscopy reveals no obvious abnormality.

4. A 68-year-old patient presents to his GP feeling generally unwell. He has recently registered at the GP practice and has not seen a doctor in years. His blood pressure is 195/100, and his blood glucose level is 10. Funduscopy reveals arterioles with a broad light reflex, flame-shaped haemorrhages, cotton wools spots and optic disc swelling in both eyes.

5. A 68-year-old patient presents to his GP feeling generally unwell. He has recently registered at the GP practice and has not seen

a doctor in years. His blood pressure is 170/95, and his blood glucose level is 10. Funduscopy reveals tortuous veins, retinal haemorrhages and 'sea fan'-shaped neovascularisation.

Q Ophthalmology Q13 – Visual impairment

A. 6/9
B. 6/12
C. 6/60
D. 3/60
E. Age-related macular degeneration
F. Cataract
G. Diabetic retinopathy
H. Galilean telescope
I. Newtonian telescope
J. Uncorrected refractive errors

From the list above, choose the most appropriate option for each of the following examples.

1. The commonest cause of registered blindness in the Western world.
2. The commonest cause of visual impairment worldwide.
3. A person can be registered as sight impaired if their visual field is normal, and their best visual acuity is less than this.
4. According to UK driving regulations, this is the absolute minimum visual acuity in the best eye required to drive a private car.
5. Used as a low-vision aid.

Q Ophthalmology Q14 – HIV eye disease

A. Carotid cavernous sinus fistula
B. Cytomegalovirus retinopathy
C. Herpes simplex keratitis
D. HIV microvasculopathy
E. Hypertensive retinopathy
F. Kaposi's sarcoma
G. Lymphoma
H. Molluscum contagiosum
I. Thyroid eye disease
J. Toxoplasma retinochoroiditis

From the list above, choose the most appropriate diagnosis for each of the following examples.

1. A 40-year-old man with a history of HIV presents to the GP surgery complaining of visual blurring and seeing dark spots in front of his right eye. He has no other significant past medical history. Visual acuity is 6/18 in the right eye, and 6/6 in the left. Funduscopy reveals a white exudative region nasal to the macula, containing large flame-shaped haemorrhages.

2. A 40-year-old man with a history of HIV presents to the GP surgery complaining of a 1-day history of a painful red right eye with visual blurring and photophobia. He has no other significant past medical history. On examination, his right pupil is small and his visual acuity is 6/18 in the right eye, and 6/6 in the left. Slit-lamp examination reveals a hazy vitreous and a pigmented retinal scar with adjacent white fluffy lesions.

3. A 40-year-old man with a history of HIV presents to the GP surgery complaining of dry eyes. He has no other significant past medical history. Visual acuity is 6/6 in the right eye, and 6/6 in the left. Funduscopy reveals numerous bilateral cotton wool spots. His blood pressure is 130/85 and his blood glucose level is 7.

4. A 40-year-old man with a history of HIV presents to the GP surgery. He is concerned about a small lump underneath his lower eyelid. His partner has noticed that the lump is getting bigger. He has no other significant past medical history. On examination, the lump is nodular and dark red in colour. It is non-tender and non-blanching on palpation. Visual acuity is 6/6 in the right eye, and 6/6 in the left. No abnormality is seen on funduscopy.

5. A 40-year-old man with a history of HIV presents to the GP surgery. He complains that his right eye is bulging out. He also complains of new double vision. He has no other significant past medical history. On examination, there is bilateral proptosis, the right more than the left. He also has tender swellings on the lateral sides of his neck and his right supraclavicular region. Visual acuity is 6/6 in the right eye, and 6/6 in the left. Visual fields are normal. No abnormality is seen on funduscopy.

Q **Ophthalmology Q15 – Ocular side effects of drugs**
- A. Amiodarone
- B. Atropine
- C. Corticosteroids
- D. Digoxin
- E. Ethambutol
- F. Hydroxychloroquine
- G. Morphine
- H. Tamoxifen
- I. Vigabatrin
- J. Warfarin

From the list above, choose the most likely culprit of each of the following stated side effects.
1. Xanthopsia.
2. Vortex keratopathy and grey skin discolouration.
3. Cataracts and glaucoma.
4. Miosis.
5. Bull's eye maculopathy.

Q **Ophthalmology Q16 – Ocular conditions in the developing world**

A. Azithromycin

B. Frequent face and eye washing

C. Ivermectin

D. Ocular lubricants

E. Phacoemulsification

F. Rifampicin, isoniazid, pyrazinamide and ethambutol

G. Valganciclovir

H. Vitamin A supplementation

I. Vitamin E supplementation

J. Will resolve spontaneously

From the list above, choose the most appropriate management option for each of the following examples.

1. A 53-year-old man attends the eye casualty clinic with a left irritable red eye. He complains of a very distressing foreign body sensation in his eye. He has noticed deterioration in his vision but otherwise he has no other ocular symptoms. He has a past medical history of malaria and hypertension. He lives in Malawi, and is currently visiting his daughter in the United Kingdom. On examination, he has marked tarsal conjunctival scarring, and ingrowing eyelashes that are rubbing against the globe. Visual acuity is 6/9 in both eyes.

2. A 49-year-old Bangladeshi woman presents to the eye casualty clinic with blurry vision in the right eye. She first noticed the blurry vision about 2 weeks ago but was too busy to see her doctor. She is now feeling generally unwell, and is worried that her vision is getting worse. She does not have any other ocular symptoms otherwise, and is normally fit and healthy. On examination, her temperature is 38.4°C. Her blood pressure, heart rate, respiratory rate and blood glucose level are all within normal limits. On funduscopy, the optic nerve appears normal, but there are white lesions with indistinct borders at the posterior pole of the eye.

3. A 46-year-old woman presents to the eye casualty clinic with a red and painful right eye. She explains that this has recently been a frequent problem for which she been seeing her doctor in Yemen. On examination, the right eye is photophobic, and there are snowflake opacities in the cornea. Visual acuity is 6/18 in the right eye and 6/9 in the left. Intraocular pressure is 16 mmHg in

the right eye and 15 mmHg in the left. You notice a number of subcutaneous nodules on her arms.

4. An 8-year-old boy is brought to eye casualty clinic by his father. The boy's father is concerned that his son is going blind. His son trips frequently when walking at night because he cannot see things clearly. Apart from dry eyes, he does not have any other ocular symptoms. He has a past medical history of ocular infections that were treated with topical antibiotics. On examination, the eyes are clearly dry, and there are a number of small triangular plaques surrounding the cornea. Visual acuity is 6/6 in both eyes.

5. A 72-year-old refugee from Zimbabwe presents to eye casualty clinic with blurry vision in the right eye. His vision is worse at night, which is debilitating, as he is irreversibly blind in the left eye because of a childhood injury. He has a past medical history of hypertension, type 2 diabetes mellitus, osteoporosis and tuberculosis. On examination, both his blood pressure and blood glucose levels are normal. Visual acuity is 6/36 in the right eye, and he can only count fingers with the left. There is loss of the red light reflex in both eyes. Funduscopy is very difficult in both eyes, because of a white dense opacity in the anterior segment. The intraocular pressure is 18 mmHg in both eyes.

Q **Ophthalmology Q17 – Ocular signs I**

A. Band keratopathy

B. Congenital Horner's syndrome

C. Fuch's endothelial dystrophy

D. Hyperlipidaemia

E. Keratoconus

F. Osteogenesis imperfecta

G. Pterygium

H. Vernal keratoconjunctivitis

I. Viral conjunctivitis

J. Wilson's disease

From the list above, choose the most appropriate diagnosis from each of the following clinical findings stated.

1. Blue sclera.

2. Giant papillae.

3. Guttata.

4. Heterochromic irides.

5. Fleischer ring.

Q Ophthalmology Q18 – Ocular signs II

A. Band keratopathy
B. Congenital Horner's syndrome
C. Fuch's endothelial dystrophy
D. Hyperlipidaemia
E. Keratoconus
F. Neurofibromatosis
G. Osteogenesis imperfecta
H. Pinguecula
I. Pterygium
J. Wilson's disease

From the list above, choose the most appropriate diagnosis from each of the following clinical findings stated.

1. Circumferential opacity around the limbus.
2. Leish nodules.
3. Small grey-white corneal deposits containing small holes.
4. Triangular-shaped yellow-white conjunctiva growth extending to the peripheral cornea.
5. Vogt's striae.

Q Ophthalmology Q19 – Pupillary disorders

A. Adie's pupil

B. Amaurotic pupil

C. Argyll Robertson pupil

D. Horner's syndrome

E. Marcus Gunn pupil

F. Occulomotor nerve lesion

G. Opiate use

H. Physiological anisocoria

I. Trochlear nerve lesion

J. None of the above

From the list above, choose the most appropriate diagnosis for each of the following examples.

1. A 48-year-old lady presents to her GP complaining of ptosis and double vision. She has a past medical history of type 1 diabetes mellitus, for which she takes insulin injections. On inspection, she has a profound left-sided ptosis. On lifting her eyelid, the left eye is looking down and out. The pupil is not dilated, and reacts normally to light and accommodation. She does not have a right-sided ptosis, and her right pupil reacts normally to light and accommodation.

2. A 48-year-old man presents to his GP complaining of unequally sized pupils. He has a past medical history of rheumatoid arthritis and psoriasis, and is on a number of medications for these conditions. His pupils are small and irregular even when the room is dark. The pupils constrict when focusing on a near object but do not react to light.

3. A 28-year-old lady presents to her GP complaining of weakness in her hands. She has a past medical history of asthma, for which she is on various inhalers. On examination, there is wasting of the hand muscles as well as loss of pain and temperature sensation in both of her hands. You also note that the right pupil is constricted and remains constricted in a dark room. The left pupil appears to be normal, and slightly dilates in a dark room.

4. A 58-year-old lady presents to her GP complaining of a severe left-sided headache. This has started yesterday and is getting worse. She has a past medical history of hypertension, for which she takes various anti-hypertensive medications. On examination, you notice an oval-looking left pupil that is poorly reactive

to light. Her right pupil has a normal round shape and reacts normally to light.

5. A 48-year-old lady presents to her GP complaining of unequal pupils. She has a past medical history of hypertension, which she is trying to control with lifestyle measures. On slit-lamp examination, her pupils show slow and incomplete constriction to light, and a sustained accommodation to a near object. Topical 0.125% pilocarpine drops result in rapid pupil constriction.

Q Ophthalmology Q20 – Paediatric ophthalmology

A. Concomitant squint
B. Congenital cataracts
C. Congenital glaucoma
D. Familial exudative vitreoretinopathy
E. Nasolacrimal duct obstruction
F. Non-concomitant squint
G. Ophthalmia neonatorum
H. Retinoblastoma
I. Retinopathy of prematurity
J. Sickle cell retinopathy

From the list above, choose the most appropriate diagnosis for each of the following examples.

1. A mother brings in her 3-year-old son, concerned that he is developing a squint. The child was born at 41 weeks' gestation via an uncomplicated vaginal delivery, and has been fit and healthy otherwise. On examination, the child has a squint in all directions of gaze. He can only fixate his left eye on a target. When the left eye is occluded, the right eye moves outwards to fixate on the target.

2. A mother brings in her 7-week-old baby to the GP, explaining that she has noticed that her baby is constantly tearing from the right eye. She has not noticed any coloured discharge or other abnormalities. The baby was born via a vaginal delivery at 34 weeks' gestation, and has been healthy otherwise. On examination, the baby has normal vital signs. Her right eye is watery with mucous accumulation over the eyelashes. There is no eye redness or purulent discharge. The pupil appears normal, and funduscopy is unremarkable.

3. An ophthalmologist examines a baby delivered at 30 weeks' gestation who weighs 1.1 kg. On ophthalmoscopy, she finds a white pupillary reflex in the right eye and peripheral proliferative retinopathy in the left eye. There is no eye redness or discharge. The baby has normal vital signs.

4. A mother brings in her 6-month-old baby to the GP, complaining that her baby is continuously tearing from his eyes. She has not noticed any eye redness or discharge. The baby was born via a vaginal delivery at 34 weeks' gestation, and has been healthy otherwise. On examination, both eyes look enlarged, with large

cloudy corneas. There is no eye redness or purulent discharge, and the pupils appear normal. Funduscopy is difficult due to the corneal haziness. The baby has normal vital signs.

5. An infant is delivered at 36 weeks' gestation via normal vaginal delivery. A physical examination reveals no abnormality, but a white fundus reflex is noted in the right eye. There is no eye redness or discharge, and the pupil looks otherwise normal. The baby's father does remember that he had a white eye as a baby, but does not know what the diagnosis was. The baby has normal vital signs, and is urgently referred to an ophthalmologist.

Ophthalmology Q21 – Ocular trauma

A. Clean the tarsal conjunctiva
B. Clean the tarsal conjunctiva and topical antibiotics
C. Intravenous steroids
D. Lateral canthotomy and cantholysis
E. Observation
F. Ocular irrigation and topical antibiotics
G. Surgical reduction
H. Topical antibiotics, padding and analgesia
I. Topical steroids
J. Topical steroids, topical antibiotics and padding

From the list above, choose the most appropriate management option for each of the following examples.

1. A 33-year-old man presents to A&E with a red painful left eye, after having splashed cement on it while at work. The ocular pain is getting worse, and he is afraid of losing his eyesight. On slit-lamp examination, there is conjunctival injection and swelling in the left eye with traces of cement as well as mild corneal oedema. Visual acuity is 6/6 in the right eye, and 6/12 in the left.

2. A 26-year-old man presents to A&E with a bruised left eye. He was playing rugby this morning when another player's knee hit his right eye. He thought all he needed was rest, but he is experiencing significantly worsening pain and blurring in his left eye. He has no significant past ocular history. On examination, his left eye has eyelid ecchymosis and an extensive subconjunctival haemorrhage. The eye is also slightly proptosed, and there is increased intraocular pressure and a relative afferent pupillary defect. Visual acuity is 6/6 in the right eye and 6/60 in the left eye.

3. A 74-year-old lady presents to her GP with double vision that is worse on looking up and down. She has a past medical history of hypertension, osteoporosis and Alzheimer's disease. On examination, there is an area of reduced sensation on the cheek underneath the left eye. Her visual acuity is 6/9 in both eyes. No abnormalities are seen on ophthalmoscopy.

4. A 39-year-old man presents to A&E with severe pain, foreign body sensation and watering in the right eye. He was on his way back home after a long day of welding when his symptoms started. He refuses to let you come close to his eye, but after instilling several drops of tetracaine into his eye, his pain almost completely

resolves. On ophthalmoscopy, there is no obvious injury or bleeding in the eye. Visual acuity is 6/9 in the right eye and 6/6 in the left. An orbital CT scan does not detect any intraocular foreign bodies.

5. A 58-year-old lady presents to A&E with sharp left eye pain, photophobia and tearing. She was having a cup of tea after gardening, when she noticed ocular pain that has since been getting worse. She has no significant past medical history. On examination, there is conjunctival injection and excessive tearing in the left eye. Visual acuity is 6/9 in both eyes. After instilling fluorescein drops, slit-lamp examination reveals vertical scratch marks on her left cornea.

Ophthalmology Q22 – Refraction

A. Bifocal lens
B. Convex lens
C. Hard contact lens
D. Laser-Assisted In Situ Keratomileusis (LASIK)
E. Laser-Assisted Sub-Epithelial Keratomileusis (LASEK)
F. Photorefractive keratectomy (PRK)
G. Prism
H. Soft contact lens
I. Toric lens
J. Varifocal lens

From the list above, choose the most appropriate management option for each of the following examples.

1. A school bus driver is becoming long-sighted and needs spectacles.
2. Can be used for refractive correction and also as an ocular bandage for a chronic epithelial defect.
3. A musician with a history of myopia now needs spectacles for presbyopia.
4. A flap of corneal stroma is incised and folded back, and the exposed cornea is lasered to alter its refractive power.
5. A medical student needs spectacles for the treatment of astigmatism.

Q **Ophthalmology Q23 – Neuro-ophthalmology**
A. Anterior ischaemic optic neuropathy
B. Chronic open angle glaucoma
C. Diabetic retinopathy
D. Optic chiasm lesion
E. Optic tract lesion
F. Papilloedema
G. Parietal lobe lesion
H. Posterior optic radiation lesion
I. Temporal lobe lesion
J. None of the above

From the list above, choose the cause of each of the following clinical findings stated.
1. Bitemporal hemianopia.
2. Bilateral central scotomas.
3. Bilateral tunnel vision.
4. Left superior quadrantinopia.
5. Unilateral inferior altitudinal field loss.

Q Ophthalmology Q24 – Eyelid disorders

A. Basal cell carcinoma
B. Chalazion
C. Cyst of Moll
D. Cyst of Zeis
E. External hordeolum
F. Internal hordeolum
G. Keratoacanthoma
H. Molluscum contagiosum
I. Preseptal cellulitis
J. Squamous cell carcinoma

From the list above, choose the most appropriate diagnosis for each of the following examples.

1. A 22-year-old woman presents to her GP with a red irritable right eye. She also complains of small lumps on her upper eyelid that she has had for months. She has not noticed any discharge, pain, photophobia or blurry vision in her right eye. Her left eye is asymptomatic. She has no significant past medical history and is on the oral contraceptive pill. On examination, she has two small pearly lesions with an umbilicated centre on the upper lid margin of her right eye.

2. A 27-year-old man presents to his GP complaining of a right eyelid lump. The lump is not tender or discharging and he has never had one in the past. He is otherwise asymptomatic and has not noticed any change in vision. He is normally fit and healthy and is not on any medications. On examination, there is a translucent fluid-filled cyst on the anterior upper lid margin of his right eye. It is non-tender on palpation and the surrounding skin looks normal.

3. A 19-year-old woman presents to her GP with a round lump on her right eyelid. The lump has been present for weeks, and she is worried that it is enlarging. It is not painful or discharging, and the overlying skin looks normal. She has not had any eyelid lumps in the past, and she is normally fit and healthy. On examination, there is a small opaque cyst on her right upper eyelid that is rubbery and non-tender. The inner eyelid looks normal on eversion.

4. A 23-year-old woman presents to her GP with a painful red lump on her left upper eyelid. She was told previously that she

has a chalazion, and that it will resolve on its own. Her left eye is tearing, and she also complains of a foreign body sensation in the eye. She has no past medical history and is not on any medications. On examination, her upper eyelid is red and swollen. The lump is tender on palpation. Visual acuity is unchanged in both eyes.

5. A 53-year-old man presents to his GP complaining of a lump on his lower eyelid. He has been overseas for a few months and has not had time to see a doctor. He first noticed the lump 4 months ago. It grew rapidly in the first few weeks, but then stopped growing for the past 2 months and has started involuting. He has a past medical history of osteoarthritis, but is otherwise fit and healthy and does not take any medications. On examination, there is an involuted lump on his lower eyelid with a crusty depression at its centre. There is no discharge or surrounding erythema.

Ophthalmology answers

A   Ophthalmology A1 – Sudden painless visual loss

1. **B – Anterior ischaemic optic neuropathy** (AION) is an ischaemic necrosis of the optic nerve head. It can be non-arteritic (90%–95%) or arteritic (5%–10%) in origin. In non-arteritic AION, there is perfusion insufficiency of the short posterior ciliary arteries, but the exact pathogenesis is not understood. The arteritic form is the result of posterior ciliary artery obstruction, which can be caused by inflammation, atheroma or emboli. The patient in the scenario has signs and symptoms most consistent with giant cell arteritis (GCA). This is an inflammatory vasculitis affecting medium and large sized arteries, and is therefore an arteritic cause of AION. It is both an ophthalmic and medical emergency requiring immediate assessment and treatment. GCA affects females more commonly than males (3:1), and is rare under the age of 60 years. Patients present with an anterior unilateral headache and profound visual loss. They may experience pain on chewing (jaw claudication) and brushing their hair (scalp tenderness). The superficial temporal artery can result in a localised headache, and may become tender, hard and pulseless. Patients often complain of systemic symptoms, such as malaise, fever, myalgia, reduced appetite and weight loss. These systemic symptoms are important to elicit, but junior doctors often do not enquire about them! Patients may have pain and stiffness of proximal muscles of the shoulder and pelvic girdle, which are classic features of polymyalgia rheumatica. This can be associated with GCA, so it is therefore important to exclude GCA in these patients. Funduscopy reveals a swollen optic disc in acute AION, which is 'chalky white' in the arteritic form. The erythrocyte sedimentation rate (ESR) is invariably elevated (>50 mm per hour), but the gold standard test is temporal biopsy done before or within a few days of starting treatment with steroids. If there is strong clinical evidence of GCA, a temporal artery biopsy should not delay treatment. It is important to note that temporal arteritis causes patchy arterial inflammation (also known as 'skip lesions'), which may result in falsely negative biopsy results. Patients should therefore commence intravenous steroid therapy as soon as there is a strong

clinical suspicion of GCA. The dose can be tapered down when erythrocyte sedimentation rate decreases and symptoms improve, but it should not be completely stopped in less than 6 months. Treatment with steroids may last for years, and many patients are elderly females. Osteoporosis prophylaxis is therefore crucial in these patients. Visual loss is not reversible, with aim of treatment being to prevent further visual loss and other ischaemic events, which can occur within hours of presentation. In this scenario, failure to promptly manage GCA can result in loss of vision in her other eye. Risk of visual loss in the other eye falls from 90% to 10% with immunosuppressive treatment. If it affects the vertebrobasilar or carotid arteries, it can result in a stroke and death. This is why GCA is a medical as well as an ophthalmic emergency.

2. **C – Central retina artery occlusion** (CRAO). Retinal arterial occlusions can affect the central retinal artery or a branch of the central retinal artery. Emboli are the most common cause of retinal arterial occlusions, usually originating from the carotid artery or heart valves. Other important causes are thrombosis and vasculitis. A CRAO results in unilateral painless loss of vision, which may be transient (amaurosis fugax) if the embolus dislodges. Visual loss in CRAO is often more severe than central retinal vein occlusion. Relative afferent pupillary defect (RAPD) is usually present (resulting in what is known as 'Marcus Gunn' pupil). During a swinging light test, normal constriction is present in both eyes when light is shone onto the unaffected eye. Pupillary constriction is reduced in both eyes when light is shone onto the affected eye. When light is swung (very quickly) from the non-affected eye onto the affected eye, the affected eye will dilate because of afferent nerve damage. The resultant oedema of the retina gives it a classic pale appearance. The retina is thinnest at the foveal region, thus making the intact choroid circulation more visible, appearing as a cherry-red spot. GCA must always be excluded. Patients must also undergo comprehensive investigation for cardiovascular risk factors. Patients should also have a carotid duplex scan and echocardiogram to find the source of the emboli. CRAO is an ophthalmic emergency, in which irreversible damage occurs after 90 minutes. Patients should be urgently referred to exclude similar presentations such as GCA. Another important management step in these patients is trying to dislodge the emboli with techniques such as lowering the intraocular pressure medically, ocular massage, paracentesis and rebreathing into a paper bag. The success rate of these techniques, however, is low. Once irreversible damage has occurred, vision cannot be restored. Management is then prophylactic, aiming to

prevent further arterial occlusions (e.g. long-term antiplatelet therapy, carotid endarterectomy).

3. **J – Vitreous haemorrhage** (VH) is the most common cause of sudden visual loss in diabetic proliferative retinopathy, resulting from a bleed of the new small friable blood vessels. The main symptoms of a VH are visual loss and an increase in floaters. Key features on examination are loss of the red eye reflex and not being able to see much with an ophthalmoscope. It is important to note that a VH does not cause an RAPD. Urgent investigation of these patients is important, as VH can be caused by retinal detachment, requiring early surgical intervention. A B-scan ultrasonography can help exclude a retinal detachment. VH may absorb a few weeks after onset; otherwise, it requires removal by vitrectomy.

4. **D – Central retinal vein occlusion** (CRVO) characteristically presents with sudden painless unilateral loss of vision. Retinal vein occlusions can affect the central retinal vein, or a branch of the central retinal vein. Risk factors for retinal vein occlusions include old age and raised intraocular pressure, as well as cardiovascular risk factors such as hypertension, diabetes and smoking. Elderly patients with CRVO should have their blood pressure, blood glucose level and lipid profile checked. Younger patients should also be screened for clotting disorders. Severe visual loss in CRVO occurs because of involvement of the macula. CRVO results in increased intravascular pressure, thus resulting in the characteristic signs of CRVO: diffuse flame-shaped haemorrhages throughout the retina and dilated tortuous veins. Other signs include cotton wool spots and papilloedema. In branch retinal vein occlusions, signs are confined to the area of the retina drained by the blocked vessel. In severe cases, a RAPD may be present. The patient in this scenario has CRVO in the left eye, and signs of background diabetic retinopathy in the right eye. The resultant ischaemia from CRVO results in macular oedema, and can also result in neovascularisation of the retina, optic disc or iris. More than 90% of patients end up with a vision of 6/60 or worse. Intravitreal injection of triamcinolone, anti-vascular endothelium growth factor agents (e.g. bevacizumab/ranibizumab) as well as intravitreal dexamethasone implants have been shown to be of benefit for treatment of macular oedema and improving vision in retinal vein occlusion. Grid laser photocoagulation treatment can reduce macular oedema in branch retinal vein occlusion. If iris rubreosis (neovascularisation) is left untreated, it can result in a painful chronic form of glaucoma known as rubreotic glaucoma.

5. **I – Retinal detachment** (RD) is a common cause of sudden painless loss of vision. It occurs when the neurosensory retinal layer separates from the retinal pigment epithelium layer. The most common cause is a tear in the neurosensory retina, which leads to accumulation of vitreous fluid in the subretinal space. This is known as rhegmatogenous RD. The other two less common types of RD are tractional and exudative. Rhegmatogenous RD is usually preceded by posterior vitreous detachment, which is when the vitreous peals away from the retina causing the patient to see flashing lights (photopsia) and floaters (black floating objects). When a rhegmatogenous RD occurs, patients describe an increase in floaters and flashing lights, and describe a grey curtain being pulled down the visual field of their affected eye. The more advanced the RD, the more profound the peripheral visual field loss. If the retinal detachment affects the macula, visual acuity will be affected. Severe loss of visual acuity, as is the case in this scenario, suggests detachment of the fovea. On funduscopy, the red eye reflex is lost and the grey retina may be seen bowing forwards. On slit-lamp examination, Shafer's sign (floating pigment cells in the anterior vitreous) may be seen. Patients with retinal detachment should be urgently referred to an ophthalmologist for surgical management. If left untreated, the eye will almost certainly become blind. Immediate surgical intervention is of more value in patients who have retained a good visual acuity than patients whose visual acuity has deteriorated. This is because in patients with good central vision, the macula has not detached and surgical reattachment of the peripheral retina can prevent this from occurring. If the macula has been detached for more than 24 hours, full visual recovery is unlikely.

A   Ophthalmology A2 – Painful eye

1. **A – Acute primary angle-closure glaucoma** (ACG) is an ophthalmic emergency that is an important global cause of blindness. Delay in treatment can lead to irreversible retinal optic nerve damage. About 90% of ACG cases present unilaterally. Known risk factors for ACG are age >40 years, female sex and hypermetropia. ACG is thought to occur due to opposition of the iris to the lens, which blocks aqueous flow from the posterior to the anterior chamber. The subsequent increase in pressure in the posterior chamber leads to anterior bowing of the peripheral iris. This then blocks the angle of the anterior chamber, preventing aqueous drainage and leading to a vicious cycle of rising intraocular pressure (IOP). This significantly raised IOP leads to corneal, iris and retinal ischaemia,

giving the clinician a narrow 4-hour window to reduce the IOP and salvage the optic nerve and the retina. ACG could also be intermittent in nature, where acute attacks spontaneously resolve. ACG can present with ocular and non-ocular manifestations, which can sometimes lead to them being admitted on medical wards and investigated for abdominal pathologies. Pain is a prominent symptom of ACG, and patients complain of pain in or around the eye, headaches and sometimes abdominal pain. Common ocular symptoms besides pain include loss of vision (due to corneal oedema) and photophobia. Patients may also report seeing halos around lights, especially at night, before the acute episode of ACG. Other prominent systemic symptoms of acute ACG include nausea and vomiting, which is a common feature of migraines, an important differential also commonly presenting with visual symptoms. It is important to be able to recognise the signs of acute ACG, which make it easy to differentiate it from other similar presentations of an acutely painful red eye. The affected pupil is oval, fixed, semi-dilated and poorly reactive to light because of iris ischaemia. The affected eye has a raised IOP (>50 mmHg), cloudy cornea (corneal oedema), ciliary congestion and a shallow anterior chamber (usually a bilateral finding). A simple quick bedside test is to gently palpate both eyes with the eyelids closed. The affected eye is tender and significantly harder than the unaffected eye on palpation. The exact IOP should be measured with a tonometer.

2. **B – Anterior uveitis** is an inflammation of the uveal tract, which consists of the iris, ciliary body and choroid. The exact mechanism of uveitis is unknown, although it is thought to be partly due to an immune reaction against foreign antigens that results in immune complex deposition in the uveal tract. Anterior uveitis refers to inflammation of the iris. The ciliary body is often also inflamed (cyclitis). Intermediate uveitis refers to inflammation of the pars plana, and posterior uveitis refers to inflammation of the choroid. Seventy-five per cent of cases are anterior in nature. Most cases of anterior uveitis are idiopathic, but it can be associated with other ocular diseases, ocular trauma, infections and a variety of systemic disorders such as ankylosing spondylitis, inflammatory bowel disease and sarcoidosis. In the present scenario, the raised red lesions on the patient's shins may be suggestive of erythema nodosum, which is associated with a number of systemic conditions. In acute anterior uveitis, patients present with an acutely painful red eye, visual loss, photophobia, lacrimation and a small pupil (due to iris spasm). Contrast this with posterior uveitis, in which patients have minimal pain and photophobia, but complain mainly

of visual blurring and floaters. The redness of anterior uveitis is most marked around the limbus (circumcorneal), in contrast to conjunctivitis in which the circumcorneal region remains clear. Slit-lamp examination reveals floating inflammatory cells and flare (protein exudates), similar to dust passing through a projector beam. This is what results in the visual blurring experienced by the patient. Accumulating inflammatory cells may form a white fluid level in the anterior chamber, known as a hypopyon; a sign of severe inflammation. Keratitic precipitates may also be seen on the corneal endothelium, particularly in the lower half, which represent clumps of inflammatory cells. Inflammatory adhesions between the iris and lens can form, known as posterior synechiae. These can cause an irregular pupil. A dilated funduscopy examination is essential to exclude posterior uveitis. It is also important to look for complications of anterior uveitis such as cataracts and secondary glaucoma. Most patients suffer from a single episode of anterior uveitis. Systemic investigations are carried out if the clinical history is suggestive of a systemic disease, or the anterior uveitis is granulomatous, recurrent or bilateral.

3. **E – Endophthalmitis** is an infection and inflammation of the eyeball contents. Acute post-operative endophthalmitis is a rare but devastating consequence of intraocular surgery (0.3% risk). This is characterised by a very painful red eye and profound visual loss 1–7 days post-operatively. The most common pathogen is *Staphylococcus epidermidis*, with the most frequent source being the flora of the eyelids and conjunctiva. Typical signs on examination are corneal oedema, conjunctival chemosis (oedema), injection and discharge, hypopyon, vitritis and relative afferent pupillary defect. Patients must be admitted, aqueous and vitreous samples aspirated and intravitreal antibiotics simultaneously administered. Topical, intravitreal or systemic steroids may be used, but there is no evidence that this improves visual acuity. If on presentation the affected eye has a poor visual acuity, i.e. perception of light only, a vitrectomy is performed.

4. **C – Bacterial conjunctivitis** is the most common cause of a red eye, and is most frequently allergic, viral or bacterial. The patient in this scenario complains of red sticky eyes that are burning or irritable but not painful, the hallmark features of conjunctivitis. Visual loss and photophobia are very rare features of conjunctivitis, although visual blurring in the morning can result because of discharge obscuring vision. If there is significant deterioration in visual acuity, alternative pathologies should be sought. Bacterial conjunctivitis starts unilaterally, but usually soon after infects

the other eye. It produces an excessive yellow/green sticky discharge, as opposed to clear/white discharge associated with viral and allergic conjunctivitis, but the distinction is not always clear. Conjunctival swelling and injection are common signs, and conjunctival papillae may also be found. The conjunctival injection is most marked away from the limbus. Most cases of bacterial conjunctivitis settle without treatment, but a topical broad-spectrum antibiotic such as chloramphenicol can hasten recovery. A conjunctival swab is not necessary, and most cases are due to *Haemophilus influenzae*, *Streptococcus pneumoniae* and *Staphylococcus aureus*. In neonatal cases of bacterial conjunctivitis, on the other hand, a swab should always be performed before starting treatment, and it is common to start broad-spectrum antibiotics before culture and sensitivity are back. A conjunctival swab is only performed in adult bacterial conjunctivitis resistant to treatment. Corneal ulceration should be excluded in all cases of bacterial conjunctivitis.

5. **G – Optic neuritis** (ON) is inflammation of the optic nerve. It is termed papillitis if the optic nerve head is affected and retrobulbar neuritis (RBN) if the optic nerve is affected posteriorly. ON does not cause a red eye. It typically affects adults aged 20–50 years, and more commonly affects females. It is typically unilateral and worsening over hours/days. In RBN, the optic nerve looks unaffected in the acute stage, with optic disc atrophy occurring a few months later. On the other hand, papillitis is characterised by optic disc swelling. It is important to note that the term papilloedema should only be used to describe bilateral optic disc swelling resulting from raised intracranial pressure. The important features of papilloedema are optic disc swelling, blurring of the optic disc margin and venous engorgement. Optic neuritis is an inflammatory condition, and the must therefore not be described as papilloedema. In RBN, the optic nerve sheath compresses the optic nerve, resulting in retrobulbar pain on eye movement, which is a common and early finding in these patients. The key clinical features are reduced coloured vision, reduced visual acuity, central scotoma on visual field testing and a relative afferent pupillary defect. The most common cause of ON is multiple sclerosis, which can be confirmed by finding demyelinating plaques on MRI scanning of the brain. Less routine tests for multiple sclerosis include examining the cerebrospinal fluid for oligoclonal bands. The risk of developing multiple sclerosis 5 years after the first episode of ON is approximately 30%. ON occurs in up to 70% of patients with multiple sclerosis. Less common causes of ON include viral infections and vasculitis. Visual recovery begins within 2 weeks, but

visual function may not always fully recover. Systemic steroids may hasten visual recovery, but have not been shown to affect the final visual outcome. Recurrent ON can lead to optic atrophy, due to loss of nerve fibres, and to permanent visual impairment.

A Ophthalmology A3 – Red eye

1. **C – Bacterial keratitis**. Keratitis is an inflammation of the cornea. The cornea is a very effective barrier against pathogens. *Neisseria gonorrhoea* is one of the few pathogens that can penetrate the corneal epithelium. A bacterial keratitis is therefore usually the result of a break of the corneal surface. Predisposing factors include contact lens wear, trauma, blepharitis and use of immunosuppressives. *Staphylococcus*, *Streptococcus* and *Pseudomonas* are the most common bacterial pathogens. The patient in this scenario is a contact lens wearer, and is therefore at increased risk of fungal keratitis. When the pathogen is not known, the term 'microbial' or 'infectious' keratitis is more accurately used. The typical clinical features are a painful red eye with foreign body sensation, photophobia and visual loss. In severe cases, a hypopyon may be present. The distinguishing feature from other causes of a painful and photophobic red eye with visual loss is anterior corneal stroma infiltration (white lesions), an overlying epithelial defect and an adherent mucopurulent exudate. When this occurs with a history of contact lens use, bacterial keratitis is the most likely diagnosis. Corneal epithelial defects can be detected by fluorescein staining and illumination with a cobalt blue light. Contact lens wear is associated with *pseudomonas* and *acanthamoeba* ulcers. The latter is a rare diagnosis, usually found in patients who use homemade saline solution or swim without removing their contact lens. Pain in *acanthamoeba* infection is characteristically out of proportion to the clinical findings. Once a diagnosis of bacterial keratitis is suspected, swabs should be taken from the conjunctiva and cornea for microbiology, culture and sensitivities. The contact lens with their solution/cases should also be sent for culture, and the patient should temporarily stop wearing contact lenses. Broad-spectrum topical antibiotics should be started until the culture and sensitivity results are back. Admission may be necessary if the infection is severe. Bacterial keratitis can lead to permanent corneal scarring, corneal thinning and perforation, which requires corneal grafting.

2. **E – Herpes simplex virus keratitis**. The cornea is composed of five layers (outermost to innermost): corneal epithelium, Bowman's layer, corneal

stroma, Descemet's membrane and endothelium. Inflammation of the cornea (keratitis) due to herpes simplex virus (HSV) can affect any one of these layers. It is usually due to HSV type 1, with which the primary infection occurs in childhood. The virus remains dormant in the trigeminal ganglion until it is re-activated. On re-activation, it travels down a branch of the trigeminal nerve to the nerve terminals at the corneal epithelium, which is why it most commonly infects the epithelial layer causing a dendritic keratitis. The pathognomonic finding in this condition is a branching epithelial defect with terminal bulbs, hence the name 'dendritic' ulcer. This can be viewed with fluorescein staining and cobalt blue light. Worsening of the ulceration can lead to a geographic ulcer. HSV keratitis is unilateral in most cases (~2% bilateral). If the patient has had previous episodes of HSV keratitis in the context of a new dendritic ulcer, the diagnosis is straightforward. Patients who have had prior episodes of HSV keratitis often have reduced corneal sensation. This is a useful sign to look for before the administration of anaesthetic eye drops. Other ocular features of HSV keratitis include ocular pain, redness, blurred vision and lacrimation. Blurred vision is a result of corneal inflammation, and is worse if there is a central corneal ulcer affecting the visual axis. Patients can also have extra-ocular features of an HSV infection, such as skin vesicles and pre-auricular lymph nodes. The diagnosis of HSV keratitis is confirmed by scraping cells from the edge of the ulcer.

3. **F – Herpes zoster ophthalmicus**. A primary infection with herpes zoster virus causes chickenpox (varicella). Similarly to HSV, the virus remains dormant in the sensory ganglion of the trigeminal nerve, and may be re-activated later in life (shingles). It is important to bear in mind the herpes zoster ophthalmicus (HZO) could be the initial manifestation of HIV. Unlike HSV infections, however, patients usually experience prodromal symptoms. This is followed by a unilateral dermatomal vesicular eruption in the distribution of the trigeminal nerve (fifth cranial nerve). A maculopapular rash develops first, followed by vesicles, papules and crusting. The ophthalmic division of the trigeminal nerve is involved in approximately 15% of shingles cases, and is known as HZO. Ocular involvement is more likely if the tip of the nose is involved (Hutchinson's sign), as both structures are supplied by the nasociliary nerve. Complications of HZO include conjunctivitis, keratitis, anterior uveitis, scleritis, episcleritis, secondary glaucoma and optic neuritis. Symptoms vary with the complications of HZO, but patients often have a red painful eye, blurry vision and a headache. Involvement of the corneal stroma and anterior uvea is common

in HZO, unlike HSV keratitis, which usually affects the corneal epithelium only. A possible long-term consequence of HZO is post-herpetic neuralgia, which is a chronic pain in the region of the rash that can be debilitating.

4. **G – Marginal keratitis** is a relatively common inflammatory condition of the cornea. It is thought to be a hypersensitivity reaction to exotoxins released from organisms colonising the lids, leading to immune complex deposition in the peripheral cornea. It is associated with chronic blepharitis, rosacea and atopy. This patient has typical clinical features of keratitis: ocular redness, pain, foreign body sensation, photophobia, lacrimation and reduced visual acuity. His history of dry eyes is consistent with chronic blepharitis. On examination, there are multiple peripheral subepithelial corneal infiltrates, separated from the limbus by a clear zone. These can coalesce and spread circumferentially. Unlike bacterial keratitis, the epithelial layer is usually intact. Marginal keratitis is treated with topical antibiotics and steroids. Steroids reduce inflammation, while antibiotics are given prophylactically to prevent an infection. It is also important to ensure adequate management of the blepharitis in this patient to minimise the risk of infections, secondary conjunctivitis (which may not be infective) and recurrence of the marginal keratitis. There are three key steps to the management of blepharitis: (1) regular lid hygiene, (2) antibiotics and (3) artificial tears.

5. **H – Orbital cellulitis** is a medical emergency that is both sight and life threatening. It is an infection of the soft tissues posterior to the orbital septum, and is more common in children. Infection can be acquired from a variety of sources, most commonly from the adjacent sinuses (usually ethmoid sinus). The commonest causative organism is *H. influenza*. It is important to be able to recognise the symptoms and signs of this condition. Patients complain of ocular pain, red eye, reduced eye movements, double vision, reduced colour vision and visual blurring. Signs to look for on examination are swelling, tenderness, erythema of the eyelids, conjunctival injection, proptosis, and restricted extraocular movements. The presence of reduced visual acuity, colour vision or a RAPD suggests that the optic nerve is affected. It also is important to look for signs of sepsis, such as fever and malaise. Orbital cellulitis should be differentiated from preseptal cellulitis, the latter being an infection of the eyelid only with no ocular involvement. If a diagnosis of orbital cellulitis is suspected, the patient should be admitted, blood cultures taken (if pyrexia is present) and

intravenous antibiotics started promptly. An orbital CT is used to detect a periosteal or sinus abscess, but should not delay start of antibiotics. If an abscess is found, it will require drainage. Orbital cellulitis is a rapidly progressive ophthalmic emergency, and can lead to a number of serious ocular (e.g. endophthalmitis, optic neuropathy) and systemic (e.g. brain abscess meningitis, cavernous sinus thrombosis) complications.

A Ophthalmology A4 – Management of red eye

1. **E – Lid hygiene, artificial tears and topical antibiotics**. This patient has the characteristic features of blepharitis, a chronic lid margin disease. Blepharitis can be bacterial or seborrhoeic. The bacterial form is often due to lid commensals, primarily staphylococci. Seborrhoeic blepharitis results from meibomian gland dysfunction, and it is commonly associated with generalised seborrhoeic dermatitis. The main symptoms of blepharitis are eye irritation, dryness and stickiness that is often worse in the morning. Common signs on examination are conjunctival injection (dilation of blood vessels), redness and scaling of the lid margins. Blepharitis can be associated with dry eyes (tear film dysfunction), secondary conjunctivitis and corneal epithelial erosions (autoimmune response to staphylococcal exotoxins). In this scenario, the patient has developed bacterial conjunctivitis on top of chronic blepharitis, which is a common scenario. There are three key steps to the management of blepharitis: (1) regular lid hygiene to remove scales, crusts and sebum and open secretory glands (this can be done with warm compresses soaked with diluted baby shampoo), (2) topical antibiotics for the treatment of infections once the area is cleaned (this is best done with topical ointments rather than drops, as they cling better to the eyes; in severe or persistent infections, systemic antibiotics and weak topical steroids could be required) and (3) artificial tear drops to treat tear inadequacy. Blepharitis can have a chronic course and patients should be made aware of this. Patients should also be educated about the importance of regular lid hygiene in minimising the risk of infections. Patient advice leaflets about blepharitis can be very useful.

2. **F – Oral NSAIDs**. A severe deep, dull pain and redness of the eye are typical features of anterior scleritis. The pain may be severe to the extent that patients cannot sleep at night. As implied by the name, scleritis is a non-infective inflammation of the full thickness of the sclera. It is associated with systemic conditions in 50% of cases, such as connective tissue diseases (most commonly rheumatoid arthritis) and herpes zoster ophthalmicus.

It is a sight-threatening condition, and is most common in middle-aged women. Fifty per cent of cases are bilateral. Episcleritis on the other hand is a much more common but less serious condition than scleritis. It is a non-infective inflammation of the episclera, a thin tissue layer superficial to the sclera, and is rarely associated with systemic conditions. It is most common in young women. Pain is a much more prominent feature in scleritis than in episcleritis in which pain is mild or absent. Furthermore, scleritis is more likely to cause hyperaemia of the entire sclera rather than the 'segmental' hyperaemia often seen in episcleritis. Other important signs of scleritis are engorged large blood vessels, swollen sclera and tenderness of the globe on palpation. Vision is not often affected in scleritis, and almost never affected in episcleritis. Application of topical vasoconstrictors (e.g. phenylephrine 10%) results in blanching of the superficial episcleral vessels in episcleritis, but does not affect the engorged deep scleral vessels in scleritis. This is a useful method to help distinguish between the two conditions. Non-necrotising scleritis is usually managed with oral NSAIDs (e.g. flurbiprofen). Topical and systemic steroids are the mainstay of treatment for more severe scleritis, with very severe cases requiring high systemic doses or the addition of other immunosuppressive agents. Inadequate treatment can lead to perforation of the sclera. Episcleritis is usually self-limiting, although topical NSAIDs or corticosteroids may alleviate symptoms.

3. **A – Advice on infection control**. Conjunctivitis is the most common cause of a red eye, and is most frequently allergic, viral or bacterial. The patient in this scenario complains of red irritable painless eyes, which are the hallmark features of conjunctivitis. Visual loss or photophobia are not features of conjunctivitis, although visual blurring in the morning can result due to ocular discharge obscuring vision. The history of the patient's husband having similar symptoms, and the fact that she has not had these symptoms before suggests an infective rather than an allergic pathology. Moreover, allergic conjunctivitis gives symptoms of itchiness rather than irritation. Viral conjunctivitis is very infective, and although it can start unilaterally, it commonly affects both eyes. The discharge is watery, in contrast to bacterial conjunctivitis in which it is more often mucupurulent (yellow/green). Viral conjunctivitis is most commonly caused by adenovirus infection. It may be preceded by prodormal symptoms, such as a sore throat, low-grade fever and myalgia. Patients may also have conjunctival follicles and tender peri-auricular and cervical lymphadenopathy, which can help distinguish it from other types of conjunctivitis. It is usually self-limiting, but advice on infection control is paramount as it is a very infective condition and can

cause epidemics. Patients should be advised on the importance of hand washing, avoiding touching of their eyes and not sharing towels or pillows.

4. **J – Topical antihistamines and mast cell stabilisers**. The seasonal nature of this patient's symptoms, along with the 'itchiness' of her eyes is most consistent with a diagnosis of allergic conjunctivitis. This is an IgE-mediated allergic reaction, and is most common in the spring and summer due to increased grass and tree pollen exposure. It can be acute (known as seasonal allergic conjunctivitis or hay fever conjunctivitis) or chronic (vernal keratoconjunctivitis in children, atopic keratoconjunctivitis in adults), and accounts for 15% of ophthalmological presentations to GP surgeries. The main symptoms of allergic conjunctivitis are itchy, red eyes and lacrimation. The common signs on examination are conjunctival injection and swelling (chemosis), and a mucous discharge. In the acute form of allergic conjunctivitis, patients frequently present with other symptoms of hay fever, such as a nasal discharge and sneezing (allergic rhinitis). In the chronic form, patients may have giant papillae on the tarsal conjunctiva. These can coalesce to form giant (cobblestone) papillae, but this is more common in allergic conjunctivitis due to contact lens use. Compare this with the conjunctival 'follicles' and more watery discharge seen in viral conjunctivitis. Diagnosis of allergic conjunctivitis is usually clinical, and it is managed with the use of topical antihistamines or mast cell stabilisers, which are very effective. Topical treatment combining both of these agents is the optimal topical treatment. Systemic antihistamines are also very effective and may be used prophylactically. More severe cases may require steroid drops, but these should only be used under the guidance of an ophthalmologist. Chronic use of topical steroids can result in cataracts and glaucoma.

5. **B – Conjunctival swab and topical antibiotics**. Neonatal conjunctivitis, also known as ophthalmia neonatorum, is conjunctivitis occurring in the first 28 days of life. It affects up to 12% of neonates in developed countries, and up to 23% of neonates in developing countries. It is a notifiable condition in the United Kingdom, and may or may not be due to maternal sexually transmitted infections. Neonates with sexually transmitted conjunctival infections have contracted the infection from their mother's vaginal tract during delivery, and a careful history and examination of parents is therefore very important. Neonates present with bilateral eye discharge and eyelid oedema. Chlamydial conjunctivitis is the most common type of neonatal conjunctivitis. There are useful clinical features

that can help distinguish the causative pathogen. Gonoccocal and chemical conjunctivitis usually present in the first week of life. Conjunctivitis due to chlamydia and herpes simplex typically presents between the first and second postnatal weeks. Other non-sexually transmitted bacterial infections present after the first week. An excessive purulent discharge is common in gonoccocal infections. Other bacterial infections, including chlamydia, cause a mucopurulent discharge. Herpes simplex conjunctivitis can produce a profuse watery discharge and vesicular lid lesions. Chemical conjunctivitis can produce a watery discharge, but frequently does not cause a discharge, which is an important feature to elicit. Neonates with a watery eye and mild or no redness may have congenital nasolacrimal duct obstruction, which is an important differential diagnosis. It is also very important to look for extraocular features in all neonates (such as pneumonitis and otitis in chlamydial infections) and to exclude corneal ulceration. The presence of lid swelling should alert you to the possibility of orbital celluitis. Swabs for gram stain, culture and sensitivity in ophthalmia neonatorum are mandatory in all cases, and should be done before starting any antibiotic treatment. Note the difference in management of adult bacterial conjunctivitis, where swabs are only indicated if the conjunctivitis does not improve with standard antibacterial treatment. Topical broad-spectrum antibiotics in neonatal conjunctivitis should be started before the causative organism is identified. Chlamydial conjunctivitis is treated with a 2-week course of oral erythromycin. Tetracycline is contraindicated in children under 12 years of age, as it stains their growing teeth. Although much rarer, gonococcal infections can lead to corneal perforation and endophthalmitis, and should be promptly treated with parenteral benzylpenicillin or cephalosporins if pending sensitivity results. Topical povidine-iodine eye drops are effective prophylactic agents against both chlamydial and gonorrheal conjunctivitis. Herpes simplex conjunctivitis is treated with topical antivirals, such as aciclovir.

A   Ophthalmology A5 – Diplopia

1. **D – Graves' ophthalmopathy**. This is also known as Graves' eye disease or dysthyroid eye disease. Ocular muscle thickening is a feature of a variety of ocular conditions. The clinical presentation of the patient in this scenario is suggestive of Graves' eye disease. Patients have ocular as well as systemic features of hyperthyroidism. Ophthalmopathy is a hallmark of Graves' disease, occurring in about 30% of cases of Graves' hyperthyroidism. An autoimmune reaction to orbital antigens results in infiltration

of extraocular muscles with inflammatory cells and oedema. Ocular features include exophthalmos (proptosis), conjunctival oedema (chemosis) and injection (redness), lid retraction (white of the sclera visible above the pupil), lid lag (lid movement lags behind globe movement on downgaze), restrictive eye movement and diplopia. Conjunctival redness and swelling are due to proptosis and lid retraction, leading to excessive corneal exposure. If left untreated, this can lead to corneal ulceration and even perforation. The ocular muscle swelling results in restricted eye movements. If severe, it can lead to compressive optic neuropathy, a sight threatening complication. Systemic immunosuppression, radiotherapy or surgical decompression may be required to prevent corneal ulceration and optic nerve damage. The inferior rectus is the most commonly affected muscle in dysthyroid eye disease, resulting in diplopia on upgaze due to mechanical limitation. The second most frequently affected muscle is the medial rectus. Reasons for this pattern of muscle involvement are unknown. This explains the clinical presentation in the scenario. A fourth cranial nerve palsy affecting the superior oblique will result in diplopia on downgaze, as it supplies the superior oblique which mainly depresses the eye. It is important to know the ocular and systemic effects of hyperthyroidism, which are commonly asked about in clinical examinations. Systemic effects are listed in medical textbooks. An increased appetite and weight loss are characteristic features of hyperthyroidism, giving the clue to a diagnosis of hyperthyroidism rather than ocular myositis in this patient. It is also important to be aware of the clinical features specific to Graves' hyperthyroidism, which is the most common cause of hyperthyroidism in the developed world. These are: ophthalmopathy, pre-tibial myxoedema and a thyroid goitre with a bruit. Additional steps in the management of thyroid eye disease include lubrication, prisms (for diplopia) and eyelid surgery (lid retraction). Smoking is a key risk factor, and smoking cessation advice should be offered. Treating the thyroid hormone dysfunction does not affect the ocular disease course.

Hint: Thyroid eye disease is the most common cause of unilateral and bilateral proptosis.

2. **B – Carotid cavernous sinus fistula** is an abnormal communication between the internal or external carotid arteries and the cavernous sinus. This occurs following trauma (75%), due to tearing of the intracavernous carotid artery, or spontaneously (25%). The patient in this scenario suffers from hypertension, which is a known risk factor. Patients may complain

of eye redness and/or bulging, diplopia, decreased vision and hearing a pulsatile buzzing sound (bruit). Findings on examination are a pulsating exophthalmos, eyelid oedema, conjunctival swelling, injected episcleral veins and a loud ocular bruit. The gold standard test to determine the site of the lesion is cerebral angiography. Patients need to undergo closure of the abnormal arteriovenous communication, which is done by balloon embolisation or by surgical repair.

3. **J – Posterior communicating artery aneurysm**. A third cranial nerve palsy with a fixed dilated pupil is a posterior communicating artery (PCA) aneurysm until proven otherwise. This is a neurosurgical emergency requiring urgent referral. A headache may or may not be present, and is a non-specific feature of PCA aneurysm. Pupil involvement, presence of pain or patient age < 50 years are urgent indications for a CT brain or magnetic resonance angiogram, and these should be performed to exclude a PCA aneurysm. The third nerve passes laterally to the PCA on its course to the eye. It supplies all of the oculomotor muscles, except for the superior oblique and lateral rectus muscles, which are supplied by the trochlear and abducens nerves respectively. In a third nerve palsy, the patient's eye is therefore depressed and abducted as a result of the unopposed action of the superior oblique (eye intorsion, depression and abduction) and lateral rectus (eye abduction) muscles. The third cranial nerve innervates the levator palpebrae superioris, which is the main muscle responsible for elevating the eyelid. This is why a third nerve palsy usually causes a complete ptosis, unlike Horner's syndrome, which causes a partial ptosis. The third cranial nerve also supplied the pupil and ciliary body, and is responsible for constriction of the pupil. In a third nerve palsy, the pupil does not constrict to light or accommodation. Anisocoria (different-sized pupils) can be noticed in bright rooms. The most common pathological causes of a third nerve palsy are microvascular ischaemia (e.g. diabetes mellitus, hypertension, vasculitis, migraine) or a PCA aneurysm. Microvascular causes spare the pupil, as the third nerve pupillomotor fibres have a different blood supply to the rest of the nerve. Other causes are idiopathic (25%), trauma, raised intracranial pressure and a congenital third nerve palsy. An aneurysm of the PCA can be occluded by interventional neuroradiology, or may require neurosurgery. Ischaemic third nerve palsy usually resolves within 3 months. The diplopia can be managed with prisms or a patch to occlude vision unilaterally.

Hint: A third nerve palsy with a fixed dilated pupil is a posterior communicating artery aneurysm until proven otherwise.

4. **A – Carotid artery dissection**. Sudden onset of Horner's syndrome with a headache, pain in the face, neck or jaw or a history of recent neck trauma is carotid artery dissection until proven otherwise. This is a life-threatening condition that can result in a thrombotic or embolic stroke, and accounts for a significant proportion of strokes in younger people. Patients should be referred for urgent imaging (e.g. CT angiogram, axial MRI, conventional angiography) and management. Aneurysmal dilatation of a carotid dissection can have a mass effect on the nearby sympathetic fibres, causing Horner's syndrome. The sympathetic fibres innervate the iris dilator muscle, which is responsible for mydriasis. Sympathetic fibres also innervate Müller's muscle, which contributes to about 1.5 mm of lid elevation. A lesion to the sympathetic nerve supply to the eye causes Horner's syndrome, which presents with the classic triad of MAP – **m**iosis, **a**nhydrosis (hemifacial) and **p**tosis (partial). Carotid artery dissection may also be associated with a funny taste in the mouth (dysgeusis). Management options include observation, anticoagulation, carotid artery stenting or ligation.

Hint: In a history of painful Horner's syndrome, think carotid artery dissection!

5. **F – Myasthenia gravis** (MG) is an autoimmune neuromuscular condition in which the body forms autoantibodies against nicotinic acetylcholine postsynaptic receptors in neuromuscular junctions. This can cause ocular symptoms, mainly ptosis and diplopia. Ptosis is bilateral and variable, increasing with fatigue. The ptosis is worse towards the end of the day. Ocular symptoms may be the earliest features of MG. Other features include facial and proximal muscle weakness, dysphagia and dyspnoea. It is important to note that MG is associated with thymoma, which is why patients should undergo CT chest scanning. If found, a thymoma should be removed because of its neoplastic potential. Investigations for MG include acetylcholine receptor antibodies – this has a sensitivity of 60%–88% and a specificity of 90%. If raised, a diagnosis of MG is established. Another useful antibody to measure is the anti-striated muscle antibody, which is more frequently positive in patients with a thymoma. Another useful investigation is the Tensilon test (rarely done in clinical practice), in which edrophonium chloride (an anticholinesterase) is injected intravenously and the patient is observed for signs of reduced weakness (e.g. resolution of ptosis). If an improvement is observed, this is diagnostic of MG. Another useful test is placing an ice pack over the closed eyelids, which can improve ptosis in MG. Treatment of MG is with an oral anticholinesterase agent, such as pyridostigmine.

A pancoast tumour is subset of **lung cancers** situated in the pleural apex, the most common type being bronchogenic cancer. It can affect the brachial plexus causing pain in the shoulder and ulnar nerve distribution of the arm and hand. It can also cause upper limb oedema and muscle wasting in the T1 myotomal distribution. A pancoast tumour can affect the cervical sympathetic chain and the left (but not right) recurrent laryngeal nerve causing Horner's syndrome and a hoarse voice respectively. As with other types of lung cancer, it can cause respiratory symptoms such as chest pain, shortness of breath, cough and haemoptysis. *Hint: In patients with Horner's syndrome and a history of smoking, look for signs and symptoms of lung cancer.*

An acute rise in orbital pressure due to direct force by an object that is more than 5 cm in diameter can cause a fracture of the thin inferior and medial walls of the orbit. The resultant oedema, muscle entrapment and nerve damage can all lead to diplopia. Clinical features of an **orbital blowout fracture** include periocular ecchymosis and oedema, enophthalmos, restricted ocular motility, diplopia (commonly vertical), cheek and teeth numbness and bone crepitus. The presentation, investigations and management of an orbital blowout fracture are discussed in Question 21 (Ophthalmology section).

Ocular myositis is an inflammatory disorder of one or more extraocular muscles. The superior and inferior rectus muscles are the two most commonly affected muscles. Patients present with painful diplopia, with pain being most prominent on ocular movement in the direction of the muscle involved. Diagnosis is usually made with orbital CT or MRI, which shows muscle thickening. A biopsy is rarely needed. Treatment is with immunosuppression.

Orbital cellulitis is a medical emergency that is both sight and life threatening. It is discussed in Question 3 (Ophthalmology section).

A Ophthalmology A6 – Management of ocular conditions

1. **I – Timolol**. The first principle in the management of acute closed-angle glaucoma (ACG) is to reduce the elevated intraocular pressure (IOP). The rapid and significant IOP rise in ACG causes corneal, iris and retinal ischaemia. This results in severe ocular pain and photophobia. If the IOP is not reduced within the narrow 4-hour window, irreversible retinal and optic nerve damage can occur leading to permanent visual impairment. Both timolol (non-selective beta blocker) and acetazolamide (carbonic anhydrase inhibitor) are used for the reduction of aqueous humour formation in acute ACG. Timolol is used topically, while acetazolamide is

given systemically. Patients often have nausea and vomiting, which is why acetazolamide is given intravenously rather than orally at first. Another agent used in the acute management of ACG is topical pilocarpine, which constricts the pupil (miosis) to reverse the pupil block. The IOP should be monitored hourly until IOP is well controlled. Symptomatic relief in the form of analgesia and anti-emetics should also be offered.

2. **E – Iridotomy**. The second principle in the management of ACG once the acute attack has resolved, is to prevent further attacks. A laser peripheral iridotomy is performed, in which a small hole is made in the peripheral iris to permit aqueous flow from the posterior to the anterior chamber, bypassing the pupil. This is also done prophylactically in the other eye, which is also at high risk of developing ACG.

3. **D – Cyclopentolate**. Patients with anterior uveitis present with intense ocular pain due to iris spasm, and it is important that pain relief is started immediately. Topical mydriatics such as cyclopentolate or atropine help relieve the ocular pain and photophobia, as well as break and prevent the formation of posterior synchiae. The definitive treatment of anterior uveitis is topical steroids to manage the inflammation. It is important, however, that these are not started until the diagnosis is confirmed, and an urgent referral to the ophthalmologist may be more appropriate. Viral or bacterial causes of a red eye can present similarly to anterior uveitis, and the infections can be made much worse by the administration of steroids. Topical steroids and mydriatics are adequate for most cases of anterior uveitis. In a severe or resistant case, steroids may need to be administered subconjunctivally or systemically. Other systemic immunosuppressives may also be tried. It is important to monitor for secondary glaucoma and cataracts, which can develop as complications of anterior uveitis or topical steroid use.

4. **B – Aciclovir**. The diagnosis of HSV keratitis is confirmed by scraping cells from the edge of the ulcer. It is treated with a topical antiviral, usually aciclovir ointment. Patients should be reviewed weekly to review resolution of the ulcer. Oral aciclovir can be used prophylactically in recurrent HSV keratitis. Topical steroids should not be used as they can delay healing of a corneal ulcer, and may significantly worsen the corneal ulceration resulting in a geographic ulcer. Inflammation of the stromal layer of cornea (with or without epithelial ulceration) is characterised by multiple ring opacities and keratitic precipitates. This can lead to corneal vascularisation

and scarring. Topical steroids and cycloplegics are used for treatment, but the topical steroids should only be administered under the guidance of an ophthalmologist, and patients must be closely monitored.

5. **C – Aciclovir and prednisolone**. Oral antivirals reduce the severity and duration of herpes zoster ophthalmicus (HZO). A possible long-term sequel of HZO is post-herpetic neuralgia, which is a chronic pain in the region of the rash that can be debilitating. Oral antivirals reduce the incidence of post-herpetic neuralgia if given within 3 days of the vesicular eruption. Involvement of the corneal stroma and anterior uvea is common in HZO, unlike HSV keratitis, which usually affects the corneal epithelium only. Topical steroids are therefore important for the treatment of severe keratitis and uveitis. Topical antibiotics may also be used over the rash to prevent a superimposed bacterial infection. HZO can cause a number of complications that need be looked out for and treated. Complications of HZO include conjunctivitis, keratitis, anterior uveitis, scleritis, episcleritis, secondary glaucoma and optic neuritis.

    Latanoprost is a prostaglandin analogue. Other examples include bimatoprost and travaprost. This is a topical medication that increases aqueous outflow via the uveoscleral route. Aqueous fluid is normally drained via the trabecular meshwork (90%) and uveocleral route (10%). Prostaglandin analogues are the first-line treatment for chronic open-angle glaucoma (the most common form of glaucoma).

    A **trabeculectomy** is a surgical procedure performed for chronic open-angle glaucoma to allow aqueous fluid in the anterior chamber to drain underneath the conjunctiva forming a subconjunctival bleb, where it is consequently absorbed. This reduces the IOP in the eye.

A   Ophthalmology A7 – Ophthalmological terms

1. **H – Hypermetropia**. Emmetropia means that the eye has a normal refractive power. Myopia, or short-sightedness, is when light rays from a distant object are brought into focus in front of the retina. This is because the eye is too long or the refractive power is too great. The opposite is true in hypermetropia (or long-sightedness), so that light rays from a distant object reach the retina before coming into focus.

2. **A – Amblyopia** is also known as a 'lazy eye' and is most commonly unilateral. It is defined as poor vision in an eye in the absence of an organic cause, which is not correctable by refraction. It is most frequently caused

by strabismus (also termed 'squint'), which is a misalignment of the two eyes. If strabismus is present during a child's visual development, it can lead to amblyopia (without double vision). Strabismus occurring during visual development (first 6 years of life) leads to amblyopia without double vision, unlike strabismus occurring after visual development is complete which results in double vision.

3. **F – Flare**. The light scattering properties of protein leaked from blood vessels results in the visualisation of a flare on slit-lamp examination. Floating inflammatory cells and flare are important signs in anterior uveitis. On slit-lamp examination, floating cells appear similar to dust passing through a projector beam

4. **C – Astigmatism** is when the cornea is aspherical or rugby-shaped instead of being spherical or basketball-shaped. This leads to variable refraction of light rays received from different directions.

5. **J – Hypopyon**. A hypopyon can be seen in severe inflammatory conditions of the eye, such as a severe anterior uveitis or keratitis. Hyphema is when a red fluid level (blood) can be seen in the anterior chamber (e.g. in trauma).

    Anisocoria refers to a difference in size between the two pupils.

    Diplopia is the ophthalmological term for double vision.

    Floaters are dark spots that can be visualised by the patient, often described as flies, spiders, and so forth. This can be a phenomenon of normal ageing, or indicative of a posterior vitreous detachment, retinal detachment or inflammation. Photopsia are flashes of light, also indicative of retinal traction. Patients notice an increase in floaters and flashing lights when a retinal detachment occurs.

    A **scotoma** is an area of decreased or no vision in the visual field, surrounded by an area of good vision. This is a common feature of some chronic diseases such as glaucoma and age-related macular degeneration.

    Binocular vision is essential for the development of **stereopsis** (three-dimensional vision). Binocular vision is the ability to see an image simultaneously with both eyes. It is important for both eyes to be aligned and to have a good visual function to achieve binocular vision. Binocular vision allows for better visual fields and visual acuity, and also eliminates the blind spots from the visual fields.

A   Ophthalmology A8 – Eye structure and function

1. **B – Cornea**. Seventy per cent of the total refractive power of the eye is contributed by the cornea, and 30% is contributed by the lens, aqueous and vitreous. The cornea is a transparent structure made up of five layers, of which the stromal layer makes up 90% of the corneal thickness. It is avascular and made up of organised small diameter collagen fibrils that keep it transparent. The cornea has two principal functions: refraction of light and protection against entry of microorganisms and trauma. The refractive power of the cornea is the result of its curvature and its higher refractive index than air.

2. **G – Orbicularis oculi**. The orbicularis oculi is a sphincter muscle that closes the eyelid. It is innervated by the seventh cranial (facial) nerve. This is why facial nerve palsy causes an inability to close the ipsilateral eye and an ectropion of the lower eyelid.

3. **F – Müller's muscle**. Sympathetic fibres innervate Müller's muscle, which contributes to about 1.5 mm of lid elevation. The main muscle causing eyelid elevation is the levator palpebrae superioris muscle, which is innervated by the third cranial (oculomotor) nerve. The sympathetic fibres also innervate the iris dilator muscle, and are responsible for mydriasis. A lesion to the sympathetic pathway causes Horner's syndrome, which presents with the classic triad of MAP – **m**iosis, **a**nhydrosis (hemifacial) and **p**tosis (partial).

4. **A – Ciliary body**. The ciliary body is made of the ciliary muscle, ciliary processes and pars plana. Aqueous humour formation occurs in the ciliary processes.

5. **J – Zonules**. The ciliary muscle is innervated by the parasympathetic fibres of the third cranial nerve. Contraction of the ciliary muscle causes the zonular fibres, which are normally under tension, to relax. This results in an increased convexity of the elastic lens, which are attached to the zonules, thus enabling the eye to focus on nearby objects. This is known as accommodation. Relaxation of the ciliary muscle is passive, increasing tension on the zonules and leading to increased lens concavity for distant vision.

    The **trabecular meshwork** is the main site (90%) of aqueous drainage in the eye. Aqueous fluid passes through the trabecular meshwork and then through the canal of schlemm. The other 10% of aqueous drainage is via the uveoscleral route. Increased resistance at the trabecular meshwork is thought to lead to open-angle glaucoma.

The **retina** is made of the neuroretina and the retinal pigment epithelium. The neuroretina contains multiple retinal layers, which has the key function of transferring refracted light into electrical impulses that are sent to the brain via the optic nerve. The neuroretina contains photoreceptor cells, which are the cones and rods. Cones are concentrated within the fovea, which is at the centre of the macula. The macula is important for high-resolution, bright and colour vision. Rods are distributed throughout the retina, and are important for night vision and movement detection.

A   Ophthalmology A9 – Features of chronic ocular disorders

1. **C – Central scotoma**. Age-related macular degeneration (AMD) is the biggest cause of registered blindness in the Western world, accounting for approximately 40% of registered cases in the United Kingdom. As the name suggests, it is an ocular disease that becomes more prevalent with increasing age. It affects the central vision, but not the peripheral vision. Hence, it affects visual acuity but not peripheral vision. This therefore impacts on activities like reading and distinguishing distant objects, but not navigational activities. This is an extremely important message to convey to the patient, as navigational vision enables a patient to maintain independence in many activities of daily living. The cause of AMD is unknown. There are two forms of AMD: dry (non-exudative) and wet (exudative). Although dry AMD accounts for 90% of total AMD cases, wet AMD accounts for 90% of registered blindness due to AMD. AMD is characterised by subretinal drusen deposits and retinal pigment epithelium focal hyperpigmentation or atrophy. Visual loss occurs gradually over months or years. In wet AMD, neovascularisation from the choroidal circulation grows through defects in Bruch's membrane to form a choroidal neovascular membrane (CNVM) in the sub-retinal pigment epithelium or subretinally. This can bleed into the subretinal space or vitreous, leading to severe rapid loss of central vision (central scotoma). Patients may alternatively experience metamorphopsia (distortion of straight lines), which can be tested using an Amsler grid. The seemingly rapid onset of visual blurring in this scenario is more in keeping with a diagnosis of wet AMD, but this needs to be confirmed with fundus fluorescein angiography. The main findings of dry AMD on funduscopy are drusen deposits (well-circumscribed yellow lesions) and loss of the foveal reflex. No effective treatment for dry AMD exists. In the wet form, CNVM, as well as

subretinal haemorrhages and hard exudates, may be seen. Subretinal (disciform) scarring leads to permanent visual loss. Fundus fluorescein angiography is important for diagnosis and treatment. Treatment options include anti-vascular endothelium growth factor (anti-VEGF) therapy and photodynamic therapy (PDT), but these are not always effective.

2. **B – Arcuate scotoma**. Acquired primary (or chronic) open-angle glaucoma (POAG) is the most common type of glaucoma. It is the second most common cause of blindness worldwide, and the leading cause of irreversible visual loss. It is defined as a chronic degenerative optic neuropathy, and the pathophysiology is thought to be multifactorial. The optic neuropathy is the result of retinal ganglion cell loss and thinning of the retinal nerve fibre layer. The key clinical features of POAG are bilateral progressive optic disc cupping, optic disc rim notching and peripheral visual field loss. The anterior chamber angle is open on gonioscopy (unlike closed-angle glaucoma). The optic disc is made up of the white optic cup, which contains no fibres, and a surrounding disc with a pink neuroretinal rim, which is made of nerve fibres. There are also blood vessels entering and leaving the optic disc. Loss of optic nerve fibres in POAG leads to the neuroretinal rim becoming thinner, paler and notched, and the optic disc becoming thinner (cupping). A normal optic disc rim usually follows the 'ISNT' rule (thickest inferiorly then superiorly then nasally and thinning temporally). The neuroretinal rim thinning in glaucoma does not follow the ISNT rule, and notching typically occurs inferiorly or superiorly. An optical coherence tomography (OCT) scan of the peripapillary retinal nerve fibre layer (RNFL) is useful for illustrating RNFL thinning. Remember to correlate these findings with the pattern of visual field loss. Patients may also have retinal haemorrhages on or around the optic disc. The normal cup:disc ratio is about 0.2–0.3. Glaucoma is suspected in the presence of a cup:disc ratio of ≥0.6 or a ratio difference of >0.2 between the two eyes. About 25%–35% of retinal ganglion cells are lost before visual field defects are detected, which is why the disease is often diagnosed late. The classic visual field defects in the early stages of glaucoma are arcuate, paracentral or nasal step scotomas. The progression of the visual field loss should be regularly monitored (automated perimetry), and should correspond to the neuroretinal rim thinning. Severe peripheral visual field loss leading to 'tunnel vision' is a very late finding in glaucoma.

POAG is associated with raised intraocular pressure (IOP >21 mmHg). This is due to impairment of aqueous drainage through the trabecular meshwork (TM), the cause of which is incompletely understood. As 90%

of aqueous drainage is through the TM, aqueous fluid accumulates, leading to elevation of the IOP. IOP can be measured by tonometry. Central corneal thickness can affect the IOP reading, and must therefore always be measured (corneal pachymetry). Thick corneas overestimate the IOP and vice versa. It is important to note that up to one-third of patients with POAG have a normal IOP, and that of all patients with raised IOP, only a third have glaucoma. Other key risk factors for POAG are family history, old age, African race and steroid use. Glaucoma leads to loss of peripheral vision, with central visual field loss occurring late in the disease process. Patients typically notice reduced vision only once severe loss of peripheral vision has occurred. Lowering IOP remains the only proven therapy for POAG, and can slow or stop the disease progress. This is done with medical, laser or surgical therapy, and is discussed in Question 10 (Ophthalmology section).

3. **A – Annular mid-peripheral scotoma**. Retinitis pigmentosa (RP) is the most common inherited retinal condition, affecting 1 in 4000 of the population. It is a degeneration of the outer retina. It may be sporadic or inherited. Inheritance is autosomal recessive (most common), dominant and x-linked. It is important, therefore, to take a comprehensive family history to determine the mode of inheritance. It presents with the clinical triad of arteriolar attenuation (due to narrowing), mid-peripheral 'bone-spicule' retinal pigmentation and waxy pallor of the optic disc. The main symptoms are decreased night vision (often night blindness, termed 'nyctalopia') and loss of peripheral vision. RP causes an annular mid-peripheral scotoma, which progresses to a small central field of vision ('tunnel vision'). The diagnosis can be confirmed with an electroretinogram, which shows markedly reduced or non-recordable signals. Decreased ERG amplitude usually precedes retinal changes. Twenty-five per cent of RP is associated with systemic diseases. In Usher's syndrome, there is a combination of RP and hearing impairment. Management of RP includes counselling, social services and low-vision aids. Vitamin A palmitate may slow disease progression. Complications of RP include cataract and cystoid macular oedema. Patients should be monitored for these complications and managed accordingly.

4. **C – Central scotoma**. The most common visual field defect in dry AMD is a central or paracentral scotoma. AMD does not affect the peripheral visual field, hence why patients maintain their navigational vision.

5. **G – Loss of red reflex**. The lens inside the eye has a clear crystalline structure. It is an encapsulated crystalline structure with an inner nucleus and an outer cortex. Cataract is an opacification of the lens, and is the most common cause of visual impairment in low- and middle-income countries. It is an extremely common condition in the elderly, but not all patients require treatment. Most cataract is due to age-related degenerative changes, known as senile cataracts. Risk factors for senile cataracts include excessive exposure to ultraviolet light, diabetes mellitus, smoking and alcohol drinking. A small proportion of cataract is due to ocular causes (e.g. trauma, uveitis, topical steroids, post-operative), systemic disease (e.g. diabetes mellitus, hypocalcaemia), or medications (e.g. systemic steroids). Cataracts can also be congenital, and this is discussed in Question 20 (Ophthalmology section). There are different types of cataract. The principal types of cataract in the senile form are nuclear sclerosis (common), subcapsular and cortical. Steroid excess is usually associated with posterior subcapsular cataract. 'Oil drop' cataract is associated with galactosaemia (most common metabolic cause of congenital cataract). The degree of opacification is also important, and cataract is divided into immature, mature, hypermature and morgagnian cataract. The latter types are rare in the developed world as patients undergo intervention before reaching these stages. Common presenting symptoms include blurring of vision (near or distant), glare (poor vision in bright light) and monocular diplopia (due to monocular cataract). On examination, visual acuity is reduced and there is dimness or loss of the red reflex on direct ophthalmoscopy. The type of cataract can be determined on slit-lamp examination. It is also important to examine the fundus for other causes of visual impairment, which may be challenging in the presence of an advanced cataract. An ultrasound scan may be carried out in these cases to exclude retinal detachment. Changing the spectacles prescription may be effective initially, as cataract alters the refractive power of the eye (can become hypermetropic, but more commonly myopic). When the cataract is significantly affecting the patient's quality of life, surgery is offered as a definitive treatment for the patient. The surgical options are discussed in Question 16 (Ophthalmology section).

A **cherry-red spot** at the fovea with a pale retina and narrowed retinal arterioles is characteristic finding in central retinal artery occlusion. A cherry-red spot at the macula also occurs in various lipid storage disorders (e.g. Tay–Sachs disease). Diabetic proliferative retinopathy is when retinal neovascularisation occurs because of retinal ischaemia, and is a sign of advanced retinopathy.

A **pigmented fundus** lesion could be due to retinal pigment hypertrophy, regions of previous chorioretinitis, choroidal naevi or a malignant choroidal melanoma. The latter is the most rare but also most serious cause, and it is the most common primary intraocular malignancy in adults. The incidence is about 6/1 000 000 and is more common in Caucasians. Clinical symptoms are variable depending on the stage of the disease, and the tumour is often found incidentally. The diagnosis is usually made on indirect ophthalmoscopy, and an ocular ultrasound scan is important to further investigate the tumour. It is important to investigate patients for metastatic spread.

Roth's spots are retinal haemorrhages with pale centres composed of coagulated fibrin. They are most commonly found in leukaemia, subacute bacterial endocarditis and diabetes mellitus.

A   Ophthalmology A10 – Management of chronic ocular disorders

1. **I – Timolol**. The patient in this scenario has primary open-angle glaucoma (POAG). The bilateral inferior optic disc rim notching corresponds to the superior visual field defects. POAG is managed with medical, laser or surgical therapy. Lowering the intraocular pressure (IOP) remains the only proven therapy for glaucoma. IOP is reduced by either decreasing aqueous production or increasing aqueous drainage. Medical treatment is the first line for IOP reduction and is sufficient for most patients. The first-line medications for POAG are topical prostaglandin analogues and beta blockers. Prostaglandin analogues are more potent than beta blockers and have fewer side effects. Beta blockers should be avoided or used with extreme caution in patients with asthma, chronic obstructive pulmonary disease, bradycardia, second or third degree heart block and congestive heart failure. Table 1 lists important information about the medical therapy of POAG. It is very important to be familiar with these medications, their mechanism of action and side effects.

TABLE 1 Medications used to lower intraocular pressure (IOP) in glaucoma

Topical medications used for lowering IOP in glaucoma

Drug	Examples	Mechanism of action	Side effects
Prostaglandin analogues	Latanoprost, travoprost	Increases aqueous drainage via the uveoscleral route	Conjunctival hyperaemia, iris pigmentation, elongation of eyelashes
Beta blockers	Timolol, carteolol, betaxolol	Decreases aqueous production	Ocular irritation, systemic side effects of beta blockers (e.g. bronchospasm, bradycardia, heart block)
Alpha 2 agonists	Brimonidine, apraclonidine	Decreases aqueous production Increases aqueous drainage via the uveoscleral route	Allergy, bradycardia, fatigue, dry mouth
Carbonic anhydrase inhibitors	Brinzolamide, dorzolamide	Decreases aqueous production	Ocular irritation, allergic blepharoconjunctivitis, metallic taste
Muscarinic agonists	Pilocarpine	Increases aqueous drainage via the trabecular meshwork	Blurred vision, headache, brow ache, sweating, gastrointestinal disturbance, bradycardia

Systemic medications used for lowering IOP in glaucoma

Drug	Examples	Mechanism of action	Side effects
Carbonic anhydrase inhibitors	Acetazolamide	Decreases aqueous production	Metallic taste, malaise, paraesthesiae, depression, electrolyte disturbance, aplastic anaemia
Hyperosmotic	Mannitol	Osmotic diffusion	Headache, gastrointestinal disturbance, hyperglycaemia

2. **E – Panretinal laser photocoagulation**. Patients with proliferative diabetic retinopathy (DR) or diabetic maculopathy should be urgently referred to an ophthalmologist, as these are conditions that can progress to blindness. Good control of the blood glucose level (HbA1c 6.5%–7%), lipid levels and blood pressure is important in reducing progression of DR and the need for laser therapy. Diabetic maculopathy normally causes a gradual loss of vision. Proliferative retinopathy can lead to a more sudden

decline in vision. Fibrous proliferation from the growth of new blood vessels can contract and cause traction on the retina, leading to tractional retinal detachment (RD). Furthermore, the new fragile blood vessels can bleed, leading to a vitreous haemorrhage (VH). The risk of tractional RD and VH can be minimised by regular screening of diabetic patients and timely intervention. If they develop, patients need urgent vitreoretinal surgical review. Treatment of proliferative diabetic retinopathy is with panretinal laser photocoagulation, which causes regression of new blood vessels, reducing the risk of tractional RD and VH. This can be performed in the outpatient clinic.

3. **C – Focal laser photocoagulation.** Treatment of diabetic maculopathy is with laser photocoagulation aimed at points of leakage, which can be identified with fluorescein fundus angiography. If the leakage is focal (microaneurysms), then focal laser photocoagulation is used. If the leakage is diffuse, then grid laser photocoagulation is used, which treats the entire macula (excluding the fovea). This reduces vascular leakage and increases reabsorption of the retinal oedema. Laser treatment of proliferative retinopathy and maculopathy halves the risk of visual loss.

4. **H – Ranibizumab.** This patient complains of distortion of straight lines, also known as metamorphopsia, which is a typical symptom of wet (or exudative) age-related macular degeneration. Other symptoms include a central or paracentral scotoma and rapid (sometimes slow) loss of central vision that can be profound. A choroidal neovascular membrane (CNVM) is the typical finding on funduscopy, and patients should have fundus fluorescein angiography. This is useful in confirming the diagnosis, determining the size and location of the CNVM, and monitoring response to treatment. If the CNVM is non-subfoveal, then thermal laser photocoagulation is used. If the CNVM is subfoveal, then PDT or anti-vascular endothelium growth factor is used. PDT is performed every 3 months for up to 2 years. This decreases vision loss but does not improve vision. Intravitreal injections of anti-vascular endothelium growth factor agents (pegaptanib, ranibizumab and bevacizumab) is a relatively new treatment that is superseding PDT. Ranibizumab has been found to improve visual acuity by three or more Snellen chart lines in 30%–40% of eyes.

5. **J – Trabeculectomy.** When medical treatment of glaucoma fails, laser or surgical methods of lowering intraocular pressure (IOP) can be tried. The two most common treatments are laser trabeculoplasty and a

trabeculectomy. In a laser trabeculoplasty, argon laser treats the trabecular meshwork to increase aqueous flow. One of the key problems with this procedure is the risk of IOP rising again. A trabeculectomy is more reliable than laser trabeculoplasty, and is the most suitable option for this patient. A trabeculectomy is when a fistula is made between the anterior chamber and the subconjunctival space. Aqueous then drains into a subconjunctival bleb, where it is then absorbed. The operation has a high success rate. Complications include intraocular infection, cataract development, failure to reduce IOP, hypotony (abnormally low IOP) and macular oedema due to over-reduction of IOP. Antimetabolites such as 5-fluorouracil or mitomycin C may be given to reduce the risk of subconjunctival scarring post-operatively.

A Ophthalmology A11 – Ophthalmic tests

1. **G – LogMAR charts**. Visual acuity, in simple terms, is the clarity of someone's vision. A Snellen chart or a LogMAR chart can be used to assess visual acuity. LogMAR charts are more accurate than Snellen charts and are increasingly used in children, patients with poor vision and research. A Snellen chart comprises of multiple lines, each containing letters. As you move down the chart, the number of letters increases, and their size decreases. Each line on the Snellen chart is labelled with a number, which is the distance in metre at which a person with normal vision is able to read this line. The patient should stand at a distance of 6 metres and cover one eye before reading the letters. The visual acuity is recorded as a fraction: the distance at which the patient is standing (i.e. 6) over the lowest line that can be read. For example, if the patient can read down to the line labelled 12, his or her visual acuity is 6/12. It is important to be able to tell the patient what this means. A visual acuity of 6/18 means that the patient can see at 6 metres what a person with normal vision can see at 18 metres. If the patient cannot read any of the lines, the test can be repeated at 3 metres and 1 metre. Visual acuity can then be recorded as the distance from the chart in metres (numerator) over the lowest row that can be read (denominator). If the patient can still not read the letters, they are assessed for ability to count fingers, see hand movements or have perception of light. If they do not have perception of light, this is recorded as no perception of light. On the LogMAR chart, the difference in letter size between each row is standardised. Furthermore, the number of letters in each row is equal throughout. This makes the LogMAR chart a more accurate test of visual acuity than Snellen charts. The patient is situated 4 metres from

the LogMAR chart, and visual acuity is recorded as a decimal, with 0.00 equating to 6/6 on the Snellen chart. The visual acuity score takes into account the number of letters the patient can see on a row, as incompletely read lines are a common finding in optometric practice.

2. **H – Perimetry** is a formal method of plotting someone's visual field, and can detect more subtle visual field defects than confrontational visual field testing. It can be static or kinetic. In static visual field testing, the patient reports when he or she can first see a stationary light of increasing brightness (e.g. Humphrey's perimetry). In kinetic visual field testing, the patient reports when he or she can see a light of a known luminance moving from a non-seeing to a seeing area (e.g. Goldmann perimetry).

3. **B – Biometry** involves measuring the corneal curvature as well as the axial length of the eye to calculate the correct refractive power of the intraocular lens to be used in cataract surgery. Keratometry allows measurement of the corneal curvature, but this is insufficient on its own for calculation of the appropriate refractive power of an intraocular lens. Keratometry measures illuminated shapes reflected from the surface of the cornea. It is important before fitting spectacles lens, before refractive surgery as well as before intraocular lens insertion in cataract surgery. The axial length (anteroposterior diameter) of the eye is measured using an A-scan (ultrasound modality).

4. **D – Gonioscopy** is a special diagnostic contact lens with an inbuilt mirror that is used for assessment of the iridocorneal (or anterior chamber) angle. This angle is closed in angle-closure glaucoma (ACG). The anterior chamber angle is usually also shallow in the contralateral unaffected eye in ACG, which is why both eyes are at increased risk of developing ACG.

5. **I – Seidel test** is used to assess aqueous leakage from the anterior chamber due to a perforation. Sodium fluorescein (2%) is applied over the potential perforation site that is then observed with the blue cobalt light of a slit lamp. If the Seidel test is positive, the fluorescein dye will be diluted by aqueous from the wound site, and appears as green (dilute) stream within the orange (concentrated) dye.

   Ishihara plates are used to assess colour vision defects, particularly red and green cone function. An Ishihara plate book consists of 13, 17 or 21 plates (depending on the book used) containing different sized and coloured dots arranged in patterns representing numbers. The first plate is a control plate, which does not test colour vision. For the purpose of the test, one eye is covered and the patient is asked to read each plate at a normal reading distance (maximum time of 5 seconds per plate is allowed). The number of plates read is then recorded as a fraction of the total number of plates. It is important to ensure that there is adequate lighting in the room, and that any reading glasses are worn. Red desaturation is another clinical test in which the patient is asked to look at a red object with each eye and report if the redness is dimmer in one eye than the next. Colour vision dysfunction is caused by macular disease (involving the cones) or anterior visual pathway disease. This is because colour vision is detected by cones and transmitted by the optic nerve.

An **Amsler grid** is used to test central macular function. It is made of multiple equally sized squares and a black dot in the middle of the chart. The patient is asked to fixate vision on the central black dot from a distance of an arm's length and is asked to report any missing (scotoma) or curving lines (metamorphopsia). It is used to detect central and paracentral scotomas indicative of macular dysfunction. A scotoma is an area of the visual field in which vision is depressed or lost. Metamorphopsia is an important finding in wet age-related macular degeneration.

Tonometry is used for the measurement of the intraocular pressure (IOP). Normal IOP range is thought to be between 10–21 mmHg. In acute ACG, IOP is substantially elevated, often above 50 mmHg.

A   Ophthalmology A12 – Ocular manifestations of vascular diseases

1. **H – Severe non-proliferative diabetic retinopathy**

2. **E – Grade 2 hypertensive retinopathy**

3. **C – Diabetic maculopathy**

4. **G – Grade 4 hypertensive retinopathy**

5. **J – Sickle cell retinopathy**

Microaneurysms, dot and blot haemorrhages, flame-shaped haemorrhages, exudates and cotton wool spots are non-specific signs of a number of acute and chronic retinal vascular diseases. They can occur in both diabetic and hypertensive retinopathy. Regardless of the underlying disease, the aforementioned changes are the result of either vascular leakage or vascular occlusion in the retinal capillaries.

Damage to the capillaries can result in leakage of blood and lipid deposits, manifesting as haemorrhages and exudates respectively. Cotton wool spots are swollen axons caused by microinfarctions of the retinal nerve fibre layer, which is the result of precapillary arteriolar occlusion. These appear as fluffy white focal lesions. Hard exudates are typically smaller, more well-defined and yellowish in colour.

The most commonly used staging system for **hypertensive retinopathy** (HR) is the Modified Scheie Classification. Staging is as shown in Table 2.

TABLE 2 The modified Scheie classification of hypertensive retinopathy

Grade of hypertensive retinopathy	Funduscopy findings
1	Generalised arterial narrowing (seen as 'copper' or 'silver' wiring)
2	Grade 1 + arteriovenous nipping
3	Grade 2 + flame-shaped haemorrhages and/or cotton wool spots
4	Grade 3 plus disc swelling

Chronic elevation of blood pressure leads to arteriosclerosis. This gives rise to arteriolar narrowing and venous nipping (constriction) at arteriovenous (AV) crossing points. AV nipping is a sign specific to HR, and is not a feature of diabetic retinopathy (DR). Arteriolar narrowing is another important feature of HR, and is due to smooth muscle contraction in the vascular wall in response to elevated blood pressure. This results in increased opacity with a resultant broadening of the arteriolar light reflex. The light reflex occupies part or all of the arteriolar width, resulting in 'copper' or 'silver' wiring respectively. Disc swelling can be a sign of malignant hypertension, which has a 90% 1-year mortality rate if untreated. HR is treated by blood pressure reduction. An acute drop in blood pressure, especially in patients with severe hypertension, can result in a stroke. HR is normally reversible once blood pressure is adequately controlled.

Around 80% of diabetic patients develop **diabetic retinopathy** 20 years after the onset of the disease. The earliest sign of DR on funduscopy is microaneurysms, which are focal capillary dilatations resulting from loss of pericytes surrounding the capillaries. Rupture of these microaneurysms gives rise to dot and blot haemorrhages. Leakage from these capillary walls and from microaneurysms results in retinal oedema and hard exudates.

Diabetic maculopathy refers to the presence of retinal oedema (pale retina) and hard exudates within the macula. Macular oedema may be very difficult to detect on funduscopy (as is the case in the third scenario), and any patient therefore with unexplained visual loss should be urgently referred to an ophthalmologist. Clinically, macular oedema appears as retinal thickening at the macular area. Ocular coherence tomography (OCT) scanning is an invaluable method for the assessment of diabetic maculopathy. A large number of cotton wool spots reflects the presence of significant ischaemia. Venous loops and venous beading (saccular bulges) occur in areas of retinal ischaemia, and are the most significant predictors of the development of proliferative retinopathy. Retinal ischaemia leads to the release of vasogenic factors, which result in the growth of new blood vessels (neovascularisation). Table 3 outlines the International Clinical Diabetic Retinopathy Disease Severity Scale.

TABLE 3 International Clinical Diabetic Retinopathy Disease Severity Scale

Stage of diabetic retinopathy	Funduscopy findings
No apparent retinopathy	No abnormalities
Mild NPDR	Microaneurysms only
Moderate NPDR	More than just microaneurysms but less than severe NPDR
Severe NPDR	No signs of proliferative retinopathy, with any of the following: • >20 intraretinal haemorrhages in each of four quadrants • definite venous beading in two or more quadrants • prominent intraretinal microvascular abnormalities in one or more quadrants
Proliferative diabetic retinopathy	One or more of the following: • Optic disc or retinal neovascularisation • Vitreous or pre-retinal haemorrhage

NPDR, Non-Proliferative Diabetic Retinopathy.

Diabetic patients should have annual funduscopy and digital retinal photography to monitor for new or progressing diabetic retinopathy. Good control of the blood glucose level is essential (HbA1c 6.5%–7%). Diabetes is also associated with cataracts, rubeotic glaucoma, extraocular muscle palsies and retinal vascular occlusions. Patients with proliferative DR or diabetic maculopathy should be urgently referred to an ophthalmologist, as these are conditions that can progress to blindness. Patients with pre-proliferative DR need a routine ophthalmologist referral. Diabetic maculopathy normally causes a gradual blurring of vision. In proliferative retinopathy, fibrous proliferation from the growth of new blood vessels can contract and cause traction on the retina, leading to tractional retinal detachment. Furthermore, the new fragile blood vessels can bleed, leading to a vitreous haemorrhage. These two conditions are important causes of rapid visual loss, and need urgent vitreretinal surgical intervention. Treatment of proliferative diabetic retinopathy is with panretinal laser photocoagulation (leads to worsening of night vision). The aim of treatment of diabetic maculopathy is to prevent foveal damage. Focal laser photocoagulation aimed at points of leakage is used for focal maculopathy. Points of leakage can be identified with fluorescein fundus angiography. Diffuse maculopathy is treated with grid laser photocoagulation. Laser treatment of proliferative retinopathy and maculopathy significantly reduces the risk of visual loss. Intravitreal steroids may also be used for treatment of macular oedema (risk of intraocular pressure rise). The US Food and Drug Administration (FDA) approved Lucentis (Ranibizumab, an anti-VEGF agent) for the treatment of diabetic macular oedema in 2012. In January 2013, Lucentis was also approved in the UK by the National Institute for Health and Clinical Excellence (NICE) for this purpose. This is particularly effective for centre-involving diabetic macular oedema, and can be used with or without combination laser treatment.

Sickle cell retinopathy, a severe retinopathy, can present in patients with sickle cell haemoglobin C and sickle cell haemoglobin with thalassemia, as a result of sickle-shaped red blood cells that obstruct the smaller retinal vasculature. Paradoxically, a milder retinopathy is seen in homozygous sickle cell (SS) disease. Two types of retinopathy are seen: non-proliferative and proliferative. In the non-proliferative form black sunburst scars, salmon-patch retinal haemorrhages and tortuous veins are seen. In the proliferative retinopathy form, neovascularisation occurs, with blood vessels forming in a 'sea fan' distribution. Patients with proliferative changes should be urgently referred to an ophthalmologist. Treatment is with laser photocoagulation. As with diabetic retinopathy, both retinal detachment and a vitreous haemorrhage can occur.

Central retinal artery occlusion is a cause of sudden severe monocular visual loss. Typical findings on funduscopy include pale retina (oedematous) with thin blood vessels and a 'cherry-red spot' at the fovea. It is discussed in Question 1 (Ophthalmology section).

A   **Ophthalmology A13 – Visual impairment**

1. **E – Age-related macular degeneration**. About 2.5% of the UK population have a visual impairment that is not correctable by refraction. Two-thirds of these patients qualify for registration as blind. Age-related macular degeneration accounts for approximately 40% of registered blindness in the United Kingdom, followed by glaucoma (13%) and diabetic retinopathy (8%).

2. **J – Uncorrected refractive errors**. Around 284 million people around the world are estimated to have visual impairment. Of these, 39 million are blind, and 245 million have low vision. More than 90% of people with visual impairment live in low-income countries. Cataract is the main cause of visual impairment in low and middle-income countries. Worldwide, uncorrected refractive errors are the main cause of visual impairment.

3. **C – 6/60**. 'Severe visual impairment' is the term now used for blindness. If a person's best corrected visual acuity is less than 3/60 with a normal visual field, they are eligible for registration as 'severely sight impaired'. If the best corrected visual acuity is better than 3/60 but less than 6/60, with a normal visual field, a person can be registered as 'sight impaired'. A person can be registered as 'severely sight impaired' or 'sight impaired' at better visual acuities than stated here if they also have certain visual field defects. Registration entitles patients to various types of home, community and financial support services. However, only one in three of the population who are eligible for partial sight or blind registration are actually registered.

4. **B – 6/12**. A private car driver must be able to read in good light (with corrective lenses if necessary) a registration mark fixed to a motor vehicle and containing letters and figures 79.4 mm high at a distance of 20.5 m. This equated to a visual acuity of between 6/9 and 6/12 on the Snellen chart. For large goods vehicles (LGVs) and passenger-carrying vehicles (PCVs), visual acuity (with corrective lenses if necessary) must be at least 6/9 in the better eye and at least 6/12 in the worst eye. If corrective lenses are used, the uncorrected acuity in both eyes must be at least 3/60. To drive a private car, the binocular visual field must be 120 degrees horizontally and 20 degrees above and below the horizontal meridian. Visual field defects bar driving of LGVs or PCVs. Monocularity and corrected diplopia are permitted for private car drivers, but not for LGV and PCV drivers.

5. **H – Galilean telescope**. The Galilean telescope was used by Galileo to observe distant celestial objects in the sky. It consists of a convex lens, which acts as the objective, and a concave lens as the eyepiece. It is used as a low-vision aid as it produces an upright magnified image (2–4× strength), and has the advantages of being light and inexpensive. A Newtonian telescope is a reflecting telescope in which the image is viewed through an eyepiece at right angles to the optical axis. It is not used as a low-vision aid.

A Ophthalmology A14 – HIV eye disease

1. **B – Cytomegalovirus retinopathy** is the most common opportunistic ocular infection in AIDS, causing a severe retinitis. Before the advent of HAART, this was present in up to 40% of patients with AIDS. Maintaining the CD4+ count above 50/mm^3 is effective prophylaxis against cytomegalovirus (CMV) retinitis. The most common symptoms are visual blurring and floaters. The characteristic funduscopy finding is a white area of exudate in the retina, containing flame-shaped haemorrhages. The appearance is said to resemble 'pizza' or 'cottage cheese'. Unlike toxoplasmosis infection, there is no vitritis or iritis. Parenteral antivirals (ganciclovir and/or foscarnet) form the mainstay of treatment. These drugs may also be by intravitreal injection.

2. **J – Toxoplasma retinochoroiditis**. The patient in this scenario has symptoms of anterior uveitis. His funduscopy findings are pathognomonic of toxoplasma retinochoroiditis. Unlike CMV retinitis, vitritis and iritis are common in toxoplasma retinochoroiditis. The infection is caused by the organism toxoplasma gondii, and may be congenital or acquired. Toxoplasmosis is the most common cause of posterior uveitis in non-HIV patients. A toxoplasma retinochoroiditis is common in AIDS patients, most frequently due to an acquired infection. Similarly to CMV retinitis, the most common symptoms are visual blurring and floaters, but patients may be asymptomatic. The eye may also be red and painful. It presents with characteristic funduscopy findings: fluffy white/yellow lesions (focal retinal necrosis) with vitreous haze (due to white cell infiltration), usually occurring on the border of an atrophic (chorioretinal) scar with a pigmented border. The diagnosis is clinical. A positive toxoplasma antibody test must be interpreted carefully as it is a frequent finding in non-infected adults. Treatment is with anti-protozoal drugs (e.g. pyrimethamine). Immunocompetent patients also require systemic steroids.

3. **D – HIV microvasculopathy** is the most common retinal pathology in HIV-positive patients (~75% of HIV patients). It is a non-infective microvascular disease affecting the conjunctiva and/or retina. Vision is unaffected. The most common sign on funduscopy is cotton wool spots (white fluffy lesions), followed by tortuous retinal vessels, intraretinal hameorrhages and microaneurysms. No treatment is indicated. It is important to exclude diabetic and hypertensive retinopathy in these patients. Cotton wool spots are indicative of advanced diabetic or hypertensive retinopathy. The patient in this scenario complains of dry eyes, which are not a feature of this condition, but are a very common finding in HIV-positive patients. They are managed with topical eye lubricants. Dry eyes may or may not be associated with blepharitis.

4. **F – Kaposi's sarcoma** (KS) is the most common malignancy in patients with HIV disease, and is an AIDS-defining illness. It presents as a non-blanching dark red/purple lesion, usually palpable and non-pruritic. It can appear anywhere, but typically occurs in the head and neck or lower limbs. Conjunctival KS is brighter red in colour. KS is commonly associated with lymphoedema, and a thorough examination of the head and neck is therefore essential. It is important to measure the CD4+ count and plasma HIV viral load if KS is suspected. Treatment is with surgical excision, radiotherapy or chemotherapy.

5. **G – Lymphoma**. This patient has a bilateral exophthalmos and signs of lymphadenopathy. Both Graves' disease and carotid cavernous sinus fistula can cause exophthalmos, but do not cause a lymphadenopathy. As thyroid eye disease is the most common cause of unilateral and bilateral proptosis, a thyroid function test is essential to exclude the disease. Orbital lymphomas (most common being non-Hodgkin's) and orbital cellulitis are the most common orbital complications in HIV-positive patients. Orbital lymphoma is treated with local radiotherapy and systemic chemotherapy.

    Carotid-cavernous sinus fistula is an abnormal communication between the internal or external carotid arteries and the cavernous sinus. This occurs following trauma (75%) or spontaneously (25%). Patients may complain of eye redness and/or bulging, diplopia, decreased vision and hearing a pulsatile buzzing sound (tinnitus). Findings on examination include ocular proptosis (which may be pulsatile), eyelid oedema, conjunctival swelling, injected episcleral veins and a loud ocular bruit. It is not associated with HIV infection or lymphadenopathy.

    Molluscum contagiosum is a white nodular lesion at the lid margin.

In HIV patients, profuse lesions can be present. It is caused by poxvirus, and can cause a chronic conjunctivitis.

Grave's thyroid eye disease and **HSV keratitis** are very important eye conditions, which are commonly asked about in written and clinical examinations. These have already been discussed in this book.

A   Ophthalmology A15 – Ocular side effects of drugs

1. **D – Digoxin**. Xanthopsia refers to a yellowing of vision. The most common causes of this are digoxin overdose and cataracts. It is important to be familiar with signs of digoxin toxicity, as digoxin is a relatively commonly used drug with a narrow therapeutic index. Other visual symptoms of digoxin toxicity are blurring of vision and seeing halos around lights.

2. **A – Amiodarone** is an anti-arrhythmic drug that can cause a whorl-like pattern of microcorneal deposits, known as whorl or vortex keratopathy. This occurs in more than 90% of patients who have been on amiodarone for 6 months. A vortex keratopathy may also occur in Fabry's disease and as a side effect of a variety of other medications including indomethacin, chloroquine, chlorpromazine and tamoxifen. The presence of slate-grey skin discolouration makes the most likely answer to be amiodarone. In 1%–2% of patients, amiodarone can cause an optic neuropathy.

3. **C – Corticosteroids**. Use of systemic and topical ocular steroids is associated with the development of posterior subcapsular cataract (a functionally debilitating form of cataracts) and secondary glaucoma.

4. **G – Morphine**. Opiates can cause pupil constriction or a sluggish pupil in overdose. These are important signs to pick up, as opiates are commonly used for pain control. Opiate overdose is not uncommon in hospital wards and can be fatal.

5. **F – Hydroxychloroquine** and chloroquine are antimalarial drugs. Hydroxychloroquine is also used as a disease-modifying anti-rheumatic drug for the treatment of rheumatoid arthritis, juvenile arthritis and systemic lupus erythematosus. Side effects include reversible corneal deposits and non-reversible 'bull's eye' maculopathy. The latter sign is associated with impaired visual acuity and central visual field disturbance. This is why patients on these medications should be monitored for visual signs and symptoms annually, preferably by an optometrist. A bull's eye maculopathy

may also occur in age-related macular degeneration, Stargardt's disease, cone dystrophy and Spielmeyer–Vogt syndrome.

Atropine, tropicamide and cyclopentolate are muscarinic receptor antagonists, often used topically as mydriatics/cycloplegics. Pupil dilation can result in visual blurring, especially on near vision as the pupil cannot accommodate. They may also precipitate angle-closure glaucoma in people with shallow anterior chambers.

Ethambutol and quinine are associated with optic neuropathy. Ethambutol is used for the treatment of tuberculosis, and quinine is used for the treatment of malaria and night-time leg cramps.

Tamoxifen is used as a hormonal treatment for breast cancer. It can cause crystalline deposits in the retina (crystalline retinopathy), and more rarely in the cornea.

Vigabatrin is an antiepileptic agent, also used for infantile spasms (West's syndrome). It can cause visual field defects. Patients should have baseline visual field testing before starting treatment, and 6-monthly reviews thereafter for 3 years. If no visual field defects are detected after 3 years of treatment, patients can be reviewed annually.

Warfarin is an anticoagulant that can cause retinal and subconjunctival haemorrhages.

A   Ophthalmology A16 – Ocular conditions in the developing world

1. **A – Azithromycin**. Trachoma is the most common infectious cause of blindness worldwide. A trachoma infection is caused by the organism *Chlamydia trachomatis* (serotypes A–C), leading to a severe chronic conjunctivitis. It is spread by flies and hand-to-eye contact, and it is endemic in areas of crowding and poor hygiene. *C. trachomatis* also affects the genital tract and respiratory system. The initial clinical features are a red sore eye with a purulent discharge and palpebral conjunctival features due to a mucopurulent keratoconjunctivitis. A commonly used clinical system of classification for trachoma is the World Health Organization classification.

TABLE 4 World Health Organization classification system for trachoma

Trachoma inflammation follicular	Trachoma inflammation intense	Trachoma scarring	Trachoma trichiasis	Corneal opacity
Five or more follicles in upper tarsal conjunctiva of >0.5 mm diameter	Papillary hypertrophy plus inflammatory thickening of the upper tarsal conjunctiva obscuring more than half of deep tarsal vessels	Tarsal conjunctival scarring	One or more ingrowing eyelashes touching the globe or epilation (eyelash removal)	Corneal opacity obscuring part of the pupil margin

Recurrent trachoma infection causes scarring and contraction, leading to a shortened and distorted upper eyelid and trichiasis. This leads to corneal ulceration and scarring, which in turn leads to corneal opacification: the cause of blindness in trachoma. A diagnosis of trachoma is made if two of following criteria are met:

- superior tarsal follicles
- limbal follicles or Herbert's pits (necrosis of follicles)
- subepithelial conjunctival scarring
- superficial corneal neovascularisation.

Swabs can be taken for immunofluorescence staining. The SAFE strategy is a public health strategy that is endorsed by the World Health Organization for the treatment and prevention of trachoma.

- **S**urgery: for entropion and trichiasis
- **A**ntibiotics: treatment is with a single dose of oral azithromycin (1 g)
- **F**acial cleanliness: to prevent disease transmission; ocular lubricants are helpful for eye dryness
- **E**nvironmental change: increased access to water and sanitation

Promotion of face washing and fly control with insecticides has been shown to reduce trachoma infection. It is important to know the difference between trichiasis and entropion, as they may be caused by different conditions and managed differently. Trichiasis refers to eyelashes growing in their normal position, but which are posteriorly directed. When the eyelashes grow from an abnormal position, this is known as distichiasis. Entropion and ectropion refer to an abnormal inversion and eversion of the eyelid respectively. The most common form of both conditions is the involutional form, which results from ageing. An entropion can lead to a pseudotrichiasis, in which the eyelashes are posteriorly directed because of the lid inversion.

2. **F – Rifampicin, isoniazid, pyrazinamide and ethambutol**. About one-third of the world's population is estimated to be infected by mycobacterium tuberculosis (TB). Each year, more than 9 million people around the world develop TB disease (when the tuberculosis bacteria is active). The incidence of ocular TB in active TB is 1.5%–5.7%, which increases to 2.8%–11.4% in patients with HIV. TB can affect the external (e.g. lid abscess, scleritis), anterior (e.g. anterior uveitis, keratitis) and posterior (e.g. vitritis, retinitis) structures of the eye. The most common ocular manifestations of TB are choroidal tubercles and choroiditis. Choroidal tubercles are detected on ophthalmoscopy as multiple small and discrete white or yellow nodules with indistinct borders in the choroid at the posterior pole of the eye. These can be as unilateral or bilateral, and are virtually diagnostic. Choroidal tubercles may be the first signs of miliary (disseminated) disease, allowing the clinician to institute anti-TB treatment earlier in the disease course. It is therefore essential to examine the fundi of a patient with suspected TB. The clinical presentation depends on the ocular structure affected. Most commonly, patients present with blurred vision, with or without a red eye and ocular pain. It is crucial that all patients presenting with active TB have an ocular examination, as they may not have ocular symptoms. The chest X-ray will show signs of TB in 50% of ocular TB cases. Characteristically there are apical infiltrates, but less specific signs include consolidation, pleural effusion and hilar lymphadenopathy. It is important to take a comprehensive history from the patient and establish the presence of any other systemic features, as TB can affect most systems in the body. One of the most important factors in determining duration of treatment is the body system affected by TB. In suspected TB, patients should have a chest X-ray, tuberculin skin test (Mantoux test) as well as multiple sputum and early morning urine samples sent for microscopy, culture and sensitivity and Ziehl-Neelsen staining. It is important to test close contacts of patients with confirmed TB. The main test for latent TB is the Mantoux test (tuberculin testing). If the Mantoux test is positive or less reliable (e.g. in those vaccinated with the Bacillus Calmette–Guérin vaccine), then interferon-gamma testing can be done. A positive interferon-gamma test means that the person has been infected with TB, but the test does not inform the physician if the patient has a latent TB infection or TB disease. More specific tests depend on the body organ affected (e.g. cerebrospinal fluid examination

in suspected TB meningitis). As TB is an AIDS-defining illness, patients at risk of co-existing HIV infection should be offered an HIV test. The standard treatment regimen for active TB is with oral rifampicin, isoniazid, pyrazinamide and ethambutol for 2 months, followed by rifampicin and isoniazid for 4 months. Baseline renal and liver function tests are done before starting treatment. Pyridoxine is co-administered with isoniazid to reduce the risk of peripheral neuropathy. Ethambutol can cause an optic neuritis, which is why all patients should have their visual acuity, near vision, colour vision and visual fields checked before commencing therapy. Patients are warned to report any visual symptoms throughout the duration of treatment. Additional treatment to the aforementioned anti-TB regimen may be required depending on the ocular structures affected. TB cases with persistent ocular TB despite the aforementioned anti-TB therapy may also require topical or systemic steroids. These patients should be treated and monitored by both an ophthalmologist and a TB specialist.

3. **C – Ivermectin**. Onchocerciasis (river blindness) affects about 20 million people worldwide. It is caused by *Onchocerca volvulus*, a helminth. The vector is a female blackfly (*Simulium* species), which breeds in areas of fast-flowing water. It is endemic in equatorial Africa, Yemen and South America. The blackfly bite transmits larvae into the skin, resulting in subcutaneous nodules (onchocercomata) in which adult worms grow. These produce microfilariae that migrate through the skin and lymphatics all over the body, but are preferentially found in the skin and eye. A hypersensitivity reaction to these microfilariae causes the clinical features of onchocerciasis. An early clinical sign is 'snowflake' punctate keratitis, in which opacities represent a reaction to the microfilarium. This advances to sclerosing keratitis, which is complete opacification of the cornea, resulting in blindness. Onchocerciasis also commonly causes a chronic anterior uveitis (may result in a pear-shaped pupil), chorioretinitis and secondary glaucoma. Less commonly, it causes optic neuritis (leading to optic atrophy). Slit lamp examination may reveal the microfilariae in the aqueous. Antibodies may be detected in blood, but do not distinguish between past and present infections. A skin-snip biopsy can confirm the diagnosis. Ivermectin, a broad-spectrum anti-parasitic agent, is the drug of choice for onchocerciasis.

4. **H – Vitamin A supplementation**. Vitamin A deficiency is a major cause of visual impairment in Africa and Latin America. Vitamin A is important for the maintenance of the epithelium. Deficiency of vitamin A results

from dietary deficiency (rare in developed countries), chronic alcoholism or impaired gastrointestinal tract absorption. It occurs most commonly in children affected by poverty in the developing world, with a peak incidence between 3 and 5 years of age. Deficiency leads to atrophy and keratinisation of epithelium throughout the body. The earliest and most common symptom in vitamin A deficiency is night blindness. Patients also complain of dry eyes, eye pain and visual loss. Therefore, it is important to differentiate this condition from other causes of night blindness (e.g. retinitis pigmentosa) and dry eyes (e.g. conjunctivitis sicca). Vitamin A deficiency causes xerophthalmia (dryness) of the conjunctiva and cornea, resulting in ulceration, necrosis and scarring of these tissues. Xerophthalmia is therefore a blinding ocular disease.

TABLE 5 World Health Organization classification of vitamin A deficiency xerophthalmia

Classification	Ocular signs
XN	Night blindness
X1A	Conjunctival xerosis
X1B	Bitôt's spot
X2	Corneal xerosis
X3A	Corneal ulceration or keratomalacia, with less than one-third of cornea involved
X3B	Corneal ulceration or keratomalacia, with one-third or more of cornea involved
XS	Corneal scar
XF	Xerophthalmia fundus

Xerosis means dryness. Bitôt's spots are grey, foamy, triangular perilimbal conjunctival plaques containing keratinised debris and saprophytic bacteria. The corneal xerosis and ulceration of trachoma is different in that it begins at the conjunctival surface of the upper eyelid. Keratomalacia, referred to in Table 5, is when the cornea becomes soft and necrotic. Xerophthalmia fundus is when white dots are detected on funduscopy around the periphery of the fundus.

Vitamin A deficiency affects many other systems throughout the body. Increased severity of xerophthalmia is associated with increased morbidity and mortality. Treatment is vitamin A supplementation, which can be oral (preferred) or intramuscular, and a protein rich diet. Highly pigmented vegetables are an excellent source of vitamin A. Vitamin A supplementation should be avoided in pregnant women because of the risk of vitamin A embryopathy. Dietary supplements with vitamin A are used prophylactically in high-risk areas to prevent vitamin A deficiency. In addition to vitamin A replenishment, intensive ocular lubrication is also required initially, as the eye dryness can be debilitating. Secondary ocular infections are common in xerophthalmia, which is why topical antibiotics ointments are usually used as prophylaxis. Measles is an important cause of visual impairment and mortality in the developing world, with the risk of both sequels being increased by vitamin A deficiency.

5. **E – Phacoemulsification**. The lens inside the eye has a clear crystalline structure. It is an encapsulated crystalline structure with an inner nucleus and an outer cortex. A cataract is an opacification of the lens, and is the most common cause of visual impairment in low and middle-income countries. The presentation of cataracts is discussed in Question 9 (Ophthalmology section). Depending on the extent of lens opacification, a cataract can be immature, mature, hypermature and morgagnian cataract. This patient has advanced opacification in both eyes, causing severe loss of vision. This is more common in the developing world, as cataract removal surgery is normally performed at a much earlier stage in the developed world. As the fundus cannot be visualised in the patient, there may also be another underlying disease in the posterior segment of the eye (e.g. diabetic retinopathy). Therefore, although his cataract can be removed, his vision may still be impaired due to other underlying conditions. Changing the glasses prescription may be effective for the management of early cataract, as the opacification of the lens alters the refractive power of the eye (may become hypermetropic, but more commonly myopic). When the cataract is significantly affecting the patient's quality of life, surgery is offered as a definitive treatment for the patient. Surgery involves cataract removal and intraocular lens insertion, usually under local anaesthesia. Cataract surgery is the most commonly performed surgery in the United Kingdom and United States. Before the surgery, biometry is required. This consists of measuring the corneal curvature as well as the axial length (anterior-posterior diameter) of the eye to calculate the correct refractive power of the intraocular lens to be used in cataract surgery. Keratometry allows measurement of the curvature of the anterior corneal surface. The axial length is measured using an A-scan (ultrasound modality). Around the world, extracapsular cataract extraction is the most commonly used technique for cataract removal. In the developed world, cataracts surgery is performed by phacoemulsification and intraocular

lens insertion. This procedure takes approximately 15–20 minutes. A small incision is made in the peripheral cornea. A circular hole is then made in the anterior part of the lens capsule (capsulorhexis), and fluid is injected into the lens to separate the capsule from the nucleus and cortex. An ultrasound (phaco) probe is then inserted, and the lens is fragmented, emulsified and aspirated. When all cortical fragments have been aspirated (to minimise post-operative inflammation), a small folded intraocular lens is then inserted into the posterior capsule. The posterior capsule is left in place to hold the lens in place and keep it separate from the vitreous humour. The patient is given a short course of topical antibiotics and steroids post-operatively. About 80%–90% of patients achieve a vision of 6/12 or better. The most common post-operative complication is posterior capsule opacification (approximately 20%). This is treated by making a hole in the posterior capsule with a Nd:YAG laser capsulotomy. The risk of posterior lens capsule rupture during the surgery is less than 4%. Other uncommon complications include cystoid macular oedema (usually mild and transient), displaced intraocular pressure and retinal detachment. The most severe complications of cataract surgery are endophthalmitis and suprachoroidal haemorrhage (~0.1% risk).

A Ophthalmology A17 – Ocular signs I

1. **F – Osteogenesis imperfecta**. Blue sclera is a characteristic finding of osteogenesis imperfecta, which is an inherited disorder causing increased bone fragility. Thinning of the sclera in this condition results in the underlying coat of the choroid to become more visible. Blue sclera is less commonly associated with other disorders such as Ehlers–Danlos syndrome, Marfan's syndrome and pseudoxanthoma elasticum. It may be acquired through the chronic use of corticosteroids.

2. **H – Vernal keratoconjunctivitis**. Giant papillae are associated with vernal keratoconjunctivitis and contact lens related giant papillary conjunctivitis. Papillae (non-giant form) can be caused by bacterial conjunctivitis, allergic conjunctivitis and blepharitis. Follicles are caused by viral conjunctivitis, chlamydial conjunctivitis and may occur due to hypersensitivity reaction to ocular drops. The different types of conjunctivitis are in Questions 2 and 4 (Ophthalmology section).

3. **C – Fuch's endothelial dystrophy**. Guttata are wart-like protuberances that form between the corneal endothelium and Descemet's membrane.

The increasing number and size of the guttata causes thinning and destruction of the corneal endothelium, which does not undergo mitotic division and therefore does not regenerate. This causes endothelial dysfunction, so that the endothelium does not perform its normal function of keeping the corneal stroma slightly dehydrated to maintain its transparency. Fuch's endothelial dystrophy is a bilateral asymmetrical slowly progressive corneal oedema in the elderly that can cause significant visual loss. The epithelial layer of the cornea can also be affected, resulting in typical epithelial blisters. Corneal oedema and loss of transparency is termed bullous keratopathy, and is treated with a penetrating (full-thickness) keratoplasty or an endothelial keratoplasty. This condition can also occur after cataract surgery due to endothelial loss resulting in pseudophakic bullous keratopathy.

4. **B – Congenital Horner's syndrome**. Horner's syndrome occurs with interruption of the sympathetic nervous supply to the eye. It is characterised by the classic triad of MAP– **m**iosis, **a**nhydrosis (hemifacial) and **p**tosis (partial). If a sympathetic lesion occurs in a child younger than 2 years, heterochromic irides occurs. The affected iris is lighter in colour (i.e. hypochromic) than the non-affected iris. This is sometimes referred to as congenital Horner's syndrome, although most cases are acquired.

5. **E – Keratoconus**. This is the most common primary corneal ectasia, estimated to affect 1 in 3000 people in the general population. It is characterised by progressive thinning of the central cornea (conus) leading to stromal thinning and protrusion, progressive myopia and irregular astigmatism. It typically presents in the second and third decades of life. A characteristic sign of this condition is a Fleischer ring, which is a pigmented ring of epithelial iron deposition encircling the base of the cone. It is best seen on slit-lamp examination with a cobalt blue filter after fluorescein staining. A Fleischer ring is often confused with a Kayser–Fleischer ring, the latter of which is described shortly. The most sensitive test for the diagnosis, grading and monitoring of keratoconus is corneal topography. The mainstay of treatment is with rigid contact lenses, although the use of spectacles or soft contact lenses may be sufficient in the early stages. Corneal collagen cross-linking is a relatively new therapy that may stabilise the progressive course of keratoconus. Severe cases require corneal transplantation (deep lamellar or penetrating keratoplasty). In about 5% of patients with keratoconus, a Descemet's membrane rupture may occur, resulting in severe sudden-onset corneal oedema (known as acute

hydrops). This usually heals within 10 weeks, but corneal scarring may occur.

An important ocular diagnostic sign of Wilson's disease is a Kayser–Fleischer ring, which is found in about 95% of patients. It is a brownish-yellow ring around the corneo-scleral junction (limbus). Wilson's disease is an autosomal recessive disorder in which copper accumulates within the body's tissues, mainly the brain and liver.

A Ophthalmology A18 – Ocular signs II

1. **D – Hyperlipidaemia**. Ocular manifestations of hyperlipidaemia are arcus senilis and xanthelasma. Arcus senilis is a bilateral narrow circumferential strip of lipid deposition in the peripheral cornea, which is extremely common. It is associated with old age, but is an important sign of hyperlipidaemia in young people. It is referred to as arcus juvenilis or arcus cornealis when affecting younger individuals. Lipid profile studies should be performed if arcus cornealis is present in someone under 50 years of age. Xanthelasma are yellow subcutaneous periorbital plaques, representing cholesterol deposits. In half of patients, these are associated with hyperlipidaemia.

2. **F – Neurofibromatosis** is an autosomal dominant disorder that causes lesions in the nervous system, bones, soft tissue and skin. Iris melanocytic hamartomas (known as 'Leish nodules') are a pathognomonic finding of NF 1, the more common form of the disease.

3. **A – Band keratopathy** is a common progressive corneal subepithelial deposition of calcium salts in the interpalpebral region. Calcific deposits are seen in the cornea, with small holes representing Swiss cheese. It can be an idiopathic finding in the elderly, or can occur with systemic conditions (e.g. hypercalcaemia) and chronic ocular inflammation. Patients may be asymptomatic, or may complain of a persistent foreign body sensation and reduced vision (with central cornea involvement). Ocular lubrication is the mainstay of treatment, although surgical removal may be required.

4. **I – Pterygium** is a triangular-shaped, non-neoplastic fibrovascular band, which represents elastotic degeneration of conjunctival collagen. It is usually asymmetric, extending from the interpalpebral conjunctiva into the cornea. Surgical excision is indicated if the lesion is on the visual axis, giving a persistent foreign body sensation or posing a cosmetic problem to the

patient. Pinguecula is an extremely common disorder that is histologically similar to pterygium, but does not involve the cornea. It may affect the temporal or nasal bulbar conjunctiva, unlike pterygium, which normally affects the nasal conjunctiva.

5. **E – Keratoconus**. An important diagnostic sign of keratoconus is Vogt's striae, which are thin vertical stress lines within the corneal stroma caused by stretching and thinning. These occur in half of patients with keratoconus, and disappear by gently applying external pressure on the globe. Other clinical signs of keratoconus include an oil droplet reflex on ophthalmoscopy and apical bulging of the lower lid on downgaze (Munson's sign).

A   **Ophthalmology A19 – Pupillary disorders**

1. **F – Occulomotor nerve lesion**. The superior oblique and lateral rectus are the only extraocular muscles that are not supplied by the occulomotor (third cranial) nerve, and are supplied by the trochlear (fourth cranial nerve) and abducens (sixth cranial nerve) respectively. This can be remembered by the acronym 'LR$_6$SO$_4$'; where LR stands for lateral rectus and SO stands for superior oblique, and the numbers represent the cranial nerve number. The main action of the superior oblique muscle is intorsion, and its secondary and tertiary functions are depression and abduction respectively. The lateral rectus muscle function is abduction. In an occulomotor nerve palsy, the superior oblique and lateral rectus cause the eye to be deviated down and out. This can be remembered by thinking of a boxer who has lost a fight, 'down and out'. An occulomotor nerve palsy results in a significant or complete ptosis. If some of the parasympathetic fibres originating in the Edinger–Westphal subnucleus of the third cranial nerve are preserved, the pupil may not be affected in an occulomotor nerve palsy. Hence, explaining the ocular presentation in this scenario. Pupil-sparing third nerve palsies are a hallmark of ischaemic lesions, often resulting from microvascular disease (e.g. diabetes mellitus).

2. **C – Argyll Robertson pupils** are a feature of neurosyphilis, which occurs in tertiary syphilis. The pupils are small and irregular. There is a light near dissociation as the pupil reacts poorly to light, but has an intact near reflex. Penicillin is an effective treatment that is being increasingly used globally in earlier stages of syphilis infection. This is why tertiary syphilis is becoming less common. It is important to differentiate this condition from other

disorders causing a bilateral light-near dissociation (e.g. diabetes mellitus, myotonic dystrophy) or small pupils (e.g. opiate use, posterior synechiae due to anterior uveitis). There is no condition in which pupils have an intact reflex to light, but no accommodation reflex.

3. **D – Horner's syndrome**. The patient in this scenario presents with hand muscle weakness, loss of pain and temperature sensation and signs of Horner's syndrome, pointing to a diagnosis of syringomyelia. This is most commonly caused by cerebrospinal fluid circulation block, which is most frequently due to Arnold–Chiari malformation. The sympathetic fibres innervate the iris dilator muscle, which is responsible for mydriasis. Sympathetic fibres also innervate Müller's muscle, which contributes to about 1.5 mm of lid elevation. A lesion to the sympathetic nerve supply to the eye causes Horner's syndrome, which presents with the classic triad of MAP – **m**iosis, **a**nhydrosis (hemifacial) and **p**tosis (partial). If a sympathetic lesion occurs in a child younger than 2 years, heterochromia irides occurs. The affected iris is lighter in colour (i.e. hypochromic) than the non-affected iris. If unsure about the diagnosis, application of 4% cocaine eye drops will dilate the normal pupil, but will not dilate the affected pupil in Horner's syndrome. Another useful test is the application of 0.1% adrenaline eye drops, which will dilate the affected pupil only in Horner's syndrome. Horner's syndrome can present in both infants and adults, and it is important to look for the underlying cause. Management is based on the cause.

4. **J – None of the above**. Acute primary angle-closure glaucoma (ACG) is an ophthalmic emergency that is an important global cause of blindness. There is significantly raised intraocular pressure (IOP) leading to corneal, iris and retinal ischaemia, giving the clinician a narrow 4-hour window to reduce the IOP and salvage the optic nerve and the retina. The affected pupil is oval, fixed, semi-dilated and poorly reactive to light due to iris ischaemia. The affected eye has a raised IOP (>50 mmHg), cloudy cornea (corneal oedema), ciliary congestion and a shallow anterior chamber (usually a bilateral finding). Gentle palpation of the eyes with the eyelids closed is a simple initial bedside examination if a tonometer is not readily available. The affected eye is harder and more tender on palpation. Pain is a prominent symptom of ACG, and patients complain of pain in or around the eye, headaches and sometimes an abdominal pain. Common ocular symptoms besides pain include loss of vision (due to corneal oedema) and photophobia. Patients may also report seeing halos around lights,

especially at night, before the acute episode of ACG. Other prominent systemic symptoms of acute ACG include nausea and vomiting. Diagnosis and management of ACG is explained in more detail in Questions 2 and 6 (Ophthalmology section).

5. **A – Adie's pupil**. Denervation of the post-ganglionic fibres supplying the sphincter pupillae and ciliary muscle results in a dilated pupil that reacts poorly to light and accommodation. This is known as an Adie's pupil. It is usually unilateral, occurring more frequently in women. The cause of denervation is not understood. There is then non-uniform re-innervation of the iris sphincter by the parasympathetic fibres that control accommodation. Characteristic features on slit-lamp examination are absent or vermiform/worm-like contractions and sectorial iris atrophy. There is denervation hypersensitivity, resulting in slow constriction and re-dilatation on accommodation. Furthermore, the application of topical 0.125% pilocarpine to both eyes results in constriction of the affected pupil only. Patients may complain of visual blurring, especially on near vision. In some patients, deep tendon reflexes may be lost (Holmes–Adie syndrome).

    Physiological anisocoria occurs in 20% of the general population. There is a normal pupillary response to both light and near reflexes, and the anisocoria does not change in bright or dim light. The difference in pupil size rarely exceeds 1 mm, and the affected individuals do not complain of visual symptoms. A useful clinical observation in anisocoria is the difference in size between the two pupils in response to changes in room brightness. In a bright room, the anisocoria will worsen in an occulomotor nerve palsy because only the affected pupil remains dilated, whereas the non-affected pupil constricts. In a dark room, the anisocoria will worsen in Horner's syndrome because the affected pupil will remain constricted, whereas the non-affected pupil will dilate. In physiological anisocoria, the difference in size between the two pupils will not change in a bright or dark setting, because both pupils react normally to light.

    A pupil with a relative afferent pupillary defect (RAPD) is also known as a **Marcus Gunn pupil**. A RAPD is caused by an incomplete optic nerve lesion, or by severe retinal disease. It is not caused by dense cataracts, corneal opacities or vitreous haemorrhage. Visual signals perceived by the eye are converted to electrical signals, which are transmitted to the brain via the optic nerve. Complete damage to the optic nerve means the afferent pathway from the affected eye is non-functional, and hence the eye is completely blind (**amaurotic pupil**). The eye does not constrict to direct light, but maintains a full consensual light reflex if the optic nerve in the other eye is not damaged. If there is incomplete damage to the optic nerve, there is a weak response to the direct eye reflex, but the consensual eye reflex is normal. This can be difficult to detect, but the swinging light reflex helps to elicit this phenomenon. When light is shown to either eye, both eyes will constrict. Light is shone into one eye for 3 seconds, and then rapidly swung to the other eye for 3 seconds. When light is swung from the non-affected eye to the eye with the RAPD, the eye with the RAPD will slightly dilate. This is because the signal from the unaffected normal eye is stronger than the signal from the eye with the RAPD. In other words, the consensual light reflex is stronger than the direct reflex. When light is then swung back to the non-affected side, the eye on the affected side will re-constrict. It is important to note that while the light reflex in the eye with a RAPD is reduced, the accommodation reflex is unaffected. The patient should therefore be looking at a distant object during the test to avoid constriction due to accommodation.

Opiate overdose presents with the clinical triad of respiratory depression, central nervous system depression and miosis. Patients may also have hypotension, bradycardia, nausea and vomiting. It is important to be aware that miosis may not always be present in opioid overdose. Respiratory depression is a more specific clinical sign, and death from opioid toxicity is usually due to respiratory failure. If the airway or breathing is compromised, the patient may require ventilation. Reversal of opiate overdose is with intravenous naloxone. It is important to be familiar with the clinical presentation and management of both acute and chronic opioid toxicity. These are common topics for exam questions, because they are preventable causes of hospital deaths.

A   **Ophthalmology A20 – Paediatric ophthalmology**

1. **A – Concomitant squint**. Ocular misalignment is known as strabismus or a squint. It is the most common cause of amblyopia, which is when there is unilateral (or rarely bilateral) reduced visual acuity, for which no organic cause can be found. Amblyopia due to strabismus (or 'squint') is called strabismic amblyopia. When the squint is convergent, as is the case in this scenario, this is known as esotropia (most common type). When it is divergent, it is called exotropia. The abnormal eye may also be higher (hypertropia) or lower (hypotropia) than the normal eye. Childhood squint is usually concomitant. This is when both eyes can move fully in all directions, but the patient has a squint in all directions of gaze. In other words, when fixating on an object, only one eye is directed towards

the fixated object. This is also known as a non-paralytic squint. It can be primary or secondary (e.g. refractive error, cataract, corneal opacity). In a non-concomitant squint, one of the eyes is not able to move fully in all directions. The angle of the squint therefore varies with the direction of gaze. In a nerve palsy, for example, the size of the squint is greatest in the field of action of the affected muscle(s). This is also known as a paralytic squint. It can be due to nerve palsy, extraocular muscle disease or tethering of the globe. It is important to exclude retinoblastoma and intracranial tumours in any presentation of a squint. A useful test to elicit ocular misalignment is the Hirschberg corneal reflex test. A pen torchlight held from an arm's length distance is shone onto the eyes. The reflex should appear symmetrically on the nasal aspect of each cornea. If there is a squint, the reflection will be asymmetrical, and will depend on the type of squint present. In esotropia, the corneal reflex in the deviated eye will appear more temporally, while in exotropia, the corneal reflex in the deviated eye will appear more nasally. The cover is another useful test to elicit a squint and the extent of a squint. The eyes focus on a target and one eye is covered at a time. When the squinting eye is covered, the normal eye should maintain fixation and not move. When the normal eye is covered, the squinting eye moves to take up fixation. The direction of movement determines the type of squint present. For example, if the eye moves laterally to take up fixation, there is an esotropic squint. If no abnormality is detected with the cover test, the alternative cover test can be tried to elicit a latent squint. However, this is not a truly abnormal condition and can be elicited in most individuals with normal binocular single vision.

Another important and reversible cause of strabismus is refractive errors. Most commonly, there is a significant difference in refractive power between the two eyes, resulting in an anisometropic ambylopia. Treatment aiming to improve the visual acuity in the ambylopic eye is only effective up to about 7 years of age, as this is the period in which visual development occurs. The mainstay of treatment of amblyopia due to refractive error is correction of the refractive error with spectacles. It is also important to investigate and eliminate any 'opacities' in the visual axis such as cataracts.

The two main types of treatment for amblyopia are occlusion or atropine penalisation. The aim of occlusion is that the patient uses the 'lazy' eye to fixate on objects. Occlusion is usually only needed for a few hours each day. The principle behind penalisation is similar: Atropine 1% drops are topically applied to the better eye, causing blurring of vision through that eye. Surgery is usually indicated for cosmetic reasons, as it is unlikely to produce any functional benefits. The two principles of surgery are extraocular muscle recession (lengthening the muscle to reduce its action) or resection (shortening the muscle to strengthen its action).

2. **E – Nasolacrimal duct obstruction** (NDO) is a cause of sticky watery eyes in the first year of life. There is a delay in canalisation of the lower end of the nasolacrimal duct or an imperforate mucous membrane at the valve of Hasner, which impairs lacrimal drainage. This results in epiphora, which is important to differentiate from lacrimation due to excess tear production. The child in this scenario is unlikely to have ophthalmia neonatorum (neonatal conjunctivitis), which presents in the first 4 weeks of life and causes a red eye as well as discharge. NDO is not associated with a red eye. Congenital glaucoma can cause lacrimation, but the baby in the scenario does not have any other features of glaucoma. The main symptoms of NDO are excessive tearing with mattering (mucous accumulation) at the eyelashes. It can also result in the formation of a mucocele, which is non-infected lacrimal sac swelling at the medial canthus. This can become infected, presenting as an acute red and tender swelling with or without a discharge (acute dacrocystitis). On examination, discharge may be expressed with finger massage over the lacrimal sac at the medial canthus. Dacrocystography (radiological examination following administration of contrast medium) or nuclear lacrimal scintigraphy is sometimes used to aid in diagnosis. NDO resolves spontaneously in about 90% of cases by one year of age. Daily finger massage over the medial canthus and eyelid cleaning with sterile saline may help. If NDO does not spontaneously resolve, a syringe and probe is used at 12–18 months of age to clear the obstruction; this is successful in 90% of cases. If unsuccessful, a dacryocystorhinostomy is required.

3. **I – Retinopathy of prematurity** (ROP) is a proliferative retinopathy that mainly affects premature infants of low birthweight. In these infants, the peripheral retina may have not been vascularised, leading to retinal ischaemia, production of vasogenic factors and neovascularisation at the junction of the vascular and avascular retina. As in diabetic proliferative retinopathy, neovascularisation is accompanied by growth of fibrous tissue, which can contract and cause tractional retinal detachment. This is the main cause of blindness in ROP. The abnormal new blood vessels may also bleed, leading to a vitreous haemorrhage. The development of ROP is associated with the use of high oxygen concentration therapy. The infant in this scenario has neovascularisation in one eye and a leukocoria in the other eye, which is most likely due to tractional retinal

detachment. The main differential is familial exudative vitreoretinopathy (FEV), which is a rare autosomal dominant inherited condition presenting with similar funduscopy findings. In sickle cell proliferative retinopathy, neovascularisation occurs, with the new blood vessels forming in a 'sea fan' distribution. However, given the history of prematurity and low birthweight with the funduscopy findings, the most likely diagnosis in this scenario is ROP. All infants who are born at or less than 32 weeks' gestation, or with a birthweight of less than <1500 g should be screened by an experienced ophthalmologist. Screening starts four weeks after birth or at 31–32 weeks' gestational age, whichever is later, and is carried out regularly until the retina has fully vascularised. ROP is classified according to the zone affected, the extent (number of clock hours or 30-degree sectors involved) and the severity (*see* Table 6).

TABLE 6 Staging of retinopathy of prematurity

Stage	Description
1	Flat demarcation line separating the vascular retina from the avascular peripheral retina
2	Ridged demarcation line
3	Extraretinal fibrovascular proliferation
4	Sub-total retinal detachment: extrafoveal (4A) or foveal (4B)
5	Total retinal detachment

Note: Features of 'Plus' disease are retinal vascular dilatation, poor pupillary dilatation, iris vascularisation and vitreous haze. This may present at any of the stages given in this table.

The treatment is based on the severity of ROP, with 'threshold' disease (extensive stage 3 changes) or 'Plus' disease being a typical indication for treatment. Laser photocoagulation to the avascular retina is now the treatment of choice, replacing cryotherapy. Cryotherapy may be used as an alternative therapy. Vitreretinal surgical intervention for retinal detachment included vitrectomy, scleral buckling, cryotherapy and laser photocoagulation, but the visual prognosis is often poor.

4. **C – Congenital glaucoma**. Primary congenital glaucoma has an incidence of 1 in 10 000 live births, and is mostly sporadic. It usually presents in the first year of life, more commonly in males, and about three-quarters of cases are bilateral. It is caused by abnormal development of the anterior chamber angle, which leads to aqueous outflow obstruction and raised intraocular pressure (IOP). Unlike adults, the infant's eye enlarges with a

raised IOP, resulting in the characteristic 'buphthalmos ('ox eye'). Other important clinical features are corneal hazing, lacrimation, photophobia, blepharospasm and Haab's striae. The latter are horizontal curvilinear lines in the cornea caused by breaks in the Descemet's membrane that have healed. Optic disc cupping is another important characteristic sign on funduscopy, and is more reversible with IOP reduction than in adult glaucoma. Early diagnosis and management of congenital glaucoma is key to optimising the visual prognosis. The main surgical options are goniotomy, trabeculotomy or trabeculectomy. Delay in surgery is associated with a poor visual prognosis.

5. **B – Congenital cataracts**. Both congenital cataracts and retinoblastoma are causes of a unilateral leukocoria. Cataracts is much more common than retinoblastoma. Furthermore, up to one-quarter of cataract are familial, compared to retinoblastoma in which only 5% of cases are familial. Hence, the most likely diagnosis in this scenario is congenital cataract. A retinoblastoma must always be excluded in a child presenting with leukocoria, as it can progress to metastasis and death. Congenital cataract has an incidence of up to 1 in 4000 live births, and two-thirds are bilateral. It is an important cause of amblyopia, as it removes visual stimulus to the eye(s). A cataract may present as a white pupil on inspection, or may be detected by a white fundus reflex. It is important to look for an underlying cause (most common is idiopathic), and to exclude other ocular pathologies. Cataract on its own does not cause a relative afferent pupillary defect. Treatment of visually significant cataract is with surgical removal. It is important that this is done as early as possible, especially in unilateral cataract, to minimise the risk of amblyopia. Parental education and compliance is crucial for achieving a good visual outcome.

   Retinoblastoma is the most common primary malignant intraocular tumour in children, with an incidence of 1 in 15000–20000. Most cases are sporadic, presenting as a unilateral focal tumour. The genetic form is transmissible, presenting as multiple tumours present in one or both eyes. Median age of presentation is about 18 months. The most common clinical sign is leukocoria. Strabismus and secondary glaucoma can also occur. Slit-lamp examination reveals a dome-shaped white homogenous mass. The imaging modality of choice is ultrasound scanning, which shows characteristic calcification within the tumour and is used to assess the tumour size. MRI scanning may be used to assess optic nerve involvement (important prognostic implications) and to detect extraocular spread. A diagnostic biopsy is not performed as it may result in spreading of the tumour. It is also important that patients undergo mutational testing to differentiate somatic and genetic cases, which has important implications for family and offspring. Treatment options include radiotherapy, cryotherapy, laser therapy and enucleation. The latter is the most effective treatment, but is reserved for advanced retinoblastoma. Chemotherapy may be used to shrink the tumour before starting one of the aforementioned treatment options. Overall, there is a 95% survival rate with treatment. If left untreated, retinoblastoma progresses to local invasion, metastasis and death.

There are two types of **sickle cell retinopathy**: non-proliferative and proliferative. In the non-proliferative form, black sunburst scars, salmon-patch retinal haemorrhages and tortuous veins are seen. In the proliferative retinopathy form, neovascularisation occurs, with the new blood vessels forming in a 'sea fan' distribution. Patients with proliferative changes should be urgently referred to an ophthalmologist. Treatment is with laser photocoagulation.

A   Ophthalmology A21 – Ocular trauma

1. **F – Ocular irrigation and topical antibiotics**. Ocular alkali burns are one of the most serious injuries to the eye, and can result in rapid blindness if there is a delay in treatment. They are generally more serious than acidic burns, because the alkali substance can cause liquefactive necrosis and penetrate the anterior structures of the eye, thus entering into the intraocular structures. It is important to be aware that most domestically used chemicals are alkali, not acidic. Examples of alkali substances include cement, plasters, lye and airbag powder. Findings on examination depend on the toxicity of the chemical, as well as the severity of the injury. Corneal epithelial defects may range from small areas of epithelial loss, to loss of the entire corneal epithelium. Ocular signs of mild burns include conjunctival chemosis, erythema and haemorrhages and mild anterior chamber inflammation. In severe burns, there may also be perilimbal blanching, corneal oedema, severe anterior chamber inflammation, scleral perforation and raised intraocular pressure (IOP). In general, increased corneal opacification, limbal ischaemia and conjunctival involvement are associated with poorer visual prognosis. The 'Roper-Hall' and 'Dua' classifications are useful methods of classifying the severity of ocular surface burns.

A chemical burn to the eye must be treated as an ophthalmological emergency. Immediate management is with eye irrigation, which is the most important factor in limiting damage to the eye. It should not be delayed by a comprehensive history and examination, or choice of irrigant.

Irrigation may be done with water or normal saline, and should be continued until the pH of the eye is neutralised to 7.0. The pH should be re-measured 5 minutes and 20 minutes after completion of irrigation, and daily from then on. It is important to ensure that all retained particulate matter is removed from underneath the eyelids, which can be missed if the conjunctival fornices are not double-everted and thoroughly cleaned. An eyelid speculum and standard intravenous tubing can be used for the irrigation, and the conjunctival fornices should also be swept with a wet cotton-tipped applicator. Necrotic epithelium should be debrided, to facilitate corneal re-epithelisation. Patients usually require topical anaesthetic, cycloplegic and lubricant agents, as well as oral analgesia. After irrigation, the eye requires patching or a bandage contact lens for epithelial healing, and an antibiotic ointment for infection prophylaxis. Oral tetracycline or doxycycline may be required in severe burns. Chemical burns can cause a rise in IOP that can occur immediately or a few hours after the injury. Therefore, it is important to monitor and to timely manage IOP elevations. Patients may also develop severe uveitis, which is treated with topical (and sometimes systemic) steroids under the care of an ophthalmologist. Long-term management of chemical burns may include limbal cell transplantation, amniotic membrane grafting, keratoplasty or even keratoprosthesis.

Hint: In any cause of ocular injury, visual acuity in both eyes must be tested and clearly documented for both medical and legal purposes.

2. **D – Lateral canthotomy and cantholysis.** Ocular trauma may be blunt or penetrating, with the former being more common (80%). The most common presentation of blunt trauma to the eye is a haematoma (i.e. black eye). As well as causing an orbital blowout fracture, blunt traumas may cause a retrobulbar haemorrhage. The patient in this scenario describes typical signs and symptoms of this complication. A retrobulbar haemorrhage may act like a space-occupying lesion and cause proptosis with limitation of eye movements. There is also ocular pain and reduced vision. As the orbital pressure rises, the orbital compartment does not increase in size to accommodate, leading to increased IOP. If left untreated, this can lead to orbital compartment syndrome, in which there is ischaemia of the optic nerve and retina. The patient in this scenario has visual acuity loss with proptosis, which is an indication for surgery. Another important indication for surgery is increasing IOP. The patient requires an emergency lateral canthotomy and cantholysis to salvage his vision. A blunt

injury may cause bleeding into the eyelids, causing an ecchymosis. In the anterior segment, bleeding into the anterior chamber causes a hyphaema, which may be microscopic or may form a fluid level. There is a risk of a secondary haemorrhage occurring a few days later, often more serious than the first haemorrhage. A secondary haemorrhage may cause a sight-threatening secondary glaucoma. If there is a vitreous haemorrhage thsi will cause a severe loss of vision and loss of the red reflex. Trauma may also cause a subconjunctival haemorrhage. Bed rest and oral tranexamic acid reduces the risk of a secondary haemorrhage. A blunt force to the eye may also cause imprinting on the anterior capsule, a dilated D-shaped pupil and formation of a posterior subcapsular cataract. The lens itself may partially or completely dislocate. The damage from a blunt force may extend to the posterior structures of the eye, leading to a traumatic optic neuropathy, optic nerve avulsion, commotio retinae, choroidal rupture and retinal detachment. A relative afferent pupillary defect is detected in traumatic optic neuropathy, while optic atrophy takes several months to develop. This condition may respond to high-dose steroids or optic canal decompression. In commotio retinae (retinal bruising), the retina has pale grey oedematous patches, most commonly affecting the temporal fundus. This resolves in most cases. Retinal tears may progress to retinal detachment and choroidal rupture, the chief causes of irreversible visual loss.

3. **G – Surgical reduction.** An acute rise in orbital pressure due to direct force by an object that is more than 5 cm in diameter can cause a fracture of the thin inferior (maxillary bone – most commonly affected) and medial (ethmoidal) walls of the orbit. The resultant oedema, muscle entrapment and nerve damage can all lead to diplopia. There is normally a history of an orbital trauma, but in elderly people with dementia, this may not be elicited. Clinical features of an orbital blowout fracture include periocular ecchymosis and oedema, enophthalmos, restricted ocular motility, diplopia, cheek and teeth numbness and orbital crepitus. Enophthalmos may occur as a result of decreased orbital volume and/or due to entrapment of orbital contents within the fracture site. It may not be apparent until oedema has settled. Inferior rectus and inferior oblique entrapment within the inferior wall can result in limited vertical ocular motility, while medial rectus entrapment can result in limited horizontal ocular movement. The former is more common, resulting in a vertical diplopia. The patient in this scenario is less likely to have a cranial nerve palsy, as this supplies the superior oblique only, resulting in diplopia on downgaze only. The infraorbital nerve, which passes through the infraorbital canal, is particularly prone to

damage. This presents as reduced sensation in the cheek and molar teeth. A fractured sinus can result in surgical emphysema, which presents as crepitus on palpation (rare). Facial X-ray may show the 'droplet' sign, in which there is soft tissue prolapse through the inferior orbital wall. A fluid level may also be seen in the maxillary sinus, representing blood. A CT scan will confirm these findings, and is more reliable in visualising a fracture. Once the diagnosis is confirmed, management depends on the site of the orbital wall fracture, neurovascular damage and extent of soft tissue entrapment. The management options include observation, high dose steroids and surgery. Because of the tethering of the extraocular muscles in this patient, release of the muscles and fracture reduction is required.

4. **H – Topical antibiotics, padding and analgesia**. Ocular exposure to ultraviolet light by welders, sunbed users and during skiing (if protective eyewear is not used) can cause acute keratitis. Patients complain of moderate to severe pain, foreign body sensation, excessive lacrimation, red eye, blepharospasm and blurred vision. Ocular symptoms are typically worse 6–12 hours post exposure. On examination, there may be conjunctival injection, chemosis and punctate epithelial defects (the latter in severe cases). Application of topical anaesthesia can cause a dramatic reduction of ocular pain. Topical antibiotics and application of a pressure patch to the more affected eye usually results in visual recovery within 24 hours. Cycloplegic drops and oral analgesia may be required for symptomatic relief.

5. **B – Clean the tarsal conjunctiva and topical antibiotics**. A corneal abrasion is a common superficial injury to the corneal surface, often caused by fingernails, contact lens and plants. The resultant corneal epithelium loss results in ocular symptoms, and increases the risk of an ocular infection. Symptoms are intense ocular pain, photophobia, foreign body sensation, discomfort on blinking and excessive lacrimation. Patients usually give a history of a scratch or other trauma to the eye. A corneal abrasion is best viewed on slit-lamp examination after the application of anaesthetic drops and fluorescein dye. An important and sometime missed part of the ocular examination is inspection of the conjunctival fornices, as the tarsal conjunctivae may contain a foreign body. This results in characteristic vertical abrasions, as evident in this clinical scenario. The eyelids should be double-everted and any foreign bodies removed. A superficial abrasion should also be differentiated from a deeper corneal laceration involving the deeper layers of the cornea. Full thickness corneal lacerations and other

anterior chamber perforations can be detected using Seidel's test. This is when topical sodium fluorescein 2% is applied to the affected eye and it is then viewed with a slit lamp to assess for aqueous leakage from the anterior chamber. One of the most important aspects of management of corneal abrasions is the prevention of microbial keratitis. Topical broad-spectrum antibiotics ointments are used for prophylaxis, and these should have pseudomonal coverage in contact lens wearers. Necrotic tissue should be debrided to facilitate corneal re-epithelialisation. Some patients develop traumatic iritis one to three days after the corneal abrasion injury, which is managed with a topical cycloplegic (e.g. cyclopentolate). Patching of the eye is rarely used for small corneal abrasions, and may delay epithelial healing. Recurrent corneal erosions syndrome is a complication of corneal injuries, which occurs due to failure of epithelial re-adhesion to the basement membrane. Patients present with recurrent ocular pain and tearing, especially in the morning. Management is with ocular lubrication, and the condition may spontaneously resolve. Severe cases are managed with patching, bandage contact lens, corneal micropuncture or excimer laser photo-therapeutic keratectomy.

Full thickness perforations can result from lacerations or the entrance of foreign bodies. Besides a positive Seidel's test, other signs of a full thickness perforation are a flat anterior chamber, irregular pupil, prolapsing iris, hyphaema, vitreous haemorrhage and reduced IOP due to aqueous leak (normal IOP: 10–14mmHg). There may be a subconjunctival haemorrhage at the site of a scleral perforation. The pain perforating injuries is usually intense, resulting in significantly reduced vision. However, small high-velocity foreign bodies may cause a mild ocular pain and blurring of vision. On examination, the anterior chamber may be flat, and the iris may be prolapsing from the wound. Aqueous leak can result in a reduced IOP (normal: 10–21 mmHg), but the IOP may be raised with the presence of a hyphaema. There may be a more subtle 'microscopic hyphaema', which is detected as circulating red blood cells with a slit-lamp microscope. Cataracts can develop rapidly following a penetrating injury.

Patients with a penetrating injury should be urgently referred to an ophthalmologist, and should lie supine and have a have a shield placed over the eye until they are examined. It is important to avoid applying pressure to the globe. Patients should also be advised not to blow their nose, and are kept nil by mouth in case surgical intervention is required. If there is any suspicion of the presence of an intraocular foreign body (IOFB), an orbital X-ray or CT scan is required. An orbital ultrasound scan by an experienced operator may be more sensitive than an X-ray for high velocity small

IOFBs. Foreign bodies in the cornea are fairly easily removed with a hypodermic needle, and the eye is then treated with antibiotic ointments and padding. Ferrous foreign bodies may have a surrounding rust ring if they have been lodged in the cornea for more than 24 hours, and this must also be removed. Deeper IOFB may cause a vitreous haemorrhage and retinal tears. The IOFB can be removed with forceps or a magnet. Cataracts need removal, but this is usually done at a later stage.

A rare (0.1%) but devastating complication of penetrating ocular trauma is an autoimmune granulomatous panuveitis that affects both the injured and the fellow healthy eye. This is known as sympathetic ophthalmia, 90% of which occurs within a year of the initial injury. It can be prevented by early (first 10 days) enucleation of the injured eye, if it has a poor and irreversible visual function. A more common complication of penetrating ocular trauma with IOFBs is endophthalmitis, occurring in 8% of cases. Patients present with an acutely painful red eye and severe visual loss. Removal of IOFBs, early primary wound repair and prophylactic antibiotics reduce the risk of this severe intraocular infection. Once endophthalmitis develops, patients must be admitted, aqueous and vitreous samples aspirated and intravitreal antibiotics simultaneously administered. Any retained IOFBs must be removed. Later complications of retained IOFB containing iron or copper are siderosis and chalcosis, respectively. This can cause significant local toxicity and may lead to permanent loss of vision.

A fourth (trochlear) cranial nerve palsy commonly results from minor closed head trauma (e.g. falling). The superior oblique muscle causes depression of the eye in adduction, which becomes limited in a trochlear nerve palsy. The affected eye is slightly more elevated than the non-affected eye when the patient is looking straight ahead. Patients complain of a diplopia that is vertical, torsional and worse on downgaze. They often also adopt a contralateral head tilt to reduce the diplopia. The main causes of trochlear nerve palsy are congenital, trauma or vascular injury.

A   Ophthalmology A22 – Refraction

1. **B – Convex lens**. In order for an object to be seen clearly, light from that object must be refracted by the eye onto the retina. Emmetropia means that there is no refractive error, and hence, light is refracted normally when looking at a distant object. The eye is too long in myopia, resulting in parallel light rays from distant objects to focus in front of the retina. This is optically corrected with a concave lens, which diverts the light rays, before they undergo refraction by the eye. When the divergent light

is refracted by the eye, the light focuses on the retina which forms a clear image. The overall effect of the concave lens is therefore to reduce refraction of light. The eye is too short in hypermetropia, causing light from a distant object to focus beyond the retina. In this case, a convex lens is used to converge light from a distance before it is refracted by the eye.

2. **H – Soft contact lens**. Soft silicone contact lenses are currently the lens of choice for contact lens bandaging. They protect the corneal epithelium from injury, facilitate healing and reduce discomfort. Contact lenses are also commonly used for refractive errors, as users often find them more cosmetically acceptable than spectacles. Contact lenses can also provide greater refractive strength for people with severe refractive errors than spectacles. There are two main types: rigid and soft. Although rigid contact lenses have less serious complications in general, most users prefer soft contact lens, as they are more comfortable.

3. **J – Varifocal lens**. Presbyopia is when the eye has a reduced power of accommodation due to loss of lens elasticity with ageing (between the ages of 40 and 60 years). The affected person finds it difficult to discriminate fine close detail, which is why they require spectacles for near vision. A convex lens will compensate for the loss of accommodation power in the eye normally provided by the natural lens of the eye. Spectacles combining lens for both near and distant vision can be used for people requiring optical correction for both. Bifocal lens contain two separate areas of different refractive power. The near vision area is usually added to the lower segment of the lens. Varifocal lens, on the other hand, have a progressive change from distant to near vision down the lens, and do not have the disadvantage of a sudden change in refractive power ('bifocal line'). Bifocal lens are suitable for activities such as reading and watching TV. Varifocals are more suitable for people who require intermediate distance vision, such as computer users or musicians. Trifocal lens have three distinct areas of refractive power: distant, intermediate and near vision. Their use is becoming limited with the advances in varifocal lens technology.

4. **D – Laser-Assisted In Situ Keratomileusis (LASIK)**. Use of photorefractive surgery is becoming more popular for the correction of refractive errors. The three most commonly performed procedures are Photorefractive Keratectomy (PRK), Laser-Assisted In Situ Keratomileusis (LASIK) and Laser-Assisted Sub-Epithelial Keratomileusis (LASEK). All three procedures are considered safe and effective for the treatment of

refractive errors in carefully selected patients. In PRK, the corneal epithelium is surgically removed, and the excimer laser is used to ablate the corneal stroma and reduce its refractive power. A bandage contact lens is then placed over the eye. PRK is being replaced by LASIK and LASEK, which offer patients reduced post-operative pain and faster visual recovery. In LASIK, a flap of superficial corneal stroma is incised and folded back, and excimer laser is then applied to the cornea. The flap is then returned to its position. LASEK works in a similar principle. The corneal epithelium is first removed as a single sheet (does not include the corneal stroma, unlike LASIK) with alcohol. The corneal stroma is then laser ablated, and the epithelium thereafter replaced.

5. **I – Toric lens**. Astigmatism is a condition in which the refractive power of the cornea is not equal in different planes. It can be treated with spectacles, contact lens or photorefractive surgery. The lenses used for optical correction are cylindrical lens, known as toric lens. This lens has different refractive power in different planes, to correct the different refractive errors in astigmatism.

   A **prism** consists of a transparent material with two non-parallel flat refracting surfaces that start at the 'base' and intersect at the 'apex' of the prism. It works by optically redirecting light. The power of a prism's correction is measured in prism dioptres. Prisms are used to eliminate diplopia and achieve single binocular vision in patients with ocular misalignment.

A   Ophthalmology A23 – Neuro-ophthalmology

1. **D – Optic chiasm lesion**. Lesions at the optic chiasm damage the nasal fibres, causing a bitemporal hemianopia. The patient therefore has loss of his or her temporal vision. The most common cause is a pituitary tumour (e.g. pituitary adenoma). Other differentials include meningioma, craniopharyngioma and a chiasmal glioma. Patients may complain of bumping into things, or hitting their car's side mirrors. A detailed history and examination of the patient is essential to identify clinical features of abnormal pituitary function.

2. **F – Papilloedema** is a term used to describe bilateral optic disc swelling due to raised intracranial pressure (ICP). It is the result of axoplasmic flow stasis. Papilloedema characteristically causes a central visual field defect. Chronic papilloedema can cause constriction of visual fields, but the early finding is enlargement of the blind spot. Other visual symptoms include

reduced visual acuity (may get transient visual blurring), reduced coloured vision, diplopia and a relative afferent pupillary defect. Non-visual symptoms that should alert the physician to the possibility of raised ICP are headache (worsened by lying down/straining), nausea, vomiting, pulsatile tinnitus and visual obscurations (transient loss of vision occurring with activities that raise ICP, such as coughing or bending down). The most common cause of papilloedema is idiopathic intracranial hypertension (previously known as benign intracranial hypertension). It is important, however, to exclude other causes of raised intracranial pressure, such as a haemorrhage, abscess or tumour. The features of papilloedema on funduscopy are commonly asked about in clinical examinations. These are swollen hyperaemic discs, blurred disc margins, disc haemorrhages, venous engorgement and obscured retinal vessels. Central scotomas can be caused by damage to the optic nerve (e.g. optic neuritis), macular region (e.g. wet age-related macular degeneration) or macular fibres at the occipital cortex (e.g. space-occupying lesion).

3. **B – Chronic open-angle glaucoma**. Tunnel vision results from severe loss of peripheral visual fields, with preservation of the central visual field. Glaucoma is one of the most common causes of tunnel vision. Patients with early glaucoma present with subtle visual field defects (e.g. small arcuate scotoma). Classic visual field defects detected by perimetry are an arcuate scotoma, paracentral scotoma or nasal step scotoma. As glaucoma advances, there is worsening of peripheral visual fields. Patients often do not notice the visual field loss until it has become significant, which is why patients present late in the course of the disease. Around 25%–35% of retinal ganglion cells are lost before visual field defects are detected. It is therefore important to regularly monitor patients at increased risk of developing glaucoma (e.g. family history). Tunnel vision results in very advanced glaucoma, and is rare in the developed world. Other causes of tunnel vision include stroke, central retinal artery occlusion, retinitis pigmentosa, bilateral panretinal photocoagulation and papilloedema. Diabetic retinopathy itself does not cause a visual field defect. Tractional retinal detachment, which is a complication of proliferative diabetic retinopathy, can result in a peripheral and/or central visual field defect. The retinal detachment is caused by fibrous contraction, which pulls the sensory retina away from the retinal pigment epithelium.

4. **I – Temporal lobe lesion**. A lesion in the optic radiation of the temporal lobe will damage fibres from the inferior quadrant of the ipsilateral

temporal retina and the contralateral nasal retina. A right temporal lobe lesion will therefore cause a left superior quadrantinopia, and vice versa. A lesion in the optic radiation of the parietal lobe will damage the fibres representing the superior quadrant of the ipsilateral temporal retina and the contralateral nasal retina. A right parietal lobe lesion will therefore cause a left inferior quadrantinopia, and vice versa. Lesions of the optic tract, posterior optic radiation or occipital lobe (visual cortex) will cause a homonymous hemianopia on the side opposite to the lesion. A lesion to the deep occipital cortex will also cause a contralateral homonymous hemianopia, but with macular sparing.

5. **A – Anterior ischaemic optic neuropathy**. An altitudinal visual field defect can be superior or inferior, so that the affected individual loses their upper or lower half of visual field. It can also be unilateral or bilateral. The most common cause of an altitudinal visual field defect is anterior or posterior ischaemic optic neuropathy. A less common cause is a branch retinal artery occlusion.

A   Ophthalmology A24 – Eyelid disorders

1. **H – Molluscum contagiosum** is a poxvirus infection causing one or multiple small pearly nodules on the lid margin with an umbilicated central punctum. It is transmitted by close contact. Patients complain of an eyelid lump and frequently present with a red irritable eye due to secondary chronic follicular conjunctivitis. More profuse lesions are seen in immunocompromised patients. The diagnosis is made clinically and the lesions are usually treated by de-roofing and curettage.

2. **B – Chalazion**. A chalazion is the most common benign eyelid lump, often on the upper eyelid. It is due to a chronic meibomian gland obstruction which causes a granuloma within the tarsal plate. The lesion is typically round and painless, and may discharge. The diagnosis can be made clinically, and no investigations are necessary. Most cases are self-limiting, requiring only warm compresses. Persistent lesions may require incision and curettage. If the lesion is atypical or recurs, it should be sent for histology to exclude a malignancy.

3. **D – Cyst of Zeis**. When examining a cyst on the eyelid, it is useful to establish whether it is translucent or opaque. An opaque cyst on the anterior lid margin is caused by blockage of an accessory sebaceous gland

and is known as a cyst of Zeis. A translucent cyst on the anterior lid margin is caused by blockage of a sweat gland and is known as a cyst of Moll (apocrine hydrocystoma). An eccrine hydrocystoma looks almost identical to a cyst of Moll, but it does not involve the lid margin. No intervention is required, but the cyst may be excised for cosmetic reasons.

4. **F – Internal hordeolum**. A chalazion can become infected to form an abscess known as an internal hordeolum. Unlike a chalazion, this lump is painful, erythematous and tender on palpation. An external hordeolum (stye) is an abscess within a lash follicle that is associated with the glands of Moll or Zeis. The diagnosis of a hordeolum is made clinically, and is usually staphylococcal in origin. Management is with warm compresses and an antibiotic ointment. As a hordeolum can develop into preseptal cellulitis, it is important to assess if the inflammation is localised or more generalised. A hordeolum is fairly well-circumscribed. A more widespread swelling, tenderness and erythema of the eyelid should alert the clinician to a diagnosis of preseptal cellulitis. An orbital cellulitis is likely in a patient with any of the following additional features: pain on ocular movement, proptosis, reduced ocular motility and diplopia. Systemic features of an infection (e.g. fever, malaise) may also be present.

5. **G – Keratoacanthoma**. This case describes a typical presentation of keratoacanthoma. It is sometimes not possible to clinically distinguish between a keratoacanthoma and a squamous cell carcinoma (SCC), which is why the tumour should be completely excised and sent for histological analysis. Keratoacanthoma is an uncommon lesion that often occurs in the lower eyelid, appearing as a pink lesion that rapidly grows for 2–6 weeks until it is 1–2 cm in size. It then stops growing and undergoes involution over a number of months. As the tumour involutes, the central part becomes hyperkeratotic. This leads to a keratin-filled central crater. The lesion usually regresses on its own. The main treatment option for keratoacanthoma is complete surgical excision. Important differentials include SCC and basal cell carcinoma (BCC). An SCC accounts for 5%–10% of eyelid malignancies and is more aggressive than a BCC. A BCC accounts for 90% of all eyelid malignancies. Ninety per cent of BCCs occur in the head and neck region and 10% occur in the eyelids. It is important to be familiar with the presentation and management of BCC and SCC, which are discussed in the Dermatology section of this book.

Section B

Dermatology EMQs

Dermatology Q1 – Dermatological terms I

A. Abscess
B. Bulla
C. Closed comedone
D. Macule
E. Nodule
F. Open comedone
G. Papule
H. Plaque
I. Pustule
J. Vesicle

From the list above, choose the most appropriate answer for each of the following examples.

1. This is the dermatological term for a blackhead.
2. This is a visible collection of clear fluid in the skin that is less than 0.5 cm in diameter.
3. This is an elevated circumscribed lesion of skin that is <0.5 cm in diameter.
4. A dome-shaped solid lump in the skin that is >0.5 cm in diameter.
5. This is a non-palpable flat area of skin discolouration that is <0.5 cm in diameter.

Q **Dermatology Q2 – Dermatological terms II**

A. Angioedema
B. Ecchymosis
C. Erosion
D. Lichenification
E. Petechiae
F. Purpura
G. Spider naevus
H. Telangiectasia
I. Ulcer
J. Wheal

From the list above, choose the most appropriate answer for each of the following examples.

1. A term describing the loss of the epidermal and dermal layers of the skin.
2. An area of thickened skin with exaggerated skin markings.
3. These are red lesions less than 3 mm in diameter, occurring as a result of blood extravasation into skin. They do not blanch on pressure.
4. Raised, pale and circumscribed areas of dermal oedema, often surrounded by an erythematous flare.
5. This is a collection of small dilated blood vessels.

Dermatology Q3 – Systemic cutaneous disorders I

A. Arterial ulcer
B. Diabetic dermopathy
C. Erythema ab igne
D. Erythema multiforme
E. Livedo reticularis
F. Lymphoedema
G. Necrobiosis lipoidica
H. Pretibial myxoedema
I. Pyoderma gangrenosum
J. Urticaria

From the list above, choose the most appropriate diagnosis for each of the following examples.

1. A 40-year-old woman presents to her GP complaining of weight loss and excessive sweating. She says she has unintentionally lost about 8 kg over the past 5 months, even though she has been eating more than she normally does. She has a past medical history of vitiligo and is on the oral contraceptive pill. On examination, her temperature is 37.3°C, heart rate (HR) is 85 bpm, blood pressure (BP) 130/75 and respiratory rate (RR) 18 breaths per minute. Her eyes look proptosed, there is non-pitting oedema in both feet, and her ankle reflexes are brisk.

2. A 43-year-old man presents to his GP complaining of an ulcer on his leg. He says this started as a blister a week ago but has now become very painful. He has past medical history of ischaemic heart disease, hypertension, hypercholesterolemia and ulcerative colitis. He is on aspirin, simvastatin and ramipril. He smokes about 40 cigarettes a day. On examination, his temperature is 36.9°C, HR is 76 bpm, BP 144/91 and RR 16 breaths per minute. He has a deep ulcer on the shin of his right leg, which has a honeycomb-like base and a bluish rolled edge.

3. A 22-year-old man presents to his GP with a dry cough and a skin rash. He says that he feels unwell, and is worried about painful skin lesions on the palms of his hands that he says look like a 'bull's eye'. The rash has been there for a few days now. He is normally fit and healthy and does not take any medications. On examination, his temperature is 38.2°C. His HR is 78 bpm, BP is 131/84 and RR is 22 breaths per minute. On chest auscultation, there is bronchial breathing in the lower left lung lobe. On both

palms, there are circular red-purple lesions that do indeed match the patient's description. The patient denies taking any antibiotics.

4. A 42-year-old man presents to his GP complaining of small, red spots on his shins. He says they have been present for weeks now, and he is worried it might be something serious. He is otherwise feeling well at the moment, having recovered from a chest infection he had 2 weeks ago. He has a past medical history of type 1 diabetes mellitus and hay fever, and is on actrapid and insultard. On examination, his temperature is 38.2°C. His HR is 78 bpm, BP is 131/84 and RR is 22 breaths per minute. His chest is clear on auscultation. He has multiple small, red-brown papules on both shins in the pre-tibial region. He has no other rashes anywhere else.

5. A 62-year-old lady presents to her GP complaining of the appearance of her legs. She feels that the skin on her legs has been becoming more red and mottled over the past few months. She has to wear long dark socks in public to conceal her legs. Her legs are rarely exposed to cold weather, and she keeps them warm at night as she sleeps close to the radiator. She has a past medical history of eczema and two miscarriages, and only takes over-the-counter multivitamins. She does not smoke and nor does she drink any alcohol. On examination, her temperature is 36.0°C, HR is 75 bpm, BP is 148/86 and RR is 16 breaths per minute. The skin on her leg is red and reticulated. Her legs are not swollen, there are no ulcers and her peripheral pulses are palpable.

Dermatology Q4 – Systemic cutaneous disorders II

A. Addison's disease
B. Adrenal metastasis
C. Cushing's syndrome
D. Diabetes mellitus
E. Gastric cancer
F. Neurofibromatosis type 1
G. Neurofibromatosis type 2
H. Pancreatitis
I. Sarcoidosis
J. Tuberculosis

From the list above, choose the most appropriate underlying disorder for each of the following examples.

1. A 45-year-old woman presents to her GP complaining of lethargy, loss of appetite, weight loss and feeling nauseous over the past few weeks. She has also developed abdominal pain over the past few days, and has recently had two falls because she felt very dizzy after standing up. She is concerned that her skin colour is changing. She has a past medical history of Hashimoto's thyroiditis and carpal tunnel syndrome, and is currently on levothyroxine. She has smoked about 15 cigarettes a day for the past 15 years. On examination, her temperature is 37.1°C, heart rate (HR) is 62 bpm, blood pressure (BP) is 106/62 and respiratory rate (RR) is 16 breaths per minute. Examination of the respiratory, cardiovascular and abdominal systems is unremarkable, although she does have mild generalised abdominal tenderness. Her skin has a dull grey-brown discolouration, with increased pigmentation of the palmar creases and axillae. She also has patches of depigmented skin on the back of her hands.

2. A 40-year-old woman presents to her GP complaining of a dry cough and a skin rash. She says that she has had a persistent cough for the past 6 weeks, and has had fevers and night sweats on and off during that period. She also complains of increased fatigue and feeling generally unwell. She is worried about a red rash that has affected her face and legs. She is normally very fit and exercises regularly. She has a past medical history of two miscarriages and two recent episodes of uveitis. On examination, her temperature is 37.2°C, HR is 65 bpm, BP 114/73 and RR 18 breaths per minute. There are red maculopapular lesions on her face. On

her shins, she has tender asymmetric red nodules. Examination of the cardiovascular, respiratory and abdominal systems is unremarkable.

3. A 54-year-old gentleman presents to his GP with severe abdominal pain and nausea. His abdominal pain started a few days ago, and he has vomited a number of times since. He describes the pain as constant, pointing to his epigastric region. He has a past medical history of irritable bowel syndrome and gallstones. He smokes five cigarettes a day and drinks about 11 units of alcohol a week. On examination, his HR is 106 bpm, BP is 154/95, RR is 19 breaths per minute, oxygen saturation is 94% on room air, and his temperature is 38.8°C. He is not jaundiced, but his skin has a purple discolouration at the flanks. He has abdominal tenderness and rigidity on palpation of his abdominal epigastric region. The abdominal aorta is pulsatile but not expansile. On auscultation, bowel sounds are absent.

4. A 67-year-old man presents to his GP complaining of abdominal pain and nausea. The pain is dull in nature and is present for most of the day if he does not take painkillers. He has suffered from peptic ulcer disease for years, but his pain has been fairly well controlled. He denies any malaise, dysphagia, vomiting, loss of appetite or weight loss. He has been opening his bowels normally and there is no blood in the stools. He has no other medical conditions, and is on lansoprazole, gaviscon and paracetamol. He has quit smoking many years ago, and drinks very little alcohol. On examination, his temperature is 36.3°C, HR is 78 bpm, BP 164/92 and RR 18 breaths per minute. The patient's axillary skin looks thickened and hyperpigmented, and there are a few overlying skin tags. No abnormalities can be detected on examination of the cardiovascular, respiratory and abdominal systems.

5. A 15-year-old boy is brought to the GP by his mother, who is concerned about his skin appearance. The mother reports that he had some patches of dark skin on his chest and back when he was an infant but they have increased in number and size. The son admits that he has noticed them increasing in number more than a year ago, and thinks they are a little bigger now. He has been avoiding sports and swimming activities as he feels embarrassed by the way he looks. He is normally fit and healthy, and does not take any medications. On examination, his temperature

is 37.0°C, HR is 62 bpm, BP 115/76 and RR 18 breaths per minute. No abnormalities can be detected on examination of the cardiovascular, respiratory, abdominal and neurological systems. He has about 12 hyperpigmented macules on his trunk, which measure an average of 2 cm each. He also has prominent axillary freckling.

Q Dermatology Q5 – Dermatological disorders I

A. Atopic eczema
B. Candidiasis
C. Contact dermatitis
D. Erythroderma
E. Guttate psoriasis
F. Keratoderma blennorrhagica
G. Palmoplantar pustulosis
H. Pityriasis rosea
I. Pompholyx eczema
J. Psoriasis vulgaris
K. Venous eczema

From the above options, select the most likely diagnosis for each of the following examples.

1. A family present to their GP with a 5-month-old boy complaining of a red rash they noticed when changing his nappies that has progressively become worse. On examination there are large areas of erythema with crease sparing. These lesions are very dry, scaly and clearly tender on palpation.

2. A 37-year-old gentleman with no past medical history presents to A&E with an asymptomatic yellow-brown pustular rash on his palms and the soles of his feet. He has also noticed pain in his left knee and a burning sensation on passing urine. There is no history of trauma to the knee.

3. A 54-year-old lady presents with scaly, itchy skin on her lower legs. There is brown staining near her ankles, and the skin is thickened and indurated.

4. A 19-year-old man presents to his GP with a widespread silver, flaky red rash affecting his legs, arms, back and torso. This started as a sudden eruption of small scaly lesions which have grown in size, some an inch in diameter, others coalesced to form larger ones. It is very itchy and the lesions bleed very easily. On further questioning the patient mentions he had an upper respiratory infection a fortnight ago.

5. A 50-year-old gentleman presents to A&E with a 24-hour history of lethargy, fever and rigors. This was shortly followed by generalised erythema and fiery sensation over the body. He is known to have severe psoriasis, which was being treated with steroids until he ran out of them.

Q **Dermatology Q6 – Management of autoimmune skin disorders**

A. Admission and IV antibiotics
B. Admission, IV antibiotics and IV corticosteroids
C. Oral contraceptive pill
D. Oral corticosteroids
E. Oral doxycyline
F. Oral erythromycin
G. Oral isotretinoin
H. Oral metronidazole
I. Topical benzoyl peroxide
J. Topical corticosteroids

From the above list, select the next line of treatment for each of the following examples.

1. A 15-year-old attends his GP with his father, complaining of acne. This is not causing any distress at the moment; however, he has seen friends with more severe cases and is worried that it may progress. On examination he has a few pustules, but multiple comedones are seen on his face and back.

2. A 35-year-old Irish lady presents to her GP stating that her cheeks are always red and sometimes they become dry and peel. She mentions that she gets flushed cheeks especially after alcohol, and when hot. On examination, her cheeks and forehead were erythematous with associated telangiectasia, and several pustules. There were no visible comedones.

3. A 25-year-old lady presents with worsening acne. She is 10 weeks pregnant and has tried all types of topical agents. On examination she has multiples pustules seen particularly on the chin and cheeks.

4. A 22-year-old gentleman presents to A&E with a sudden outburst of acne on the face, upper back and chest. He is complaining of joint pains and was noted to be pyrexial on presentation. On examination he has severe ulcerating acne on his face, chest and back. He has always had mild acne, but was never bothered by it.

5. A 23-year-old lady presents to her dermatologist with persistent acne despite topical agents and oral antibiotics. She is currently not taking any medications. She has read about 'Roaccutane' and says that she does not want to use it because of its side effects and a friend's personal experience.

Q **Dermatology Q7 – Manifestations of sexually transmitted diseases**
A. *Candida albicans*
B. *Chlamydia trochomatis*
C. Epstein–Barr virus
D. Haemophilus ducreyi
E. Herpes simplex virus type 1
F. Herpes simplex virus type 2
G. Human immunodeficiency virus
H. Human papilloma virus
I. *Neisseria gonorrhoea*
J. *Treponema pallidum*

From the list above, choose the most likely organism responsible for the patient's presentation in each of the following examples.

1. A 32-year-old man presents to his GP with a rash on his palms and soles of his feet. The rash developed a week ago, and is not itchy or painful. On further questioning, he reveals that he developed an ulcer on his penis 6 weeks ago. He is extremely anxious about having caught a dangerous disease, as he has had sexual intercourse with three different male partners over the past year. On examination, his temperature is 37.7°C. He has an intense red maculopapular rash on his palms and soles of his feet. He also has a generalised lymphadenopathy and moist perianal papules.

2. A 27-year-old man presents to his GP complaining of white patches on his tongue. He first noticed these a few days ago as he felt ridges on the sides of his tongue. He does not have any pain, and is otherwise fit and healthy. On examination, his temperature is 37.1°C. He has white hairy plaques on the lateral aspects of his tongue. You try to scrape off the lesions, but you are unable to. On examination, there is no evidence of lymphadenopathy or other abnormalities.

3. A 25-year-old female presents to her GP complaining of ulcers in her genital area. She states that these started as small red lumps that are now rupturing into very painful ulcers. She is distressed by the ongoing genital pain, and complains of a burning sensation on urination. She confides that she recently met someone, and is concerned that she may have a serious sexually transmitted infection. On examination, her temperature is 36.9°C. She has small red vesicles and multiple ulcerations on her labia, extending

all the way to her cervix. She also has a bilateral inguinal lymphadenopathy.

4. A 20-year-old lady presents to her GP complaining of a brown rash on her vagina. She says that these lesions started as small pink projections, but these are now larger and are similar in shape to cauliflower. On further questioning, she states that she is sexually active and has had sex with more than one partner over the past year. She is asthmatic, and is on inhalers and the oral contraceptive pill. On examination, her temperature is 37.2°C. There are cauliflower-like lesions clearly visible on her vagina and extending to her inner thighs. There is no regional lymphadenopathy, and there are no apparent rashes anywhere else on her body.

5. A 17-year-old female complains to her GP of a green vaginal discharge, and a burning sensation when she urinates. On further questioning, she also reveals that many of her joints have been aching over the past few days. She also has pain in her hands and a rash. She is extremely anxious about having caught a sexually transmitted infection, as she has had sexual intercourse with different partners over the past few months. She is normally fit and healthy, and is only on the oral contraceptive pill. On examining the vagina, the GP sees a green vaginal discharge. He also notices a red rash on the patient's hands.

Q **Dermatology Q8 – Cutaneous ulcers**

A. Arterial ulcer

B. Basal cell carcinoma

C. Erythema nodosum

D. Infective ulcer

E. Marjolin's ulcer

F. Necrobiosis lipoidica

G. Neuropathic ulcer

H. Pretibial myxoedema

I. Pyoderma gangrenosum

J. Venous ulcer

From the list above, select the most appropriate option for each of the following examples.

1. An 82-year-old lady is referred to the dermatology outpatients with a slowly growing painless ulcer. Upon further questioning it appears that the area affected is the site of previous radiotherapy. She has a past medical history of systemic lupus erythematosus, coronary artery disease and osteoarthritis.

2. A 52-year-old male is referred to the dermatology outpatients urgently due to a fast-growing ulcer affecting his right leg. He explains that the lesion started as a small boil. His past medical history includes Crohn's disease and asthma, and he is not currently on any medications. The lesion appears 'dirty', with exudate seeping from it.

3. A 78-year-old lady is referred to the dermatology outpatients with an ulcer on her left leg. She has first noticed it about a fortnight ago, and is unsure if it is changing in size. She has a past medical history of ulcerative colitis and diabetes mellitus. Her current body mass index is 32. On examination, she has a round, shallow and painless ulcer superior to her medial malleolus. She has peripheral oedema. The rest of the cardiovascular and neurological exam of the legs is unremarkable.

4. A 63-year-old gentleman is referred to dermatology outpatients with a large waxy lesion that is yellow in colour and affecting his shin. On questioning, he reports that the lesion began as a small red lump. He has a past medical history of rheumatoid arthritis, diabetes mellitus and Graves' disease.

5. A 72-year-old gentleman presents to his GP with a painful non-discharging deep ulcer affecting his right foot. He has a past

119

medical history of hypertension and type 2 diabetes mellitus, and a 30-pack-year smoking history.

Q **Dermatology Q9 – Cutaneous lesions I**
  A. Campbell De Morgan spots
  B. Dermatofibroma
  C. Furunculosis
  D. Hidradenitis suppurativa
  E. Kaposi's sarcoma
  F. Psoriatic patch
  G. Sebaceous cyst
  H. Seborrhoeic keratosis
  I. Subcutaneous lipoma
  J. Telangiectasia

From the list above, select the most appropriate option for each of the following examples.

1. A 38-year-old man presents to his GP anxious about a purple-coloured skin lesion on his left ankle. He does not have any past medical history, and explains that he is worried about sexually transmitted diseases because he has had unsafe sex with multiple male partners. On examination, there is a firm violaceous papule behind the left lateral malleolus.

2. A 28-year-old man presents to his GP with a large bump on his right forearm. He explains the bump is smooth and rubbery, and does not cause him any pain or discomfort. He has never had any skin conditions in the past, but his sisters have had cysts in the skin. On examination, the lump is 5 × 3 cm in size, smooth, soft and fluctuant with no erythematous change on the overlying skin. The lump is not pulsatile and does not transilluminate with a pentorch.

3. A 74-year-old lady presents to her GP with multiple skin lesions on her body. They vary in colour and the largest of them are about 3 cm in diameter. The lesions have mainly affected her neck and thorax. She has decided to seek medical attention now as some of them are itchy and have bled recently. On closer inspection, they are well-defined patches and papules with a scaly appearance.

4. A 56-year-old lady presents to the dermatology outpatients clinic with multiple small bright red papules between 1 and 5 mm in diameter on her trunk. They are asymptomatic, and the dermatologist reassures the patient that they are benign and can be treated if they are aesthetically unappealing for the patient.

5. A 24-year-old lady presents to the general surgery outpatients with recurrent painful swellings in her armpits. She has similar lesions in the groin; however, the axillary lesions have discharged recently. There are also grouped blackheads on her axillae. The lady explains that she is extremely agitated by this condition. Conservative management has failed previously and the lesions have recurred even after incision and drainage.

Q Dermatology Q10 – Cutaneous lesions II

A. 2 mm
B. 4 mm
C. 5 mm
D. Basal cell carcinoma
E. Bowen's disease
F. Keratoacanthoma
G. Lentigo malignant melanoma
H. Marjolin's ulcer
I. Squamous cell carcinoma
J. Superficial spreading malignant melanoma

From the list above, select the most appropriate option for each of the following examples.

1. A 64-year-old farmer presents with a growing lesion on the bridge of his nose. He has never had any skin cancers in the past, but his wife is very concerned about this being a cancer. On closer inspection the lesion is 1.8 cm in diameter and appears as a papule with a shiny translucent appearance.
2. A 72-year-old lady has a confirmed basal cell carcinoma. The lesion is 1.6 cm in diameter. What is the recommended excision margin for such a lesion?
3. An 82-year-old lady is diagnosed with a subtype of malignant melanoma. The lesion overlies her right zygomatic arch. She reports that the lesion has been slowly growing for years.
4. A 78-year-old man presents with a painful and rapidly growing skin lesion on the lower lip. On closer inspection the lesion appears hyperkeratotic. There is crusting at the surface of the lesion, as well as formation of a cutaneous horn.
5. This is a pre-malignant cutaneous lesion that may lead to the development of cutaneous squamous cell carcinoma.

Q **Dermatology Q11 – Management of malignant melanoma**
A. 95%–100%
B. 80%–96%
C. Level 2
D. Level 3
E. Stratum corneum
F. Stratum granulosum
G. T3N2M0
H. T3N3M0
I. Wide local excision with 2 cm margin
J. Wide local excision with 3 cm margin

From the list above, select the most appropriate option for each of the following examples.

1. Breslow's depth is one of the most important prognostic indicators in malignant melanoma. From which layer of the epidermis is the thickness measured?
2. A histopathology report states that a patient's breslow depth is 1.8 mm; what is the approximate 5-year survival rate?
3. A histopathology report indicates that a patient with malignant melanoma has a tumour that has spread into the papillary dermis-reticular dermis junction. What Clark's level does this correspond to?
4. A patient with malignant melanoma has a tumour with a thickness of 3 mm, spread to three lymph nodes and no metastatic spread. What is the patient's stage according to tumour, node and metastasis staging?
5. A patient with confirmed malignant melanoma and no clinical evidence of nodal or distant metastasis is planned for elective surgery. What surgery would you offer the patient?

Q **Dermatology Q12 – Infective cutaneous lesions I**
   A. Group A streptococcal impetigo
   B. Group B streptococcal impetigo
   C. Molluscum contagiosum
   D. Pox bacteria
   E. Recurrent herpes simplex virus 1
   F. Recurrent herpes simplex virus 2
   G. Secondary herpes simplex virus 1
   H. Secondary herpes simplex virus 2
   I. Smallpox
   J. *Streptococcus aureus* impetigo
   K. Varicella zoster virus (chickenpox)
   L. Varicella zoster virus (shingles)

From the list above, choose the most likely diagnosis for each of the following examples. Answers may be used once, more than once or not at all.

1. A 4-year-old boy is brought to the GP by his mother after noticing a strange patch near his mouth that appeared a few days ago. On examination, there is a seropustular well-defined erythematous lesion with an overlying gold honey-coloured crust. The child is otherwise well; he is afebrile and his observations are stable.

2. A 19-year-old lady goes to see her GP having noticed a small lump on her bottom lip. On examination, there are small erythematous-based sores with vesiculation and ulceration. She reports that her lip began to tingle and itch prior to vesicle eruption and she has had this lesion several times in the past. The patient is otherwise well; she is afebrile and her observations are stable.

3. A mother has brought her 3-year-old son to the GP as she has noticed a widespread rash. She reports that her child had a fever to begin with and she then noticed 'spots' initially appearing across his back, which he complained were 'itchy'. On examination, there are some macules, scattered papules and some vesicles, and a few have crusted over. The child has no other conditions. His temperature is 38.1°C and his observations are stable.

4. A mother brought her 5-year-old daughter to see their GP as she is concerned about a rash that looks like 'small pearls'. On examination, there are multiple pink papules with umbilicated

centres located in a non-specific distribution across the child's neck. The child is otherwise well; she is afebrile and her observations are stable.

5. An 86-year-old lady came to see her GP as she noticed some strange, painful spots on her back. On examination, there are clear vesicles on an erythematous base extending from the midline of the back to the centre of the chest. The lesions are only on the left side of her back and front. Her co-morbidities consist of hypertension, hypercholesterolaemia and type II diabetes.

Q **Dermatology Q13 – Infective cutaneous lesions II**

A. Drug-induced reaction

B. Epstein–Barr virus

C. Measles

D. Mumps

E. Parvovirus 6

F. Parvovirus B16

G. Parvovirus B19

H. Rubella

I. *Staphylococcus aureus*

J. *Streptococcus pyogenes*

From the list above, choose the most likely diagnosis for each of the following examples. Answers may be used once, more than once or not at all.

1. An 18-month-old boy was taken by his father to see his GP. The father complained that the boy is feeling very hot to touch and has a cough. It was noted that the child had a rash behind his ear that is extending down his body. On further examination, he has a glassy conjunctival appearance and white spots on his inner cheek. The child has a temperature of 38.2°C.

2. A 6-year-old girl was brought to the GP as her mother felt the girl just wasn't well. Her mother also reported that she has developed a rash at the same time. On examination, the child has a macular rash on her face and trunk and there is suboccipital lymph node enlargement. The child is not a UK resident; she recently immigrated to the United Kingdom with her family from Afghanistan. The child's observations are stable and she is afebrile.

3. A 12-year-old boy was brought to the GP as his mother felt he just wasn't well; she also noticed a developing rash on her son's limbs. On examination, the doctor additionally noticed a slapped cheek appearance. The child's observations are stable and his temperature is 37.5°C.

4. A 5-year-old boy was taken to the emergency department by his parents, as he has been feverish with a rash for a few days and he's just not getting better. His mother reports that he complained of a sore throat initially. On examination, the patient is listless. He has a generalised exanthem on his trunk and a positive pastia sign. On closer inspection the tongue is red with oedematous papillae, and there is circumoral pallor. The child has a temperature of 38.8°C,

heart rate is 122 bpm, blood pressure is 118/68, respiratory rate is 18 breaths per minute and saturations of 98%.

5. An 8-year-old boy was taken by his mother to see his GP again for the second time this week. Mum reports he was given penicillin a couple of days ago for his sore throat but it has not gotten any better and he is now notably feverish and lethargic. On examination, the child has enlarged cervical lymph nodes, kissing tonsils and an oedematous uvula. He also has a faint developing maculopapular rash over his torso. The child's observations are stable and his temperature is 37.3°C.

Q Dermatology Q14 – Infective cutaneous lesions III

A. Amelanocytic melanoma

B. *Candida*

C. Common wart

D. Pitiryasis rosea

E. Pityriasis versicolor

F. Pityriasis rosea-like drug-induced eruptions

G. Plane warts

H. Secondary syphilis

I. Tinea capitis

J. Tinea corporis

From the list above, choose the most appropriate diagnosis for each of the following examples.

1. A 63-year-old morbidly obese lady was seen by the GP on a home visit as her daughter is concerned about a rash that she noticed under her mother's breasts. The patient has not been caring for herself recently as she is mourning the death of her cat and is just recovering from a recent chest infection for which she is taking antibiotics. On examination, there is a red macerated rash with ill-defined margins, accompanied by neighbouring satellite papulopustules. The patient also reports that she has lost weight despite maintaining her appetite and is always thirsty. The patient has hypertension and hypercholesterolaemia. She is currently taking bendroflumethiazide and simvastatin.

2. A 33-year-old gentleman presented to his GP complaining of an itchy red rash on his legs. On examination, there are annular lesions with raised scaly edges and a healing region in the centre. The patient has no medical history of note and is not on any medications. The patient is otherwise well.

3. A 21-year-old girl came to see her GP as she has a 'horrible skin rash' on her upper chest. She said she was on holiday with her friends and noticed that some patches of her skin were just not tanning. The patient is very distressed and recalls her aunt having similar lesions last year. On examination there are depigmented faint scaly macules scattered over her trunk. The patient is otherwise well.

4. A 26-year-old gentleman came to see his GP after work as he noticed a strange lesion on his shoulder 2 weeks ago that is still there. It is occasionally itchy. On examination, there is a large

pink well-demarcated scaly patch. There are a few oval pink scaly patches on the patient's back in line with his ribs. The patient is otherwise well. The patient has history of gastritis and is taking omeprazole as and when it is required.

5. A 24-year-old lady presented to the GP complaining of a strange growth on her finger. She denies any pain, itchiness or change in colour of the growth. On examination, there are two 1 cm sized dome-shaped papules on the radial surface of the index finger. They are cauliflower-like in appearance. They are both rough surfaced, one of which has two black dots and the other has reddish dots superficially. She is irritated by the lumps, as they are getting in the way of her writing. She admits to sustaining a cat-scratch around the similar area a few days ago. The patient is otherwise well.

Q   **Dermatology Q15 – Dermatological emergencies**
A. Cellulitits
B. Erysipelas
C. Extensive third-degree burn
D. Gas gangrene
E. Staphylococcal scalded skin syndrome
F. Stevens–Johnson syndrome
G. Toxic epidermal necrolysis
H. Toxic shock syndrome
I. Type II necrotising fasciitis
J. Type III necrotising fasciitis

From the list above, choose the most appropriate diagnosis for each of the following examples.

1. A 45-year-old gentleman presented to A&E complaining of severe pain and discolouration in his leg. He describes the pain coming on suddenly and worsening over the past few days with a heavy sensation in his leg. He also reports having a recent road traffic accident with an open fracture to the same limb. On examination, there is an oedematous exuding tender lower left leg, with a blue-black region on the lateral aspect. There are also two haemorrhagic bullae present; crepitus can be felt.

2. A mother brought her 2-year-old boy to A&E as he has developed a generalised macular erythematous rash. The child was seen immediately; on examination the child was febrile, had a widespread tissue paper-like rash and had a positive Nikolsky's sign. He also developed bullae in his axillae.

3. A 33-year-old gentleman was seen in A&E with an extensive rash. On examination the patient is found to have raised erythematous plaques with a necrotic centre. The patient's palms have denuding skin. The patient has red gritty eyes and ulcers in his mouth. His temperature is 38.8°C, heart rate is 122 bpm, blood pressure is 100/58, saturations 98% and respiratory rate is 19 breaths per minute.

4. A 21-year-old university student visited her GP as she noticed the latter aspect of her right calf to be swollen, red, hot and painful. She also admitted to recently suffering a cut to this area.

5. A 52-year-old morbidly obese gentleman presented to A&E complaining of intense pain in his right leg. He describes his skin initially looking red and then quickly becoming swollen. On

examination, the patient looks generally unwell and clammy. He is exquisitely tender on the right lateral thigh, where the patient reports it being the most common site for his insulin injection. There is an open deep wound with surrounding erythema, and necrotic changes at the peripheral edges. On further questioning, the patient admits to rarely changing his injection site. The patient is a type II diabetic and currently on insulin. His temperature is 38.9°C, heart rate is 136 bpm, blood pressure is 92/48, saturations 98% and respiratory rate is 22 breaths per minute.

Q **Dermatology Q16 – Burns**

A. 36% burn
B. 37% burn
C. 15 000 mL
D. 17 000 mL
E. Debridement of affected area
F. Deep partial thickness burn
G. Escharotomy
H. Full thickness skin graft
I. Split thickness skin graft
J. Superficial partial thickness burn

From the list above, select the most appropriate option for each of the following examples.

1. A 62-year-old female was brought to the burns unit with extensive burns affecting the posterior aspect of her torso, posterior aspect of her right lower limb, the right upper limb in entirety and her perineum. What is the total body surface area affected?
2. A 28-year-old male suffers burns affecting 48% of his body after a tragic accident. The patient weighs 78 kg. Using the Parkland formula, what is the total fluid requirement over 24 hours?
3. On assessment of a patient's burn, the area appears white, doesn't blanch under pressure with minimal pain sensation. What is the thickness of the burn?
4. A 68-year-old lady attends the burns unit with 50% burns. Upon inspecting the right lower limb, the burn extends to the entire circumference of the thigh. After initial stabilisation and management what is the most appropriate surgical intervention?
5. A 42-year-old lady with 45% burns is clinically stabilised then taken to the operating theatre. After extensive debridement of the affected tissue, what type of skin graft should be used for coverage?

Dermatology Q17 – Dermatological drug reactions

A. Exanthematic eruptions
B. Nikolsky's sign
C. Paracetamol
D. Photosensitivity
E. Pigmentary changes
F. Stevens–Johnson syndrome sign
G. Toxic epidermal necrolysis sign
H. Type I hypersensitivity
I. Type II hypersensitivity
J. Type IV hypersensitivity

From the list above, choose the most appropriate answer for each of the following examples.

1. Ms Hailey, a 23-year-old woman, presents to her physician with red and itchy skin over her torso which started two days ago. She is otherwise well but was on ampicillin a week earlier for treatment of a urine tract infection. This is the first time Hailey has used the antibiotic. She has no significant medical history and everyone at home is well. On examination, she was noted to have a macular rash over her chest and back and enlarged lymph nodes. She had no obvious oropharyngeal swelling and no wheeze. Observations showed a low-grade fever. Hailey was promptly advised to stop taking the antibiotics. She returns to her physician 3 weeks later, who finds that the rash has fully resolved. What is the most likely diagnosis?

2. A 67-year-old woman presents to the rapid access clinic with an itchy painful 'eye'. On examination both upper and lower eyelids are visibly swollen and erythematous with scaling on the skin. There is no obvious conjunctivitis. Her eyesight remains unchanged and there are no visible lesions on the rest of her body. She has not recently changed her cosmetics. However, her ophthalmologist gave her new eye drops for her glaucoma a few days ago. From the list of options given, what type of reaction has been described?

3. Ms Apleby presents with what she describes as 'sunburn' on a day out at the beach. She is surprised because she does not normally burn. Her face became bright red and swollen. On examination, she also has areas of erythema of her shoulders, chest and forearms with areas of normal-looking skin where she

wore a swimsuit. Some scaling, and crusting over exposed areas are visible. On general questioning, Ms Apleby has recently been diagnosed with rheumatoid arthritis. From the list of options given, what best describes this type of reaction?

4. Nicholas is a 6-year-old boy with asthma and eczema. His parents took him to a Thai restaurant where he had soup that contained peanuts. His parents have avoided nuts in his diet and were unaware of the ingredients of the soup. Nicholas' mother notes that he starts to become restless, scratching himself feverishly. He has developed skin-colored plaques over his arms and neck. His lips and eyelids are beginning to swell. Promptly they call an ambulance. From the list of options given, what type of reaction has been described?

5. An urgent call is placed to the dermatology registrar. A 47-year-old patient has rushed into the high dependency unit. He has a medical history of hypertension and has recently been diagnosed with gout. His wife reports that he was feeling unwell about 3 days ago with flu-like symptoms and started to complain of pins and needles and a burning sensation on his skin as well as a sore mouth. Over the day he developed blisters and his skin started to peel off his back and buttocks 'as though he had been burnt'. The high dependency unit nurse tells you that he also has a macular eruption. Also they are not sure how to care for him as the blisters 'break' and erode his skin with the slightest touch. What is the clinical sign called?

Dermatology Q18 – Dermatological investigations

A. Allergy patch testing
B. Dermoscopy
C. Diascopy
D. IgE quantification blood test
E. Intradermal allergy test
F. Radioallergosorbent test
G. Skin scrapes
H. Skin prick test
I. Tzanck preparation smear
J. Wood lamp examination

From the list above, select the most appropriate answer for each of the following examples.

1. A 23-year-old lady is referred by her GP to a dermatology clinic to review a 'mole on her back', that her medical student boyfriend warned her about. She is particularly worried as he says that malignant melanoma is common in her age group. On inspection there is an 8 mm, asymmetrical naevus on her lower back. What bedside investigation can be performed to better evaluate the lesion?

2. A lady brings her 5-year-old son to a dermatology clinic. He developed a 'red rash' on his head and eyebrows that has progressed into a larger, scalier lesion associated with loss of hair. On examination there is a 2 cm lesion on the frontal region on the scalp coalescing with a smaller 5 mm lesion on the right eyebrow, and there are numerous papules forming a ringed border. Her son has no past medical history. She mentions that they have recently arrived from a holiday in Mexico. On epiluminescence microscopy, there is a negative exclamation mark sign. What bedside investigation will help conclude the diagnosis?

3. A 13-year-old boy is referred to your dermatology clinic to investigate his asthma exacerbation. He has noticed that over the last 2 years his asthma has been progressively worse with no particular trigger identified. The patient has no known allergies. What is the first line investigation to identify if there is a specific trigger?

4. A 28-year-old gentleman presents to his GP with a 2-day history of multiple very painful ulcers on his penis. He also complains of pain on passing urine. He has no previous history of sexually

transmitted diseases. What is the next line investigation to diagnose this condition?

5. A 35-year-old student nurse presents to your dermatology clinic complaining of red, swollen and blistering hands. This started when she started working on the wards. She states that she has not been exposed to any new substances, and always wears gloves when handling medication or patients' body fluids. She has been using moisturisers frequently, with little benefit. What investigation can best identify the causative substance?

Dermatology Q19 – Connective tissue disorders
A. Dermatomyositis
B. Diffuse cutaneous scleroderma
C. Henoch-Schönlein purpura
D. Limited cutaneous scleroderma
E. Meningitis
F. Meningococcal septicaemia
G. Polymyositis
H. Raynaud's disease
I. Reactive arthritis
J. Systemic lupus erythematosus

From the list above, choose the most appropriate diagnosis for each of the following examples.

1. A 24-year-old Afro-Caribbean lady presented to her GP as she was feeling increasingly tired and is complaining of aches in her joints, particularly her hands. During the consultation, you notice an erythematous rash over her cheeks and nasal bridge.

2. A 44-year-old lady presented to her GP complaining of strange changes in her hands when she goes out in the cold; initially her fingers become pale, then become blue and finally turn red. On examination, there is no skin discolouration of the patient's hands. However, there is tightened, shiny, thickened skin and the fingers taper. There are also palpable subcutaneous swellings. The patient is otherwise well.

3. A 53-year-old gentleman previously fit and well presents to his GP complaining of feeling increasingly weak and tired. He is finding it particularly difficult to get up from his chair. The patient has lost his appetite in the past few months and he has lost almost 2 stones within that time period. On examination you notice an erythematous rash over the cheeks and heliotrope discolouration around his eyes. There are palpable subcutaneous swellings located on the patient's hands.

4. A 7-year-old boy is brought by his mother to see the GP as she feels he is just not right. His mother is increasingly concerned as she has noticed a strange rash over her son's legs that has been changing in appearance over the past few days. On examination, there is a purpuric, palpable non-blanching rash that is tender, over the extensor surfaces of the lower limbs. The mother reports a fever earlier of 38.2°C and upon questioning, the child

reports having a headache and knee pain. The GP contacts the paediatrician on duty for further advice. The child is previously fit and well.

5. A 27-year-old gentleman presents to his GP complaining of a lesion on his penis. On examination, there is inflammation and superficial circular red plaques and ulcers around the penile meatus. The GP notices from the record that the patient was seen 2 weeks ago complaining of symptoms of gastroenteritis. On further questioning, the patient admits to having right knee pain but this has subsided since he started frequent painkillers.

Dermatology Q20 – Pharmacology in dermatology
A. Dithranol
B. Erythrasma
C. Liver enzyme inducer
D. Liver enzyme inhibitor
E. Nappy rash
F. Nil major known
G. NSAIDs
H. Steroid cream
I. Teratogenic
J. Urticaria

Note corresponding table summarising some dermatological conditions, possible treatments and the main side effect. From the list above, complete the table with the most appropriate answer for each of the examples. Each answer may be used once, more than once or not at all.

	Disease/Condition	Treatment	Caution/Side effect
1	Ezcema	Emollients	
2	Mycosis of the nail	Itraconazole	
3		Clotrimazole cream	Nil major known
4	Psoriasis		Skin staining
5		Antihistamines	Sedation
6	Acne	Retinoids	
7	Lupus erythematosus	Corticosteroids	

Q **Dermatology Q21 – Bullous disorders**

A. Chemical injury
B. Congestive cardiac failure
C. Direct immunofluorescence – basement membrane IgG deposits
D. Direct immunofluorescence – intercellular IgG deposits
E. Direct immunofluorescence – linear IgA deposits along basement membrane
F. Hereditary epidermolysis bullosa
G. Pemphigoid
H. *Staphylococcus aureus*
I. *Streptococcus pneumoniae*
J. Toxic epidermal necrolysis

From the list above, choose the most likely diagnosis for each of the following examples.

1. A 50-year-old patient with no significant medical history presents with blisters and sores. It started a few months ago with painful blisters in her mouth making eating very difficult. She has noticed that she has started to lose weight. There is no itching. Now there are mostly 'sores' where the blisters were on her back and groin. On examination, the patient has flaccid blisters with an erythematous base, and multiple areas of erosion involving the mouth and torso. Light pressure on a blister causes its extension and erosion. A biopsy is taken. What is the most likely finding?

2. A 70-year-old patient presents to the dermatology clinic with blisters on his legs. He has a past medical history of hypertension and insulin-dependent diabetes mellitus. He mentions it started with redness and itching and later developed blisters. On examination there are multiple tense dome-shaped blisters, some haemorrhagic. The underlying skin is erythematous. The patient has no significant mucosal involvement. A biopsy is taken. What is the most likely finding?

3. Mrs Morse has been visiting the dermatology clinic for many years. She has very sensitive skin and is prone to blistering with the slightest pressure and is always very careful. Recently she went on a long hike and her right toenails have started to fall off. What is the most likely diagnosis?

4. A 3-year-old presents with blisters. Her mother reports that she has been unwell recently with a chest infection and fever. On examination she has thin-walled bullae on her thighs that

rupture with minimal pressure. Where previous bullae have been ruptured, discrete areas of erosion have appeared. The underlying skin is erythematous and appears to be sloughing off. Of note there is a larger bulla on her thumb with surrounding erythema. She finds this very tender. What is the most likely causative organism?

5. A 64-year-old gentleman presents with blisters on his legs. They have been developing over the last month and he has noticed that his legs are becoming increasingly swollen. On further questioning you note he suffers from shortness of breath, worse on lying down. He has a past medical history of two myocardial infarctions and diabetes. On examination he is obese and has dependent oedema with pitting to the knees. The blisters appear to leak clear fluid. Smaller tense vesicles are also present. Oxygen saturations are 90% on air; otherwise, he is stable. What is the most likely diagnosis?

Q Dermatology Q22 – Pruritus

A. Anogenital pruritus
B. Dermatitis herpetiformis
C. Eczema striae
D. Lichen simplex
E. Linear IgA dermatosis
F. Pre-tibial myxoedema
G. Primary biliary cirrhosis
H. Psoriasis
I. Seborrhoeic dermatitis
J. Wickham's striae

From the list above, choose the most appropriate diagnosis for each of the following examples.

1. A 32-year-old computer programmer presents with 'extremely intense itching around the anus'. His past medical history includes a long struggle with recurrent haemorrhoids and contact dermatitis. On examination, there is an obvious haemorrhoid with serous discharge and small areas of excoriation around the anal sphincter.

2. An 18-year-old man presents to the dermatology clinic with plaques on his shins. He reports he has been suffering from a chronic itch on his legs for many years and has been investigated without a diagnosis as yet. He has no significant medical history and is not on any medication. He has not changed soaps or shower gels in recent years. This itch is starting to cause him great frustration and depression. On examination of his shin, he has a discrete raised brown 4 cm discoloured plaque with excoriation marks. On general inspection, he has similar plaques on his forearms. It is also noted that his fingernails appear 'polished'. On further questioning, he has started university and feels under a lot of pressure.

3. A 40-year-old patient presents to the dermatology clinic with 'horribly itchy blisters' on his elbows and knees, now spreading to his trunk. He has a past medical history of eczema. On examination he has symmetrical erythematous plaques. Small vesicles are noted but mostly erosions where they have been scratched off. He is clearly distressed. On further questioning, he mentions he has digestive problems when he eats oats and drinks beer. A biopsy is taken and the results are as follows:

Rupert Saleem 07/04/1970

EMQ Hospital Pathology Dept

Sample: Blister from left elbow

Findings: Histology of new blisters shows small pockets of neutrophil microabcesses in tips of dermal papillary. Immunofluorescence: IgA antibodies are seen bound to intermyofibril substance of smooth muscle.

4. A 27-year-old Afro-Caribbean woman presents to the dermatology clinic with itchy purple patches on her wrists and chest. She has no significant medical history and has not started on any new medications. On close examination, the papules are sharply defined with white lines. Dabbing oil on the lesions make them more visible.

5. A 43-year-old Caucasian woman with a history of rheumatoid arthritis presents to the dermatology clinic. She has had intractable generalised itching for weeks not responsive to traditional treatments. On examination she has no obvious lesions on her skin, but many excoriation marks. You however note that she has jaundiced sclera and palpate hepatosplenomegaly.

Q **Dermatology Q23 – Skin infestations**

A. *Candida albicans*

B. *Cornybacterium minutissimum*

C. Pediculus humanus capitis

D. Pediculus humanus corporis

E. Pediculus pubis

F. Scabies

G. *Staphylococcus aureus*

H. Topical antifungal

I. Topical antifungal and steroid cream

J. Topical antifungal and zinc lotion

From the list above, choose the correct answer for each of the following examples.

1. Colin, a 17-year-old keen basketball player, presents to his GP with cracked and itchy feet. It started a few weeks ago and has become progressively worse and tender. On examination of his feet, at the interdigital spaces there are erythematous and scaly lesions. They appear to be weeping and spreading to the dorsum of his feet. His toenails however appear healthy. On general examination, there are no other lesions on his body and he is otherwise fit and well. From the list of options given, what is the most effective treatment?

2. A 45-year-old gentleman presents to the dermatology clinic 'with redness under his belly and between the thighs'. It is occasionally itchy and has been going on for a long while, but he thought nothing of it until he noted scaling of the skin around it. He feels otherwise well in himself and is on regular medication for diabetes and hypertension. On examination, the patient is notably obese. Under his stomach fold you note a large shiny erythematous area between the opposing skin surfaces. There are also isolated lesions with scaly margins. The same is noted in the groin and sub-mammary areas. From the list of options given, what is the most effective treatment?

3. Mr Simpson presents to the clinic with 'red patches' on his groin. They have been there for long while and he has tried steroid creams to no avail. They do not itch and they are not painful, but he finds them unsightly and embarrassing. On examination, the patient is overweight. He has symmetrical, reddish-brown, well-defined, erythematous lesions on his groin with areas of mild

scaling. There are no isolated lesions. The dermatologist turns off the main lights and shines a Wood's lamp over the lesion. It becomes a fluorescent coral-red colour. The patient is very anxious and wants to know if he has a flesh-eating disease. What is the likely causative organism?

4. A 20-year-old cleaner presents to her GP with severe itching that is worse at night. Over the last few days she has also noted lesions on her hands and around her breasts. On examination, she has multiple skin-coloured burrows in her finger-webs, and mamillary region. There are also areas of eczematous eruptions, crusting and punctate erosions. Her flatmates have had similar symptoms. An area of burrows is scraped and sent for microscopy. What is the diagnosis?

5. The following letter is sent to parents of children attending Early Birds Kindergarten:

> Dear Parent,
>
> Our school doctor has made the following recommen-dations with regard to the recent outbreak:
> - Anti-parasitic medication is available for collection at the infirmary
> - Once treatment is complete, your son/daughter may not return to school if lesions are visible.
> - Hair should be washed in diluted vinegar (1 part water to 1 part vinegar) and then wrapped in a towel soaked in diluted vinegar for 30 minutes.
> - Wash daily with medicated shampoo until the hair is clear.
> - Hair should then be brushed while wet with a fine-tooth comb.
> - It is essential to thoroughly examine your household to prevent epidemic spread.

What is the outbreak?

Q Dermatology Q24 – Hair and nails

A. Alopecia with punctuate leukonychia
B. Cirrhosis with punctuate leukonychia
C. Hyperthyroidism with onycholysis
D. Hypothyroidism with alopecia
E. Hypothyroidism with hirsutism
F. Koilonychia
G. Polycystic ovaries
H. Psoriasis of the nails
I. Thyroid acropachy
J. Tinea unguium

From the list above, choose the most appropriate diagnosis for each of the following examples.

1. A previously fit and well 23-year-old lady presented to her GP complaining of hair loss. On examination, there is an oval area of balding over the right parietal region. Her hair and nails appear brittle. She is also reporting gaining weight despite having a normal appetite. She is taking Movicol and occasionally senna when needed for constipation. Upon questioning, her periods have recently become irregular in the past few months and have always been heavy.

2. A 19-year-old university student presented to her GP complaining of irregular periods: 'last year I only got my period four times!' The patient has no other complaints. On examination, the patient is found to have excessive hair on her chin and on the sides of her face.

3. A 78-year-old gentleman came to see his GP complaining of right knee pain. On examination, the GP examined the joint above and below and noted an extremely tender right hip and reduced range of movement in the hip joint. When examining the joint below, i.e. the ankle, the GP noticed the patient's toenails (on the left) to be thickened and crumbling at the outside edges. There is no pitting of the nails. The nails also had a yellow-based colour. The patient has hypertension and osteoarthritis. He is taking bendroflumethiazide.

4. A 29-year-old lady came to see her GP as she is feeling very down. She is finding it difficult to deal with the loss of her mother 11 months ago. She has been drinking excessively for the past 10 months and it is getting worse. She also admits to losing her

job as she came in drunk to work a few days ago and was verbally abusive to a customer. On general examination, the patient looks unkempt. The patient's nails are surfacing from their bed and there are round white spots on the nails. She is also balding and has typical exclamation-mark hairs. There are no other physical findings.

5. A 32-year-old lady presented to her GP complaining of weight loss. She is so surprised because she is eating normally if not more. She also complains of feeling on edge and 'restless' like she has the shakes. On examination, there is hand tremor. On closer inspection, there is clubbing and the patients' distal digits are swollen. The patient has a history of pernicious anaemia.

Q Dermatology Q25 – Dermatological disorders II

A. Cavernous haemangioma
B. Hypertrophic scar
C. Keloid scar
D. Lichen planus
E. Lichen sclerosis
F. Pemphigoid
G. Pemphigus
H. Polymorphic eruption of pregnancy
I. Prurigo of pregnancy
J. Strawberry haemangioma

From the list above, choose the most appropriate diagnosis for each of the following examples.

1. A 51-year-old lady presented to her GP complaining of superficial pain during sexual intercourse with her husband. She describes a tightened feeling and that her husband is finding it difficult to achieve initial penetration. On examination, there are white lesions on the medial labia minora and peri-genital skin.

2. A 74-year-old lady was in hospital for a community-acquired pneumonia. During the ward round, the consultant noticed the patient had large tense blisters across her arms and legs on an eczematous base, none of which had ruptured. Nikolsky's test was negative. Patient is otherwise well. Immunofluorescence results show linear deposition of IgG and complement along the basement membrane.

3. A 24-year-old Afro-Caribbean lady came for a follow-up appointment 9 months post lipoma removal from her upper back. She is upset that her scar is so large and extending far beyond the size of the lump. On examination, there is a tough, raised, irregularly shaped scar. The scar is the same colour as her skin but shinier. She admits that it was fine about 5 months ago but it has started getting progressively larger since.

4. A mother gave birth to a 3.4 kg female baby. The paediatrician is called by request of the mother, as she is concerned of a lump on her newborn's head. On examination, there is a compressible red swelling on the right side of the forehead. The baby is otherwise well.

5. A 26-year-old nullipara lady who is currently 36 weeks pregnant with dichorionic diamniotic twins attends the antenatal clinic

for her routine follow-up and complains of an 'unbearably itch tummy'. On examination, there is a globular looking uterus, consistent with a multiple pregnancy, with prominent striae gravidarum. There are generalised papules located across the abdomen, although there are no skin changes around the umbilicus. She is otherwise well.

Dermatology answers

A Dermatology A1 – Dermatological terms I

1. **F – Open comedone**. This is the dermatological term for a blackhead. A closed comedone is closed by skin, giving it the appearance of a whitehead. Blackheads and whiteheads are lesions that occur in acne due to blockage of secretions caused by abnormal keratinisation of the pilosebaceous follice.

2. **J – Vesicle**. This is a small collection of fluid (blister) that is less than 0.5 cm in diameter (e.g. herpes zoster). The term 'bulla' is used when the blister is more than 0.5 cm in diameter (e.g. bullous pemphigoid).

3. **G – Papule**. An elevated circumscribed lesion of the skin, which is <0.5 cm in diameter (e.g. molluscum contagiosum). A plaque is an elevated flat-topped area of skin that is usually more than 2 cm in diameter (e.g. psoriasis).

4. **E – Nodule**. A dome-shaped solid lump in the skin that is >0.5 cm in diameter (e.g. nodular prurigo).

5. **D – Macule**. This is a non-palpable flat area of altered skin pigmentation that is <0.5 cm in diameter (e.g. pityriasis versicolor). When this area is >0.5 cm, the term 'patch' is used.

   A pustule is visible collection of pus in skin (e.g. pustular psoriasis). In contrast, an abscess is a localised collection of pus in a cavity that is more than 1 cm in diameter.

A Dermatology A2 – Dermatological terms II

1. **I – Ulcer**. An ulcer is defined as a break in an epithelial surface. When referring to skin it is an area of skin from which the epidermis and dermis have been lost. If the epidermis only is lost, the term 'erosion' is used (e.g. pemphigus). An erosion heals without scarring, whereas an ulcer leaves a

scar. A fissure is a split in the epidermis and dermis. Skin atrophy is due to thinning of the epidermis or dermis. Ulcers can occur on any epithelial surface – for example, oral ulcers in Behçet's, Crohn's disease and recurrent aphthous stomatitis, gastric and duodenal ulcers, gastrointestinal ulcerations in inflammatory bowel disease, respiratory ulcerations in toxic epidermal necrolysis, venous and arterial ulcers in peripheral vascular disease.

2. **D – Lichenification**. Lichen means tree moss in Greek. In dermatological terms it refers to an area of thickened skin with exaggerated skin markings. This is due to repetitive trauma (e.g. scratching) that leads to hypertrophy of the epidermal layer.

3. **E – Petechiae**. Extravasation of blood into skin causing bruising is termed as petechiae (pinhead-sized, <2 mm), purpura (~2 mm) or ecchymosis (large, >2 mm). This must be distinguished from erythema, which is redness due to increased local blood flow. Petechiae are most commonly secondary to trauma but may be a manifestation of an underlying disorder (e.g. thrombocytopenia). Telangiectasia is a visible dilatation of superficial blood vessels. Erythema and telangiectasia will blanch on compression, whereas petechiae, purpura or ecchymosis do not blanch.

4. **J – Wheal** is a well-circumscribed papule (circumscribed area of raised skin) that is usually secondary to an allergy as often seen in acute urticaria. Uritcaria (also known as 'hives') is a vascular reaction causing the formation of wheals. These are raised, pale and circumscribed areas of dermal oedema, often surrounded by an erythematous flare. They normally resolve within a few hours. Angioedema is a rapid swelling due to oedema below the upper dermis layer, extending to subcutaneous tissue. Both conditions usually occur as part of an allergic reaction.

5. **H – Telangiectasia**. This is a dilatation of superficial blood vessels, becoming visible at the surface of the skin. These are present in many healthy individuals, but can be associated with several diseases (e.g. limited cutaneous form of systemic scleroderma 'CREST' syndrome: **c**alcinosis, **R**aynaud's syndrome, o**e**sophageal dysmotility, **s**clerodactyly and **t**elangiectasia).

Spider naevus is a telangiectatic arteriole of which the shape resembles a spider; there is a central feeding vessel and fine radiating vessels. Between 10% and 15% of healthy individuals will have spider naevi. The presence of more than five spider naevi in a superior vena caval distribution (especially at the upper trunk) and palmar erythema are signs of chronic liver disease. Spider naevi in chronic liver disease occur due to increased portal hypertension.

A   Dermatology A3 – Systemic cutaneous disorders I

1. **H – Pretibial myxoedema** (also known as 'thyroid dermopathy') occurs in 0.5%–4.5% of patients with Graves' disease, usually after about 2 years of the diagnosis of Graves' disease. It commonly affects hyperthyroid patients with high levels of long-acting thyroid stimulator. It is characterised by induration of the skin of the shins and, less often, the dorsum of feet bilaterally, due to the deposition of excessive amounts of mucopolysaccharide in the subcutaneous layer. The skin develops bilateral, asymmetrical erythematous or flesh-coloured waxy indurated plaques or nodules. Pretibial myxoedema usually has an inflammatory appearance that gradually subsides to develop the classic rough and indurated appearance. Unlike cellulitis, the skin is not warm or tender. Pretibial myxoedema may also present as a non-pitting oedema that resembles lymphoedema, resulting in elephantiasis. Diagnosis is made clinically in the presence of thyroid-stimulating hormone antibodies (present in 80% of patients) and other features of Graves' disease. Most patients with pretibial myxoedema also have Graves' ophthalmopathy. No treatment is required for mild pretibial myxoedema, but more advanced cases may benefit from topical or intralesional corticosteroids. Topical steroids are applied under a polythene occlusion dressing to hasten the treatment.

   Hint: Pretibial myxoedema, thyroid acropachy (triad of nail clubbing, swollen fingers and periosteal reaction), thyroid goitre, thyroid ophthalmopathy and raised thyroid-stimulating hormone receptor antibodies are characteristic findings of Graves' disease.

   Hint: Non-pitting oedema is due to lymphoedema or myxoedema. A pitting oedema is usually due to increased venous pressure or decreased oncotic pressure.

2. **I – Pyoderma gangrenosum** (PG). The appearance of the ulcer and the patient's past medical history of inflammatory bowel disease makes PG the most likely diagnosis in this patient. It is a condition of an inflammatory nature that is characterised by the histological presence of ulceration, vasculitis and necrosis. Typically, PG presents on the limbs and trunk and

only in 5% of cases does it present atypically in the head and neck area. PG is characterised by an inflamed pustule, nodule or blister that breaks down centrally to form a deep discharging ulcer with a honeycomb-like or cribiform base, and a characteristic purple-blue undermined rolled edge. The ulcer(s) is intensely painful and expands rapidly (up to 2 cm per day). The most common site is the legs. The pathogenesis of PG is unclear, but is unlikely to be bacterial. About 50% of cases are associated with systemic conditions. It may be one of the initial signs of diseases such as rheumatoid arthritis, Crohn's disease, ulcerative colitis, and some monoclonal gammopathies such as myeloma. A diagnosis of PG is made clinically, once other causes (e.g. vascular insufficiency, cutaneous infections) have been excluded. Biopsies do not show diagnostic features that are specific to this condition. However, a biopsy does help in excluding other conditions such as infections, vasculitis and malignancy. A diagnosis is reached upon the presenting condition meeting the two major criteria and at least two minor criteria listed in Table 7.

TABLE 7 Criteria for diagnosis of pyoderma gangrenosum*

Major criteria	1. Rapid[a] progression of a painful[b] necrolytic cutaneous ulcer[c] with an irregular, violaceous, and undermined border
	2. Exclusion of other causes of cutaneous ulceration
Minor criteria	1. History suggestive of pathergy[d] or clinical finding of cribriform scarring
	2. Systemic diseases associated with PG[e]
	3. Histopathologic findings (sterile dermal neutrophilia ± mixed inflammation ± lymphocytic vasculitis)
	4. Treatment response (rapid response to systemic glucocorticoid treatment)[f]

[a] Characteristic margin expansion of 1 to 2 cm/d, or a 50% increase in ulcer size within 1 month

[b] Pain is usually out of proportion to the size of the ulceration

[c] Typically preceded by a papule, pustule or bulla

[d] Ulcer development at sites of minor cutaneous injury

[e] Inflammatory bowel disease, polyarthritis, myelocytic leukemia or preleukemia

[f] Generally responds to a dosage of 1–2 mg/kg/d, with a 50% decrease in size within 1 month

Adapted from: Su WP, Davis MD, Weenig RH, Powell FC, Perry HO. Pyoderma gangrenosum: clinicopathologic correlation and proposed diagnostic criteria. *Int J Dermatol*. 2004 Nov; **43**(11): 790–800.

While PG is the most likely diagnosis in this patient, it is important to exclude peripheral vascular disease, as there are multiple cardiovascular risk factors. There is no gold standard treatment for PG. However, immunosuppression is the essence of treatment and clinicians use ciclosporin and corticosteroids to achieve that. Regarding topical treatment, topical corticosteroids are popular among clinicians in conjunction with some adjunctive therapy with triamcinolone injections. Most patients require more vigorous treatment, such as systemic corticosteroid treatment (e.g. oral prednisolone, starting with a high dose of 60–120 mg). If initial treatment with corticosteroids fails, other immunosuppressants such as ciclosporin can be used; patients show improvement in just 3 weeks at a dose of 3–5 mg.kg.day-1. Ciclosporin is used as an alternative because of some of the severe side effects such as hypertension and nephrotoxicity that ensue. Other immunosuppressive agents such as azathioprine and infliximab, an anti-tumour necrosis factor drug, have been used as well. Infliximab is highly specific for tumour necrosis factor-alpha and doesn't interfere with other factors such as tumour necrosis factor-beta, and has fewer side effects than other drugs of the same category. An initial dose of 5 mg.kg-1 is recommended followed by other immunosuppressive agents depending on the response. Rapid progression from this condition has been witnessed; hence the management of such condition is a matter of high urgency.

Hint: A diagnosis of PG should only be made once other causes (e.g. vascular insufficiency (when PG affects the lower limbs), cutaneous infections) have been excluded.

3. **D – Erythema multiforme** (EM). Mycoplasma pneumonia is a common cause of community-acquired pneumonia, particularly in young healthy patients. Mycoplasma pneumonia has a classically gradual onset, with preceding constitutional symptoms (e.g. headache, malaise, fever) being common. Patients usually also have a gradually worsening dry cough. Mycoplasma pneumonia is a common cause of EM. Other common causes of EM include herpes simplex virus infections (most common cause of EM) and drugs (particularly sulphonamides). As described by the patient in this scenario, the hallmark feature of EM is circular erythematous macules or papules with a purplish centre that expand peripherally and clear centrally, forming a concentric 'target lesion' (resembling a bull's eye). These target lesions are characteristically painful and are at variable stages of development (multiform). They occur most frequently on the palms,

back of hands, forearms and soles. Patients may also have oral ulcerations and crusted, bleeding lips. A commonly confused differential diagnosis is urticaria. Unlike urticaria, the lesions of EM last for more than 24 hours and are typically more purple than red. EM is usually self-limiting and resolves between 2 and 4 weeks. Mild cases require symptomatic relief (antihistamines) and more advanced cases may benefit from oral steroids; however, evidence is lacking on its efficacy. It is important to identify and treat the underlying cause; aciclovir may be used if the eruption is caused by herpes simplex virus. Stevens–Johnson syndrome (or 'erythema multiforme major') is a more severe and generalised form of erythema multiforme, in which patients have constitutional upset, fever and involvement of mucosal-lined tissues (e.g. eyes, genitals). The most common cause is drugs, particularly penicillins and sulphonamides drugs. Patients require hospitalisation and intensive input from multiple healthcare teams.

4. **B – Diabetic dermopathy** (or 'shin spots') is the most common cutaneous condition in diabetes associated with diabetic microangiopathy. It occurs in about 50% of patients with type 1 diabetes mellitus. It is not specific for diabetes, however. It manifests as multiple small, round, red-brownish papules that progress to hyperpigmented atrophic scars. They occur most frequently on the shins bilaterally. Diabetic dermopathy is associated with microvascular complications. There is no specific treatment, and the lesions resolve spontaneously. As with all diabetic complications, good control of blood glucose levels is imperative to reducing the risk of microvascular and macrovascular complications.

   Necrobiosis lipoidica is another dermatological condition that usually occurs on the shins and is strongly associated with diabetes mellitus. However, about 50% of patients with necrobiosis lipoidica are not diabetic. The condition presents as shiny and smooth, brown-yellow, oval plaques with an atrophic centre and well-circumscribed erythematous border. The plaques are smooth, well defined and telangiectatic. The associated skin atrophy allows the underlying small blood vessels to be visualised. They expand slowly and evolve into annular lesions. They are normally asymptomatic unless they ulcerate. Topical and intralesional steroids have shown disappointing results.

5. **C – Erythema ab igne** is a relatively common skin disorder. It has a very similar dermatological appearance to livedo reticularis, but differs in that it is caused by chronic infrared radiation such as local exposure to heat (e.g. hot water bottle use, heating pads or laptops), and is more red than

purple in colour. Erythema ab igne initially presents as localised blanching reticular erythema with occasional scaling which evolves with chronic heat exposure to become a reticulated non-blanching hyperpigmentation. It is less prevalent in the United States than northern Europe due to use of central heating in the United States. There is no definitive treatment for the condition, although eliminating heat exposure can reverse the condition in the early stages. It is imperative to mention that it is a premalignant skin change that may progress to squamous epithelial carcinoma. In contrast, livedo reticularis is net-like (reticular) pattern of purple-red skin discolouration due to sluggish venous blood flow in the superficial dermis. It may be physiological, typically occurring in the legs of young women in winter. It disappears on skin re-warming and limb elevation. Livedo reticularis can also occur secondary to hypercoagulable disorders (e.g. antiphospholipid syndrome), vasculitides, connective tissue diseases and cholesterol emboli. Diagnostic biopsies are important in livedo reticularis, and all patients should be screened for the aforementioned underlying disorders.

Hint: Erythema ab igne is caused by chronic exposure to heat, while physiological livedo reticularis is triggered by cold exposure.

A   **Dermatology A4 – Systemic cutaneous disorders II**

1. **A – Addison's disease**. This patient has both vitiligo (depigmented skin macules) and Hashimoto's hypothyroidism, both of which are autoimmune diseases. The most likely cause of her symptoms is therefore autoimmune adrenalitis. This is strongly associated with other autoimmune conditions, and is the most common cause (>80%) of primary adrenal failure. The resultant clinical features are due to autoimmune destruction of the entire adrenal cortex, causing reduced mineralocorticoid (aldosterone), glucocorticoid (cortisone) and sex hormone production. Less common causes of primary adrenal failure include infections (e.g. tuberculosis), haemorrhage, adrenal metastases and surgical adrenalectomy. The patient in this scenario has the typical insidious clinical features of Addison's disease (adrenal failure), which include progressive lethargy, muscle weakness/pain, hypotension, gastrointestinal symptoms (e.g. nausea, vomiting, abdominal pain, anorexia, weight loss), axillary/pubic hair loss, postural hypotention, depression, reduced libido (men) and amenorrhoea. About 60% of patients see two or more doctors before they are diagnosed with Addison's disease. Excess adrenocorticotropic hormone (ACTH) production causes hyperpigmentation of the skin in these patients, which is a

hallmark of Addison's disease. This occurs as ACTH shares the common precursor of pro-opiomelanocortin with the melanocyte-stimulating hormone. The similar structures of those two hormones cause ACTH to increase general melanin production in the skin. It is present in more than 90% of patients with Addison's disease, and often precedes other symptoms by a few months or even years. It is therefore an important sign to recognise. Hyperpigmentation is most marked but not limited to areas exposed to sunlight, skin creases, pressure points, axillae and buccal mucosa. Diagnosis of Addison's can be confirmed by the short synacthen test. Treatment with lifelong hydrocortisone and fludrocortisone should be started before the diagnosis is confirmed if there is strong clinical suspicion.

Vitiligo is a common acquired skin disorder in which areas of the skin become depigmented due to autoimmune destruction of melanocytes. It affects about 2% of people worldwide. The cause is not clear, but it is strongly associated with other autoimmune disorders (particularly thyroid disease, which is reported in up to 30% of patients) and a family history of vitiligo. It is also linked to pernicious anaemia, diabetes and hypoparathyroidism. Patients present with well-defined, smooth, depigmented macules or patches. The most common type of vitiligo is the generalised type, in which there are symmetrical depigmented macules that most frequently affect the back of hands, face and flexures. Some clinicians advocated the use of topical steroids and psoralen with ultraviolet A treatment; however, evidence is lacking. Many patients resort to using makeup to conceal the patches of vitiligo. It is important to avoid sun exposure or apply high SPF sunscreen to avoid the tanning of surrounding skin, which will make the vitiligo patches more apparent.

Hint: Suspect Addison's disease in patients with unexplained abdominal symptoms, especially if they have other autoimmune disorders.

2. **I – Sarcoidosis** is a chronic multisystemic granulomatous disorder of unknown aetiology. It is characterised by the development of non-caseating epithelioid granulomata. The lungs are most frequently affected (>90% of cases), followed by skin (up to 35%) and eyes (>20%). Many cases are asymptomatic and only detected incidentally on a chest X-ray (CXR). About a third of patients present with non-specific symptoms of constitutional upset (e.g. fatigue, fever, night sweats, malaise). Pulmonary involvement causes a dry cough, progressive dyspnoea and reduced exercise tolerance. Acute sarcoidosis is more common in whites, and typically

presents with erythema nodosum (described below) and polyarthralgia. The most common skin manifestation of sarcoidosis is maculopapular red-brown lesions, most frequently affecting the face. A less common but pathognomonic dermatological manifestation of sarcoidosis is lupus pernio, which are indurated violaceous plaques on the nose, cheeks, ears and fingers (areas exposed to cold). These lesions are associated with more severe pulmonary disease. The patient in this scenario has had attacks of uveitis, which occur in about 20% of sarcoidosis. Other common ocular manifestations of sarcoidosis include conjunctivitis and keratoconjunctivitis sicca. Patients suspected to have sarcoidosis should be carefully examined, have a CXR (bilateral hilar lymphadenopathy, lung infiltrates or fibrosis), respiratory function tests (showing a restrictive respiratory picture) and blood tests (looking for raised erythrocyte sedimentation rate, calcium and angiotensin converting enzyme levels). A CXR is abnormal in 90% of cases, and is important for the staging of sarcoidosis. The main differential diagnosis for this patient's clinical presentation is tuberculosis, which should be excluded.

Erythema nodusum is an autoimmune reaction causing the formation of tender subcutaneous nodules as a result of inflammation of the subcutaneous fat (panniculitis). The nodules most frequently occur on the shins but may occur on the forearms. It is more common in women (3–6:1), occurring most frequently between the second and fourth decades. Erythema nodosum can be caused by systemic conditions (e.g. sarcoidosis, inflammatory bowel disease) and infections (e.g. streptococci, tuberculosis), or less commonly by drugs (e.g. sulphonamides, oral contraceptive drugs, dapsone). In about a third of cases, no cause is found. The condition presents as tender red/blue subcutaneous nodule(s). These lesions are often bilateral, and usually resolve in 6–8 weeks. They change in colour from being red/purple to yellow/green, resembling healing bruises. Treatment is aimed at the underlying cause. All patients presenting with erythema nodosum should therefore be comprehensively assessed for an underlying cause, and treated accordingly. Patients may also require oral analgesia.

3. **H – Pancreatitis**. The most likely diagnosis in this patient is acute pancreatitis. Gallstones and alcohol excess account for most cases in the Western world. Patients typically present with severe upper or central abdominal pain, which may radiate to the back, requiring strong analgesia (e.g. pethidine, tramadol, buprenorphine). Sitting forward may alleviate the pain. Nausea and vomiting typically accompany the pain. Jaundice may

be present if the common bile duct is obstructed. Ecchymosis around the umbilicus (Cullen's sign) and in the flanks (Grey Turner's sign) are signs of severe necrotising pancreatitis. This indicates a poor prognosis and may require surgical intervention. It occurs due to subcutaneous tracking of peripancreatic exudate from the retroperitoneum. Cullen's sign less commonly occurs in ectopic pregnancy. Grey Turner's sign may also occur with a ruptured abdominal aortic aneurysm or severe abdominal trauma (e.g. road traffic accident). The patient's abdominal aorta feels normal on examination, and he has an elevated blood pressure, making the diagnosis of a ruptured abdominal aortic aneurysm unlikely. Hypoxaemia is a known feature of acute pancreatitis. In severe pancreatitis, bowel sounds may be absent due to paralytic ileus. The diagnosis of acute pancreatitis needs to be confirmed with serum amylase levels (typically four times normal), serum lipase (lipase is more sensitive and specific than amylase – amylase levels may be normal in severe pancreatitis especially if the patient presents late) and a contrast-enhanced spiral CT scan (to look for pancreatic necrosis). Management involves intravenous fluids, prophylactic antibiotics and parenteral nutrition, usually through a nasojejunal tube. Intravenous nutrition if paralytic ileus is confirmed. Severe acute pancreatitis (severity can be deduced using a severity score – in the United Kingdom the modified Glasgow criteria is commonly used. A score of 3 or more indicates severe pancreatitis) should be managed in a high dependency or intensive therapy unit. Investigation and treatment of the underlying cause, which in this case is likely to be gallstones, is fundamental to the management of this patient. Early endoscopic retrograde cholangiopancreatography with a sphincterotomy should be performed within 72 hours of onset of pain. The mortality rate is up to 30% in severe acute pancreatitis.

4. **E – Gastric cancer**. The patient's worsening abdominal pain with the axillary thickening and hyperpigmentation points to a possible diagnosis of gastric cancer. This cancer is known for its non-specific presentation, and is often diagnosed at an advanced stage. The incidence of gastric adenocarcinoma is about 20 per 100 000 population in the United Kingdom. Risk factors include *Helicobacter pylori* infection, smoking, pernicious anaemia, Type A blood group, lower socio-economic status and gastric polyps (associated with adenomatous polyps). Abdominal pain similar to peptic ulcer pain is the most common symptom in gastric cancer. Other symptoms that often present at an advanced stage of the disease include malaise, nausea, indigestion, dysphagia, loss of appetite and weight loss. On clinical examination, patients may have a palpable epigastric mass, a

palpable left supraclavicular lymph node (Virchow's node – referred to as Troisier's sign), acanthosis nigricans or periumbilical metastasis (Sister Mary Joseph nodule). These features are also found in advanced gastric cancer. Acanthosis nigricans presents as thickening and hyperpigmentation of the flexures (particularly axillae, posterior neck and groin skin), giving it a velvety appearance. Skin tags may also develop. The condition may occur in normal individuals. In children, acanthosis nigricans is associated with diabetes mellitus and obesity. In adults, it is associated with internal malignancies. The most common underlying malignancy in acanthosis nigricans is gastric adenocarcinoma (60%–70% of malignant acanthosis nigricans). The patient in this scenario should therefore be thoroughly investigated for an underlying malignancy. Investigations include an urgent gastroscopy, with biopsies of any gastric ulcers. Blood sugar levels should also be checked. This patient's blood pressure is elevated (164/92), but he does not have a background of hypertension. This may simply be due to the so-called 'white coat' effect. Under the new National Institute for Health and Clinical Excellence hypertension guidelines (2011), this patient should be offered ambulatory or home blood pressure monitoring to confirm the diagnosis of hypertension before antihypertensive drug treatment is initiated.

5. **F – Neurofibromatosis type 1** (NF 1). This patient presents with typical features of NF 1 (also called von Recklinghausen's disease), which accounts for 90% of cases of neurofibromatosis. The prevalence is 1 in 3000 births. NF 1 is an autosomal dominant disease caused by a mutation in the NF 1

TABLE 8 Diagnostic criteria for neurofibromatosis type 1 (NF 1)

Criterion
≥ Six café au lait or hyperpigmented macules (≥0.5 cm in prepubertal individuals or ≥1.5 cm in postpubertal individuals)
≥ Two neurofibromas or one plexiform neurofibroma
≥ Two Lisch nodules (iris hamartomas)
Optic glioma (tumour of optic pathway)
Axillary or inguinal freckling
Bony dysplasia (sphenoid wing dysplasia, bowing of long bone ± pseudarthrosis)
First-degree relative with NF1

Reference: Neurofibromatosis. Conference statement. National Institutes of Health Consensus Development Conference. *Arch Neurol.* 1988; **45**(5): 575–8.

gene on chromosome 17, resulting in skin, nervous system and skeletal lesions. A diagnosis of NF 1 is made if two or more of the criteria outlined in Table 8 are present.

NF 2 affects the central nervous system, and accounts for less than 10% of cases with a prevalence of 1 in 30,000–40,000 births. The gene mutation is on chromosome 22. The condition causes neural tumours. Bilateral acoustic neuromas are a hallmark of the condition.

A   Dermatology A5 – Dermatological disorders I

Eczema (also known as dermatitis) is an inflammation of the skin that presents as a red, scaly itchy rash, less severe and well demarcated than psoriasis. Eczema can be atopic (most common form), hypersensitive, or caused by irritants or venous stasis.

Atopic eczema (or atopic dermatitis) is a multifactorial (genetics, infection, allergens, diet) chronic inflammation of the skin. Atopic eczema affects about 15% of children, but two-thirds of these children grow out of it by puberty. More than 90% of children are affected before 5 years of age. There is a higher prevalence of asthma and hay fever in patients with eczema. Hanifin and Rajka developed the most commonly used diagnostic criteria for atopic eczema. The UK working party diagnostic criteria is a refined and more simplified version of these criteria. According to the UK criteria, atopic eczema is likely if the following criteria are fulfilled. Must have an itchy skin condition over the past 12 months, plus three or more of the following:

- past involvement of the skin creases, such as the bends of the elbows or behind the knees
- personal or immediate family history of asthma or hay fever
- tendency towards a generally dry skin
- flexural eczema (visible or from history)
- onset below the age of 2 years (this criterion should not be used in children aged under 4 years of age).

Patients present with flare-ups in which the skin becomes erythematous and oedematous, and may become blistered, crusted, and pustular in more severe cases. Scaling of the skin is seen in less acute lesions. Excoriations (scratch marks) are a common finding. Persistent scratching/rubbing of the skin because of itchiness can lead to lichenification (thickening of the skin with attenuation of normal skin markings) and hyperpigmentation. Scratching damages the skin, therby making it more susceptible to secondary bacterial infections, which is a common complication. Management involves symptoms control and not cure. Emollients are an important cornerstone of treatment, and should be used liberally on all skin areas (but particularly dry skin as this is more susceptible to irritation) on a daily basis (you cannot overdose!) to keep the skin moist. The best emollient is the one that the patient finds most suitable. It is also important to avoid contact with irritants (e.g. soaps or biological detergents). In severe disease greasy emollients are needed. Other techniques to minimise itching include wearing cotton clothing, avoiding temperature extremes, wet wrapping and tar-medicated bandaging. Topical corticosteroid therapy is the mainstay of treatment, and a short course (7–14 days) can control most mild to moderate eczema flare-ups. They are applied mainly in the form of ointments (usually for dry skin) and creams (moist skin). The use of varying potency steroid ointments depends on the severity of the lesion, the size and age. The general rule of thumb is that the eczematous skin is treated with the weakest steroid potency required to control the disease. Mild potency steroids should be used for the face. Unlike emollients, steroids should only be used on areas of skin affected by eczema. Parental education about the benefits and risks of steroids treatment is paramount (and a common clinical examinations station!), as a false perception of the risks of steroids can lead to steroid therapy not being used and preventable suffering for the patient. Most patients require short courses of topical steroids, which do not cause side effects in most patients. Topical antibiotics may be used in combination with emollients/steroids to prevent secondary skin infections, which can develop following skin damage caused by scratching. An established skin infection is treated with systemic antibiotics (e.g. flucloxacillin). Bandaging can help prevent scratching. Sedative antihistamines may be prescribed for use at night to minimise itching.

Contact dermatitis includes irritant contact dermatitis (80%) and allergic contact dermatitis (20% of cases). The former is due to skin irritation leading to inflammation (e.g. washing detergents), while the latter is due to a delayed hypersensitivity (type IV) reaction to a specific allergen (e.g. nickel in cheap jewellery). Contact dermatitis presents with itching, erythema, papules, plaques, vesicles and scaling. Irritant dermatitis mostly affects the hands causing erythema, weeping and possibly dry fissuring. The area of the body affected can give a clue to the irritant (e.g. make-up agent affecting the face). Nappy rash is a form of irritant dermatitis with a distinctive feature of sparing of the creases, as these areas are not in contact with the irritant. It is one of the most common dermatological disorders in children under 12 years of age, but it is also seen in incontinent adults. Management is by avoiding the irritants (in the case of nappy rash, this involves longer air exposure on changing nappies as well as more frequent nappy change), use of moisturisers and temporary use of a topical corticosteroid in more advanced cases. Systemic steroids may be required in severe cases. Patch testing is useful for cases in which the specific allergen is not clear.

Seborrhoeic dermatitis is a very common red, dry scaly rash that affects the scalp, eyebrows, nasolabial folds, cheeks, upper trunk and flexures. It is typically gradual in onset and has a symmetrical distribution. Unlike other forms of dermatitis, seborrhoeic dermatitis is characteristically non-itchy. Aetiology is unknown, but may be related to overgrowth of skin yeasts (*Malassezia furfur*). This can be very severe in HIV-positive patients. Treatment depends on the area affected and is aimed at symptom control, as cure is not yet possible. Along with application of moisturisers, the mainstay of treatment is with combined topical steroid/antifungal therapy and medicated shampoos (e.g. containing tar or ketoconazole).

Venous eczema is a cutaneous manifestation of venous hypertension resulting from local venous stasis. This occurs in conditions in which there is dysfunction of the valves in the veins (e.g. varicose veins), or mechanical obstruction (e.g. venous thrombus). Varicose veins are defined as dilated, tortuous superficial veins that result from high pressure due to incompetent valves. Excessive pooling of venous blood leads to oedema, itchiness and dermatitis. If not treated early, it can progress to haemosiderosis (brown pigmentation), lipodermatosclerosis (thickening and induration of skin) and ulceration (most commonly above the medial malleolus; 'gaiter area'). Venous insufficiency can be investigated with a colour duplex venous ultrasound scan. Treatment can be targeted to the dermatitis and/or to the veins themselves. Local emollients and steroid creams can be used for the dermatitis and the itchy symptoms. Management of the veins can be conservative (compression therapy – but make sure there is no co-existent arterial insufficiency first), or surgical (sclerotherapy, avulsion therapy, endovenous ablation).

Pompholyx eczema (also known as dyshidrotic eczema) affects people aged 20–40 years, it may be acute, chronic or recurrent, and its aetiology is unknown. Patients present with severe pruritus of the palms, sides of digits and soles, with sudden-onset vesicle eruption that may transform to bullae. It is known to be poorly responsive to treatment. Treatment options include potassium permanganate or aluminium subacetate soaks, topical corticosteroids and phototherapy (e.g. psoralen with ultraviolet A treatment).

Psoriasis is a common chronic hyperproliferative inflammatory skin disorder that affects 2% of people living in temperate zones, peaking in the 20s and 50s. It affects males and females equally. There are two pathologies (epidermal proliferation and inflammatory infiltration of the dermis and epidermis). There is a strong family history, as 30% of patients have a family member with psoriasis. Stress, infection, skin trauma, drugs, alcohol, obesity, smoking and climate all act as triggers to developing lesions. The most common type is psoriasis vulgaris (also known as chronic plaque psoriasis). Patients present with symmetrical, well-demarcated, salmon-pink plaques with silvery scaling on extensor surfaces of the elbows and knees, scalp and sacrum. Removing the scales results in tiny bleeding points. Flexures are frequently affected (flexural psoriasis) but they are not scaly. Psoriatic plaques may also appear in areas of trauma; this is known as Köbner's phenomenon. Nail changes are seen in 50% of patients and these include onycholysis (separation of the nail from the underlying nail bed), pitting, thickening and subungal hyperkeratosis. Guttate (or small plaque psoriasis) occurs most frequently in young patients with a preceding streptococcal infection. Numerous small, scaly papules or plaques appear acutely on the trunk and limbs. Palmoplantar pustulosis is another type of psoriasis in which well-demarcated erythema and scaling with yellow pustular lesions develop on hands and feet. It can be identical to keratoderma blennorrhagica. Erythroderma or generalised pustular psoriasis presents with widespread erythema and scaling. Clinical presentation is referred to as 'red man', as the erythema affects most of the body surface. Patients present with constitutional symptoms of rigors, lethargy and pyrexia. Erythroderma can be triggered by abrupt withdrawal from corticosteroids. There are five types of arthropathy that psoriasis can produce (7% of psoriatic patients develop seronegative arthropathies): monoarthritis, asymmetric oligoarthritis (most common type), psoriatic spondylitis, asymmetrical polyarthritis, arthritis mutilans and rheumatoid-like polyarthritis.

Initial management of psoriasis involves patient education, avoidance of triggers and topical therapy (emollients, vitamin D_3 analogues, steroids, tar, dithranol, salicylic acid), phototherapy (e.g. ultraviolet B). For more extensive or unresponsive disease, systemic therapy may be required. This includes systemic corticosteroids, biological immune-modulating agents (e.g. anti-tumour necrosis factor-alpha), other immunosuppressives (e.g. methotrexate), retinoids (e.g. acitretin) and psoralen with ultraviolet A treatment.

1. **C – Contact dermatitis**. As discussed earlier, nappy rash is a form of irritant dermatitis, which falls under the umbrella term of contact dermatitis. Candidiasis presents similarly but also affects the creases in the groin that are spared in contact dermatitis. *Candida* rash also has satellite lesions around the edges of the skin affected. Treatment of nappy rash is to keep the area as dry and clean as possible and possibly keeping the area exposed to warm, dry air for a few hours a day. Emollients are very useful in keeping the skin from getting too dry and cracking. In severe disease low dose steroid creams can be effective. In cases of candidiasis antifungals are prescribed.

2. **F – Keratoderma blennorrhagica**. This patient has reactive arthritis (previously known as Reiter's syndrome). It is classified as an autoimmune disease which develops secondary to an infection elsewhere. Commonly, by the time the patient presents with symptoms, the trigger infection has been self-eradicated. The classic triad constitutes arthritis, conjunctivitis and urethritis. Cutaneous lesions are associated with reactive arthritis: circinate balanitis and keratoderma blennorrhagica to name a few. Reactive arthritis is a type of seronegative arthropathy. The most common triggers are sexually transmitted chlamydial infections, and less common causative organisms are *Neisseria gonorrhea*, *Salmonella*, *Shigella* and *Campylobacter*. Reactive arthritis mostly affects males between the ages of 20 and 40 years. It is more prevalent in the Caucasian population owing to the high frequency of HLA-B27 gene (strong association with reactive arthritis) in the Caucasian population. Keratoderma blennorrhagica describes erythema and crusty, yellow-brown pustular lesions on the soles of the feet that are clinically and histologically indistinguishable from pustular psoriasis. It emerges in 15% of men with reactive arthritis. In this case the presence of the classic triad makes keratoderma more likely despite the fact that alone it is indistinguishable from psoriasis. Another differential is pompholyx eczema; however, this is more of an itchy, dry, scaly rash comprised of weeping vesicles. Treatment for keratoderma is to eradicate the underlying infectious cause (if still present) with appropriate antibiotics. Otherwise treatment is symptomatic with NSAIDs and corticosteroids.

3. **K – Venous eczema**. The patient in this example has obvious varicose veins with skin changes. The brown staining is haemosiderosis due to leaking proteins from the vessel into the skin. Treatment has been discussed in the eczema section above. The 'Revised Venous Clinical Severity Score' published by the American Venous Forum is a very useful guide to the signs of chronic venous insufficiency and how the severity can be graded.

4. **E – Guttate psoriasis**. Guttate or eruptive is a type of psoriasis that presents with small lesions over the trunk, arms and legs. It is frequently found in young adults. The most common trigger is an upper respiratory tract infection, particularly streptococcal. A few weeks later, lesions erupt, initially small and itchy; then in the weeks that follow these grow to around 1 inch in diameter, some of which coalesce to develop larger affected areas. Management is discussed above.

   Pityriasis rosea is a relatively common dermatological disorder (~0.75 per 100 dermatological patients). It classically presents in young adults (between 10 and 30 years of age), beginning with a single 2–10 cm oval pink plaque ('herald patch') most commonly on the trunk, followed by generalised body rash (1–2 weeks later) consisting of smaller lesions with overlying scales. It lasts for a total of about 6–8 weeks. Pruritis is not common. Similar to guttate psoriasis, there may be a preceding upper respiratory tract infection. Other differentials include secondary syphilis and tinea. No treatment is required, however symptomatic relief from itching may be necessary (antihistamines, steroids). Direct sunlight has proven to speed up remission. Both guttate psoriasis and pityriasis rosea are differential diagnoses in this case. Nevertheless, this patient's symptoms fit the classic presenation of guttate psoriasis better than pityriasis rosea as evidenced by the traditional silvery plaques, marked pruritis and the absence of a herald patch.

5. **D – Erythroderma**. Also known as exfoliative dermatitis or red man syndrome, this describes an inflammatory skin condition that affects 90% or more of the entire cutaneous surface with erythema and scaling. Thirty per cent of erythroderma is due to unknown causes (idiopathic), 10%–30% is drug-induced reaction, 15%–20% due to dermatitis, 15% due to lymphoma or leukaemia, and only 8% is due to psoriasis. Erythroderma presents as a sudden-onset pyrexia, lethargy and rigors quickly followed by burning sensation throughout the body with associated erythema, cutaneous oedema, pruritis and pustule formation (may coalesce). Generalised superficial lymphadenopathy is a common finding. Patients suffer various systemic complications, including heart failure, hyporthermia, dehydration, hypoalbunaemia and renal failure, among other disorders. In this case this patient has psoriasis and suddenly stopped his oral steroid therapy. Sudden withdrawal of steroids can lead to erythroderma. Patients with erythroderma should be admitted and nursed in a warm room. Treatment is aimed at the underlying cause, so in this case re-starting corticosteroids should alleviate the condition. Treatment also involves use of emollients,

wet compresses, antihistamines, topical steroids and antibiotics for secondary bacterial infections. The prognosis is poor.

A   Dermatology A6 – Management of autoimmune skin disorders

In order to comprehend the answers more thoroughly it is important to understand the following conditions.

Acne vulgaris: the pathogenesis of this disorder is not fully understood, but there is increased sebum production (stimulated by androgens), blockage of follicular ducts, bacterial colonisation of sebaceous follicles and inflammation. Patients present with non-inflammatory open (blackheads) and closed (whiteheads) comedones and inflammatory papules, pustules, nodules and cysts (which can lead to scarring) – these appear most commonly on the face, neck, chest and back. Classically, different lesions are present at the same time. The skin is greasy because of increased sebum production. Acne occurs in most teenagers and can lead to significant scarring in about 20% of patients. There is a strong genetic factor: if both parents had acne vulgaris, there is a 75% chance that their child will suffer from it; if one parent had acne then there is a 25% chance. What is inherited is the tendency for follicular epidermal hyperproliferation. This subsequently leads to the plugging of the follicle (formation of comedones, which are non-inflammatory lesions). Other exacerbating factors of acne include the presence of *Propionibacterium acnes* and excess sebum production. *P. acnes* is a normal commensal organism that flourishes in the anaerobic conditions of a plugged comedone. Inflammatory response to *P. acnes* creates these typical inflamed lesions of acne, which can progress into nodules, cysts and eventually scars. The treatment is as follows.

- *Mild acne*: main line of treatment for mild acne (e.g. comedones only) is topical therapies, such as topical benzoyl peroxide (commonly used keratolytic), antibiotics (e.g. clindamycin, erythromycin), topical sulphur and topical retinoids (e.g. isotretinoin) or retinoid-like agents (e.g. adapalene). Topical therapies can be tried separately or in combination (e.g. topical benzoyl peroxide and a topical antibiotic).
- *Moderate acne*: in the presence of multiple papulopustular lesions with or without some nodules, or when topical therapy has failed, oral antibiotics are tried, usually in combination with topical agents. Antibiotics should be continued for at least 4 months for their effect to be optimal. Commonly used antibiotics are oxytetracycline and minocycline. Erythromycin can be used in pregnant women and children under

12 years of age. Oral contraceptives containing antiandrogens, such as co-cyprindiol (Dianette) has proved to be useful.

- *Severe acne*: isotretinoin (retinoid – vitamin A analogue) is the drug of choice (20 weeks) in patients who have failed to respond to the aforementioned therapies, or those with severe nodulocystic acne. It is usually taken for 4–6 months and is effective in clearing acne in more than 90% of cases. Roaccutane must not be taken by pregnant women, as it is associated with teratogenicity and increases the risk of miscarriage. Pregnancy tests should therefore be done before, during and 5 weeks after treatment. Female patients should use contraception during treatment to avoid pregnancy and for 1 month after cessation of treatment. Patients should be informed about side effects of isotretinoin (e.g. dry eyes/mouth). Intralesional corticosteroids (e.g. triamcinolone) are also a treatment option for large nodules or cysts. All cases of severe acne should be managed by a dermatologist.

It is important to explain to patients that treatment for acne often takes several months to reach optimal effect, which is why treatment should not be stopped for at least 4 months after starting.

Rosacea (also known as acne rosacea) is the chronic relapsing and remitting disorder that most commonly affects the convex surfaces of the face in fair-skinned individuals with chronic flushing. It accounts for 1% of dermatological outpatient cases, and is most common in middle-aged women. Chronic flushing can be aggravated by alcohol, hot drinks, spicy food, sunburn and heat. On examination, patients will have fixed erythema on the chin, nose, cheeks and forehead; with associated telangiectasia, papules and pustules. Comedones are *not* seen in acne rosacea. Rhinophyma (soft tissue overgrowth of the nose) may occur in males. There is ocular involvement in about 50% of patients, such as blepharoconjunctivitis (most common) and rosacea keratitis. Conservative management involves avoiding sun exposure and activities in hot weather, using sunblock, avoiding skin irritants and limiting spicy foods, hot beverages and alcohol. Use of topical metronidazole (first line) or topical azelaic acid for 2–4 months is indicated in mild to moderate disease. If there is no response to therapy or in more advanced cases, oral tetracycline containing antibiotics can be tried for 4 months. It is common to use oral antibiotics in combination with topical therapy. Isotretinoin may be beneficial in unresponsive cases, but this should be started by a dermatologist.

Acne fulminans is a rare systemic disease also known as acne maligna, most commonly affecting males between the ages of 13 and 22 years with a history of acne. The process is believed to be triggered by *P. acnes*. High levels of testosterone and anabolic steroids increase sebum excretion and the population density of this bacteria species. This in turn may activate an immunological reaction leading to acne fulminans. Paradoxically, isotretinoin has been reported to cause acne fulminans. Patients would present with sudden-onset, severe, ulcerating nodulocystic acne with overhanging borders surrounding exudative necrotic plaques that become confluent. Lesions most commonly affect the face and back. The patient may also present with systemic symptoms such as pyrexia, malaise, myalgia and arthralgia, and they can have raised inflammatory markers. On examination, painful splenomegaly and erythema nodosum may be present. Antibiotics do not have any benefit in the treatment of acne fulminans, but it is important to take skin swabs to exclude secondary infections. The first-line treatment is high-dose systemic corticosteroids, which is weaned down over 6 weeks. Topical antiseptics can be used to prevent secondary infections. By the fourth week, isotretinoin is started. If isotretinoin is contraindicated, dapsone can be used as an alternative.

1. **I – Topical benzoyl peroxide**. This patient has mild acne vulgaris, as he presents with mainly comedones with a few pustules. Therefore, the treatment is with topical agents. Benzoyl peroxide is a commonly used topical therapy, but it can cause contact dermatitis, and bleaches clothing. Topical steroids are not used for the treatment of acne vulgaris.

2. **E – Oral doxycycline**. This patient has a classic history of acne rosacea, i.e fair skin, flushed, pustules but no comedones. The initial recommended treatment is with a topical antibiotic, usually metronidazole or azelaic acids. Alternatively, sulphur-containing topical therapy (e.g. sodium sulfacetamide) can be used, with or without sunblock. Topical corticosteroids make this condition worse. Some dermatologists prefer oral therapy as initial treatment as it is more effective. Oral tetracycline-containing antibiotics are the recommended oral therapy for rosacea, but erythromycin can be used in patients intolerant to tetracycline. It is important to explain to the patient that the aim of treatment is symptom control and that none of the treatment options available can cure the disease.

3. **F – Oral erythromycin**. This patient has moderate acne vulgaris and is pregnant. Topical agents have not helped at all; therefore, oral medication is indicated. Tetracycline is contraindicated in pregnancy, breastfeeding and children under the age of 12 years, as it can cause staining of the fetal

teeth and bones and can lead to skeletal abnormalities. Isotretinoin is teratogenic and also contraindicated. The oral contraceptive pill should not be used for obvious reasons. In these cases, erythromycin is indicated. Penicillin is non-fat soluble and is therefore of no use in the treatment of acne.

4. **D – Oral corticosteroids**. This is a case of acne fulminans. This 22-year-old has severe, sudden-onset, ulcerating acne. This autoimmune disease is treated with systemic steroids, not antibiotics. The patient should be admitted for treatment.

5. **C – Oral contraceptive pill**. This patient has moderate acne and has tried topical agents as well as oral antibiotics. The next possible options are Roaccutane (isotretinoin) and the oral contraceptive pill, both of which can only be taken if the patient has no intention to become pregnant. Although the patient has read about Roaccutane (isotretinoin) and does not want to start it, it is important for the specialist to ensure accurate understanding and dispel any myths so that the patient is able to make a fully informed decision. The oral contraceptive pill can be used if the patient is not planning to become pregnant. The oral contraceptive pill has been shown to be of benefit in patients with acne and should be taken for at least 6 months before the response to treatment is fully assessed.

A **Dermatology A7 – Manifestations of sexually transmitted diseases**

1. *J – Treponema pallidum*. This patient is suffering from secondary syphilis. Syphilis is a chronic systemic disease caused by the spirochaete *T. pallidum* with an incubation period of 9–90 days. It can be transmitted via multiple routes; the most important being through sexual intercourse. It can also be transmitted via blood transfusions, in utero and via direct contact with breaks in the skin. The incidence of syphilis has been increasing in the past decade, particularly in men who have sexual intercourse with men. The skin is affected in all stages of syphilis. Table 9 summarises the cutaneous and systemic features of syphilis. Diagnosis can be confirmed by dark-field microscopy of the cutaneous lesions or serological tests. The latter include *T. Pallidum* antibodies, *T. Pallidum* haemagglutination assay, rapid plasma regain, Wassermann's reaction and Venereal Disease Research Laboratory slide test. Treatment of choice is with penicillin (treatment lasts for 1 month). Doxycycline, erythromycin or tetracycline are alternatives for patients with a penicillin allergy. Of note, the Jarisch–Herxheimer reaction

is a recognised reaction that occurs after the initial dose of antibiotics; here the patient becomes febrile, tachycardic and hypotensive. The reaction is most commonly associated with individuals with secondary disease. A careful history must be taken as contact tracing is of great importance in limiting the spread of disease.

TABLE 9 Staging of syphilis

Stage of syphilis	Clinical features
Primary	Hard, painless and ulcerated button-like lesion, often in genital area
	Approximately 1 cm in diameter, appearing on average 3 weeks after sexual contact and healing spontaneously within 3 weeks
	Accompanied by painless regional lymphadenopathy
	Depressed atrophic scar once healed
Secondary	Non-itchy, symmetric red/brown maculopapular rash on face, trunk, palms and soles of feet
	Presents 1–2 months after the chancre (painless ulceration found in primary syphilis), settles within 1–3 months
	Accompanied by generalised lymphadenopathy
	Condyloma lata (moist papules in ano-genital area) may occur
	Non-skin features: headache, low-grade fever, malaise, sore throat, arthralgia, hepatitis, meningism, uveitis
Tertiary (late)	Occurs more than 2 years after the initial presentation
	Circinate arrangement of skin nodules
	Gumma: painless rubbery nodules that ulcerate and scar (commonly occur in skin, bones, lungs and testes)
Quaternary	Cardiovascular manifestations in the form of aortic regurgitation, aortitis and aortic aneurysms
	Neurosyphilis (meningovascular disease, cranial nerve palsies, tabes dorsalis, general paralysis of the insane, Argyll Robertson pupil)

2. **G – Human immunodeficiency virus** (HIV). Oral hairy leukoplakia is more likely to occur in HIV patients than non-HIV patients. The condition occurs due to Epstein–Barr virus infection of the mucosa in immunodeficient patients. It is characterised by white hairy plaques with vertical ridging that occur on the lateral edges of the tongue. These lesions cannot be peeled off, unlike the lesions of oral candidiasis, which can be peeled off to reveal underlying raw areas. Diagnosis is clinical, and treatment is with systemic aciclovir. HIV should be excluded in all patients.

AIDS should be considered in patients with atypical, refractory severe or frequently relapsing skin diseases. Other dermatological conditions occurring in HIV disease include thrush, molluscum contagiosum, herpes simplex virus infection, herpes varicella zoster infection, scabies, seborrhoeic dermatitis, itchy folliculitis, cryptococcosis and Kaposi's sarcoma. The latter is the most common malignancy in HIV disease, occurring most frequently in homosexuals. It manifests as non-blanching purple lesions that most commonly affect the head and neck and lower limbs. It is important to measure the CD4+ count and plasma HIV viral load if Kaposi's sarcoma is suspected. Treatment is with surgical excision, cryotherapy, radiotherapy or chemotherapy.

3. **F – Herpes simplex virus type 2** (HSV-2). HSV infection of the genitals is usually caused by sexually transmitted HSV-2, although HSV type 1 transmitted via orogenital contact can be the cause and is now overtaking HSV-2. Genital infection with HSV-2 is characterised by erythematous vesicles that rapidly rupture to form multiple painful genital or perianal ulcers that usually heal in 3 weeks. These ulcers are round in shape and have a red areola. Patients also complain of genital pain, itching, urethral discharge, burning or dysuria. Urinary retention may occur. HSV infection may affect body systems other than the genitourinary system, and a comprehensive history and examination is therefore essential. EBV is an important differential. Swabs can be taken in a viral culture medium if the diagnosis is in doubt. Standard treatment is with oral valaciclovir or famciclovir, as well as oral and topcical (lidocaine gel) analgesia for the genital pain. HSV infection may be recurrent, and often affects the same area on recurrence. Patients can be reassured that recurring attacks are usually shorter, less painful and occur less frequently with time. Patients should be prescribed topical antiviral to apply at first signs of recurrence. Long-term antiviral prophylaxis may be needed in some patients to prevent recurrence.

4. **H – Human papilloma virus** (HPV). Genital warts (or condyloma acuminatum) is caused by infection with HPV, and is the most common viral sexually transmitted infection in the developed world. It affects females more frequently than males (1.4:1), and is most common in the 15–25-year age group. Genital warts affect infected individuals after several months of inoculation, and appear as pink/brown papillomatous lesions on the genitalia, perineum, anus, cervix or rectum. They may coalesce to form larger cauliflower-like lesions, which are characteristic in appearance. Diagnosis

is usually clinical. It is important to differentiate these lesions from condylomata lata (secondary syphilis). The acetic acid test or histopathology is used for diagnosis of suspicious cases. Genital warts can be caused by about 40 different subtypes of HPV, of which subtypes 16, 18 and 33 are most strongly associated with cervical and anal cancer. Infected females therefore need regular cervical screening. Patients should be referred to a genitourinary medicine specialist for screening of other sexually transmitted infections and tracing of sexual contacts. In children, it is important to bear in mind that anogenital warts can be transmitted by both sexual abuse and non-sexual contact. Treatment options for anogenital warts include imiquimod cream, cryotherapy, trichloracetic acid or podophylline paint. Both partners need treatment.

HPV vaccines have been introduced to protect against infection with genital warts and reduce the incidence of cervical cancer. Since September 2008, girls aged between 12 and 13 years have been offered the HPV vaccine in the United Kingdom, which is given in the form of three injections over a period of 6 months. In the United States, girls aged 11–12 years are offered the vaccine. Ideally, all three doses should be taken before any sexual activity. Young women aged 14–17 years in the United Kingdom and 13–26 years in the United States are also offered the vaccine if they did not receive it at a younger age. The vaccine is also approved for males aged 9–15 years in the United Kingdom and 9–26 years in the United States for prevention of genital warts and anal cancer.

Hint: Do not confuse condyloma acuminata, which is anogenital warts, with condyloma lata, seen in syphilis.

5. **I – *Neisseria gonorrhoea*.** Sexually transmitted gonococcal infection is the second most common sexually transmitted infection in the United Kingdom. It is caused by the Gram-negative diplococcus *N. gonorrhoeae* with an incubation period of 2–10 days. It may affect the columnar epithelium in the rectum, conjunctive, urethra, pharynx and cervix. The infection may disseminate and affect joints, causing a gonococcal arthritis. This is most common in young women. It presents as a localised septic arthritis, or more commonly an arthritis–dermatitis syndrome. The latter classically presents as a mild migratory polyarthritis, dermatitis and tenosynovitis. The skin lesions are grey-red vesicopustules that usually affect the hands and/or feet. Patients may have a fever, and the inflammatory markers are raised in most cases. The diagnosis can be confirmed by culturing of Gram-negative diplococci from the blood or joint aspirate. Complications

can be local (e.g. epididymitis, bartholinitis, prostatitis, salpingitis, cystitis) and systemic (septicaemia and reactive arthritis). Parenteral cephalosporins (e.g. ceftriaxone) are the treatment of choice. It is important to treat a co-infection with chlamydia (usually with a 1-week course of doxycycline or a single dose of azithromycin), which is not uncommon. Contact tracing is an important aspect of management of this sexually transmitted infection.

Chlamydia infection is the most common cause of reactive arthritis, commonly called chlamydia-induced reactive arthritis. It is important to know the skin features of chlamydial disease, as chlamydia trachomatis is the most common cause of sexually transmitted infections in the developed world.

Reactive arthritis is a sterile arthritis that is thought to be due to cross-reaction with bacterial antigens. It most commonly affects young men. The condition typically occurs as an oligoarthritis with malaise and fever 2–4 weeks post urethritis (chlamydia or ureaplasma) or dysentery (*Campylobacter*, *Salmonella*, *Shigella* or *Yersinia*). It also commonly causes conjunctivitis, keratoderma blennorrhagica (brown, raised plaques on palms and soles), circinate balanitis (superficial penile ulceration), enthesitis (plantar fasciitis, Achilles tendonitis). Reiter's syndrome is a triad of urethritis, conjunctivitis and arthritis. Inflammatory markers are usually raised, and joint aspirate reveals a sterile neutrophilia. Active infections with the causative organism are treated with antibiotics. Anti-inflammatory agents or local steroids injections are of benefit for the acute and/or chronic inflammation. The term 'Reiter's' is no longer used, because of Reiter's Nazi membership and involvement in criminal Nazi activities during World War II.

Chlamydia trachomatis types LGV 1, 2 and 3 can cause lymphogranuloma venereum. It is characterised by infection in the lymphatic system/ lymph nodes. The disease is endemic in tropical areas, but outbreaks have occurred in Europe and the United States predominantly in men having sex with men. The primary lesion is a small painless ulcerating papule on the genitalia, manifesting 1–3 weeks after exposure. The primary lesion is transient, healing rapidly. About 2–6 weeks later, patients develop a tender inguinal lymphadenopathy, which is usually unilateral. Multiple draining sinuses and abscesses (buboes) may also develop. An infection of the rectal mucosa may lead to an acute ulcerative proctitis. The chronic inflammatory reaction can lead to rectal strictures, genital lymphedema and genital/ano-rectal fistulas. Treatment with doxycycline is important early in the course of the disease to prevent progression to the chronic phase (it is continued until all lesions have started to heal). Azithromycin or erythromycin are alternatives. Syphilis and genital herpes must be excluded in all patients. Contact tracing is an important aspect of management.

Chancroid is a sexually transmitted infection caused by the Gram-negative bacteria **Haemophilus ducreyi**, with an incubation period of 1 day to 2 weeks. It is characterised by painful ano-genital ulceration and tender suppurative inguinal adenitis progressing to bubo (swelling of lymph nodes) formation. The following US Centers for Disease Control and Prevention criteria for the probable diagnosis of chancroid is a useful method of learning the diagnostic features of this disease.

- The patient has one or more painful genital ulcers.
- The patient has no evidence of **T. pallidum** infection by darkfield examination of ulcer exudate or by a serologic test for syphilis performed at least 7 days after onset of ulcers.
- The clinical presentation, appearance of genital ulcers and, if present, regional lymphadenopathy are typical for chancroid.
- A test for HSV performed on the ulcer exudate is negative.

All of these criteria have to be met for a probable diagnosis of chancroid to be made. The World Health Organization recommends a 7-day course of high-dose erythromycin for the treatment of chancroid. Other treatments include azithromycin, ceftriaxone or ciprofloxacin.

A   Dermatology A8 – Cutaneous ulcers

1. **E – Marjolin's ulcer**. This type of a cutaneous ulcer is a subtype of squamous cell carcinoma. It is an aggressive variant that arises from areas of skin that have been subject to trauma, burns, scar tissue, chronic inflammation or radiotherapy. Furthermore, they may even arise from longstanding venous ulcers. A Marjolin's ulcer grows slowly and is characterised by being painless. Wide local excision is the treatment of choice.

2. **I – Pyoderma gangrenosum** (PG). This condition is explained in detail in Question 3 (Dermatology section).

3. **J – Venous ulcer**. The ulcer in the scenario described is characteristic of a venous ulcer. The area affected is commonly known as the gaiter region – distal medial third of leg down to lower border of medial malleoli. Venous ulcers are more common in women. Deep vein thrombosis, varicose veins and obesity are known predisposing factors. There is often a histroy of minor local trauma. Venous ulcers are usually shallow and large and

characteristically painless with a 'sloping' edge. Furthermore, associated symptoms present in this patient, such as brown discolouration (hemosiderin deposition) and oedema, should further support the diagnosis of a venous ulcer. Other associated signs include eczema and lipodermatosclerosis (fibrosis of skin causing firm induration). Thickening of the skin along with proximal oedema, lead to the commonly mentioned inverted champagne bottle appearance. Medical therapy consists of treating the underlying chronic venous insufficiency, with complete healing of a venous ulcer often taking several months. Various dressing with active agents delivering growth factors have been proven to be of objective benefit in speeding up healing. Compression bandaging can be used if co-existing arterial insufficiency has been excluded. Topically applied growth factors and the use of lower-molecular-weight heparin are also evidence-based management options. Surgical therapy aims to revascularise the affected region and ligate incompetent perforators. Furthermore, debridement and coverage with skin grafts and local flaps is a viable treatment option. Amputation is also used as a last resort in patients with chronic ulcers refractive to conventional treatment.

Hint: Always biopy suspicious or treatment-resistant ulcers to exclude malignancy. Swabs are an important step in management to exclude co-existing infections.

4. **F – Necrobiosis lipoidica** (NL). The description of the lesion in this scenario is typical of NL. The history of diabetes as well should trigger your thinking of NL. It typically starts as a small red lesion that slowly grows and becomes waxy in appearance with a yellow or reddish brown colour. The exact aetiology of NL is not known, but because of its strong association with diabetes, theories have postulated that the disorder follows a similar pathophysiological mechanism as diabetic microvascular changes. Glycoprotein deposits abnormally in diabetic microvascular disorders and that is also seen in subcutaneous tissue of affected areas. NL usually appears on the pretibial area but may also occur in other parts of the body. Despite its association with diabetes, only a small percentage (<2%) of diabetics have NL lesions. Surgical excision and laser therapy can treat the affected area, however this doesn't treat the cause and they may re-appear.

5. **A – Arterial ulcer**. The painful nature of the ulcer makes it more likely a result of arterial insufficiency rather than diabetic nephropathy. The latter are characteristically painless. Arterial ulcers can result from both a

chronic (atherosclerosis) or acute (arterial emboli) process. They are usually located on the dorsum of the toes, foot and mid-chin. They are much less common than venous ulcers, and are commonly associated with an underlying systemic disease (e.g. diabetes mellitus, vasculitis). Smoking is a strong risk factor for arterial disease. In contrast to venous ulcers they are exquisitely painful (disproportional to size of ulcer), deep and have punched-out, sharply defined edges. Patients usually suffer from other features of arterial disease including hair loss, cold peripheries, toenail damage, absent or weak peripheral pulses and cyanosis. The base of the ulcer usually contains granular tissue. It is important to measure the ankle brachial pressure index of all patients with suspected arterial ulceration. An ankle brachial pressure index of 0.8 or below is indicative of arterial insufficiency and patients must not have compression bandaging. Further investigations include arterial Doppler scans of the legs, CT/MR angiograms and conventional angiography. Treatment of such ulcers is similar to venous ulcers – dressings, revascularisation and debridement with skin coverage.

Hint: Be aware of the signs and symptoms of acute arterial insufficiency, summarised by the 6 Ps: pallor, pain, pulseless, paraesthesia, perishingly cold, paralysis. Don't forget to measure to the capillary refill time!

Neuropathic ulcers are found in patients with longstanding diabetes mellitus, and are the result of diabetic neuropathy. Patients most commonly have a loss of sensation in a stocking and glove distribution (peripheral neuropathy) and may have other types of neuropathies (e.g. autonomic neuropathy). The American Diabetes Association recommendations in 2012 include that all diabetic patients should have an annual examination of: (1) pinprick sensation, (2) vibration perception (128 Hz tuning fork), (3) 10 g monofilament pressure sensation, (4) ankle reflexes and (5) signs (history and examination) of autonomic neuropathy.

A   Dermatology A9 – Cutaneous lesions I

1. **E – Kaposi's sarcoma** (KS). The description of the lesion in the scenario is characteristic of KS. Moreover, the patient's HIV status makes the diagnosis of KS even more likely. Lesions are typically erythematous/violaceous papules or macules, occurring most frequently in lower limbs, head and neck, genitalia and oral mucosa. Over time the lesions become firm, with a dark purple discolouration, and may coalesce to form large plaques.

Sometimes the lesions ulcerate and become nodular. Infections with HIV and human herpesvirus 8 have been implicated as causes for the development of KS. Other factors such as iatrogenic immunosuppression play a role. Further investigations of patients presenting with KS is essential. If the HIV status is unknown it is imperative to offer testing. Furthermore, in known patients with HIV it is essential to measure CD4 counts and HIV viral-load. Patients should also be screened for pulmonary involvement of KS using plain film radiographs and the use of gallium or thallium scans. Definitive tissue diagnosis should be obtained by a punch biopsy. In patients with HIV-related KS, optimal treatment of HIV with HAART (highly active anti-retroviral therapy) is the mainstay of treatment. The use of HAART has markedly reduced the incidence of KS. Treatment is with surgical excision, cryotherapy, radiotherapy or chemotherapy.

2. **I – Subcutaneous lipoma** (SL). Lipomas are the most common benign tumour of soft-tissue origin. They are soft, rubbery and mobile tumours of subcutaneous mature fat cells, usually appearing on the lower extremities and the back. Lipomas can also be found in the gastrointestinal tract, spermatic cord, thorax and in gynaecological adnexa. The main differential for a SL is a sebaceous cyst or abscess. However a SL differs from the former by the absence of a punctum and by the latter by the absence of signs of local inflammation. Cystic lumps transilluminate when illuminated from the side with a pentorch. An SL can be acquired or congenital, single or multiple (multiple lipomatosis – hereditary condition in which individuals develop multiple lipomas). Most SLs are asymptomatic; however, symptoms may manifest secondary to local compression (e.g. dyspnoea secondary to tracheal compression from intrathoracic lipomas). SLs do not require further investigation; however, more complicated lipomas in the thorax and abdomen may require CT scanning, MRI scans or ultrasounds to determine the extent of involvement of local structures and to provide much needed information for pre-operative planning. Treatment of SL involves surgical excision for cosmetic or functional reasons, or if there is diagnostic doubt. Excised lesions must be sent for histology to exclude other diagnoses.

3. **H – Seborrhoeic keratosis** (SK). These cutaneous lesions are benign epidermal tumours of unknown cause, and are extremely common in the elderly. They are also known as seborrhoeic warts or basal cell papillomas. SK affects males and females equally. They are often described as 'stuck on' papules, with a greasy scaling on the surface. They have

well-defined borders and are either flat or more often raised above surrounding skin resembling a patch. They are most often multiple, and are seen most frequently on the face, neck and trunk. The colour of SKs is usually uniform, and may vary from pale to deeply pigmented, and they are often 0.5–3 cm in diameter. Patients usually present when lesions itch, bleed, become aesthetically unpleasant or catch on clothing. Traumatised lesions look inflamed and may bleed or have overlying crusting. Diagnosis of SK is made clinically, but sometimes it is difficult to differentiate dark or traumatised lesions from more sinister differential diagnoses such as a melanoma. Straightforward cases of SK do not need to be treated, as the tumour is common and benign. Cryotherapy, curettage, shave biopsies and surgical excision can be used to remove an SK.

4. **A – Campbell De Morgan spots**. These were named after a British surgeon, Campbell Greig De Morgan, and are sometimes also referred to as cherry angiomas or capillary haemangiomas. They are small bright-red papules that are 1–5 mm in diameter and occur in more than 50% of adults, most frequently occurring in the trunk. They arise from surface capillaries that cluster and form a papule. The lesions are benign. Treatment is therefore reserved for cosmetic reasons and includes cryotherapy or laser ablation.

5. **D – Hidradenitis suppurativa** (HS). The scenario in this question typically describes a case of HS, otherwise known as acne inversa. HS is a chronic condition that is thought to occur when apocrine glands associated with eccrine glands are blocked and unable to drain normally, leading to severe inflammation. Individuals with HS sometimes have an inherent abnormality in the normal development of the glands. Blockage of normal secretion leads to the accumulation of bacteria and subsequent infection. HS affects areas of the body with abundant apocrine glands – namely, in the groin, axilla, areola, peri-anal and peri-umbilical regions. The condition is more common in females, affecting up to 4% of women. The axilla is more commonly affected in females, while the groin and perianal regions are more affected in men. HS present as recurrent tender nodules or 'boils' in the aforementioned regions. They can often be multiple and may discharge. Patients may be misdiagnosed with furunculosis, which is an acute pustular infection of a hair follicle and its surrounding tissues (i.e. deeper infection than folliculitis) usually with *Staphylococcus aureus*. A useful diagnostic sign of HS is the presence of open comedones (blackheads) in the affected skin, as is the case in this scenario. Conservative treatment in the form of dietary changes, weight loss and using warm baths are

recommended for asymptomatic lesions. Incision and drainage is required for large lesions that are painful, but this may lead to dissecting tunnels and fistulas between lesions. Broad-spectrum antibiotics are required if there is cellulitis. Chronic lesions can be treated with more extensive surgery. Here a surgeon will look for evidence of sinus tract formation. Wide surgical excision is employed for larger lesions that have recurred. Split thickness grafts can be used for covering the defect left after excision.

Hint: A useful diagnostic sign of HS is the presence of open comedones (black-heads) in the affected skin.

A **dermatofibroma** is one of the most common benign skin tumours. They are asymptomatic, solitary, brown-red dermal nodules, usually up to 1 cm in diameter. They are most common in young adults, appearing on the extremities in 80% of cases. The tumour is firm and 'dimples' if pinched from both lateral sides. This is known as the 'buttonhole sign'. No treatment is required, but diagnostic doubt necessates excision and histological examination.

Telangiectasia are small, dilated blood vessels at the surface of the skin.

A   Dermatology A10 – Cutaneous lesions II

1. **D – Basal cell carcinoma** (BCC) is the most common malignant skin tumour affecting humans, accounting for 80% of all skin cancers. The estimated lifetime risk is 28% in Caucasians. BCCs are sometimes referred to as rodent ulcers. The most common sites are the head and neck (especially the nose) and the trunk. The description in this scenario is characteristic of BCCs. Typically the lesions have a pearly texture, rolled edges and associated telangiectasia. Because of the absence of an epidermis in a BCC, surface breakdown leads to the formation of a central ulcer. The risk of metastasis is around 0.5%; however, urgent intervention is essential, as BCCs can grow rapidly and erode adjacent structures.
   - Nodular: most common form of BCC. Some appear cystic and are described as cystic nodular BCCs.
   - Superficial: least aggressive form. Appears like a scaly patch similar to eczema or a psoriatic patch. They are differentiated from the more benign differentials by their increasing size and the fact that they are not usually itchy.
   - Pigmented: characteristic features of a BCC with associated pigmentation due to the presence of melanocytes.

- Morphoeic/sclerosing: the most aggressive form of BCC. Superficial in appearance and resembles an atrophic scar. The loss of boundaries to this subtype of BCC makes surgical excision more difficult with higher chances of local recurrence because of inadequate excision margins.

Risk factors include fair skin, increasing age, intense ultraviolet radiations exposure, family history of BCC, personal history of BCC, radiation and immunosuppression. The aim of treatment is complete removal. If the lesion is small, an excision biopsy is carried out and the histological sub-type and the extent of the clear margins are described. If a lesion is large, a shave biopsy could be performed to determine the histological subtype. Recurrent or aggressive lesions are best excised using Mohs micrographic surgery. Some clinicians advocate the use of a punch biopsy if a lesion has features resembling those of a malignant melanoma, in order to obtain a deep biopsy.

2. **B – 4mm**. A 4mm excision margin is recommended for lesions <2 cm in diameter. Various studies have shown that this margin will achieve more than 95% cure rates. Larger lesions will require more extensive margins and the use of various reconstructive skills. If a lesion is small, direct clos-ure after excision is possible. However, larger excisions may require the use of full-thickness skin grafts, split-thickness skin grafts for coverage or the use of local flap techniques to cover the lesion. There are various other methods to treat a BCC; the following is an outline:
   - Curettage plus or minus electrodesiccation – reserved for superficial BCC .
   - Curettage plus laser ablation – effective for nodular and superficial BCC.
   - Mohs micrographic surgery – BCCs without defined borders (mor-phoeic BCC) will benefit from this specialised technique. The procedure entails removing the lesion and a small perimeter of normal appearing tissue. The sample is then immediately examined under the microscope using frozen sections. Further excision is carried out if the close inspec-tion reveals evidence of insufficient clear margins. Such technique yields the lowest recurrence rates.

3. **G – Lentigo malignant melanoma**. Malignant melanoma (MM) is an invasive malignancy arising from melanocytes. It accounts for only 5% of cutaneous cancers; however, it is responsible for 75% of skin cancer-related deaths. The incidence of MM has increased dramatically

worldwide, particularly in the developing world. Risk factors for developing an MM include ultraviolet radiation exposure (particularly short spells of intense exposure in childhood), fair skin, female gender, family history (10%–20% of cases), personal history, increasing age and congenital disorders (e.g. xeroderma pigmentosum). It is believed that around half of MMs arise from pre-existing moles. A useful guide for monitoring suspicious moles is the use of the 'ABCDEF' approach.

- **A**symmetry: this can be assessed by looking at two halves of the mole and seeing if an asymmetry in shape exists.
- **B**order: irregular outlines are suspicious of an MM.
- **C**olour: heterogeneous colouration of a mole may indicate an MM and warrants further investigation.
- **D**iameter: Moles >6mm are more likely to be MM.
- **E**volution: this refers to a changing mole in any aspect (size, prominence, itchiness, bleeding). Although many moles grow in childhood and adolescence, growth in an individual over the age of 30 warrants further investigations.
- **F**unny-looking: a mole or naevi that looks different from the others; the 'ugly duckling' sign.

The lesion in this question is a lentigo malignant melanoma. The following summarises the major forms of MM.

- Superficial spreading melanoma: this is the most common subtype of MM in Caucasians (~70%). As the name suggests, the malignant cells spread in the epidermis (slowly enlarging pigmented plaques) and invasion occurs at a later stage. It is most common on the legs in women and the trunk in men.
- Nodular melanoma: this subtype accounts for 10%–15% of MMs. This subtype has a male preponderance and usually affects individuals in their fifth to sixth decades. The lesion appears as a dark nodule. It has a poor prognosis, as vertical growth of the lesion occurs from the start of the malignancy.
- Lentigo malignant melanoma: this malignancy develops from a lentigo maligna (pre-malignant lesion – melanoma in situ). It usually occurs in elderly patients, most commonly affecting the face. A lentigo maligna is usually present for years before a malignant change occurs.
- Acral melanoma: this subtype affects the palms and soles of individuals. It is also used to describe MMs that affect the nail bed. It is more common (35%–75% of MMs) in dark-skinned individuals.

- Amelanotic melanoma: this refers to MMs that lose their ability to produce melanin secondary to dysplastic changes in the cells and poor differentiation of cells.

It is important to clinically exclude other MM lesions – 'in transit' or 'satellite' lesions – and other signs/symptoms of regional or distant metastasis. In-transit lesions are skin or subcutaneous metastases >2 cm from the primary lesion, while satellite lesions are within 2 cm of the primary lesion. The most important prognostic determinant of the primary MM is Breslow's thickness. It is measured vertically, in millimetres, from the top of the granular layer to the deepest extension of the tumour, using an ocular micrometer. Ulceration of an MM is the second most important prognostic sign, indicating a poor prognosis. The mainstay of treatment of MMs is wide local excision with sentinel lymph node biopsy or lymph node dissection. Wide local excision is performed with a 1 cm margin in tumours ≤1 mm deep, and with a 2–3 cm margin in tumours 1–4 mm in depth.

4. **I – Squamous cell carcinoma** (SCC) is the second most common type of skin cancer in Caucasians. The major known risk factor for SCC is ultraviolet radiation exposure. In addition to the risk factors associated with BCC, human papilloma virus infection plays a role in the development of SCC. This is particularly the case in immunosuppressed patients. Furthermore, tobacco use has also been associated with SCC. SCCs are most common in the elderly, occurring most frequently in the head and neck. Patients usually present with an ulcerating, flesh-coloured to pink lesion with an indurated edge that is rapidly growing and hyperkeratotic. They are often covered by a plaque and may sometimes have a cutaneous horn. An SCC can also arise from pre-existing scars or chronic wounds and is termed a Marjolin's ulcer. Examination of local lymph nodes is important to assess the extent of the carcinoma and if metastasis is suspected. There is a role for CT scanning and MRI in determining the extent of disease. Biopsies that involved full thickness of the skin affected are important to determine the histological subtype. There is a high risk of local destruction, recurrence and metastasis if SCCs are not diagnosed and managed early. As with BCCs, the aim of management is complete removal of the lesion. Medical management includes radiotherapy, photodynamic therapy, cryotherapy, and systemic/topical chemotherapy. In terms of the surgical management, lesions <2 cm are excised with a 4 mm margin and lesions >2 cm with a 6 mm margin. SCCs that are >2 cm in diameter, poorly differentiated or

deeply invasive have a greater risk of metastasis and recurrence. Mohs micrographic surgery is effective for high-risk SCCs.

5. **E – Bowen's disease** (BD). Squamous cell carcinoma in situ is referred to as BD. The malignant cells are confined to the epidermis. This is a pre-malignant condition and invasive SCC develops in about 3%–5% of cases. The lesion is typically a very slowly growing erythematous and well-defined plaque with overlying scaling or crusting. This is sometimes confused with discoid eczema, ringworm or superficial BCC (latter has a raised border). BD is most common on the head and neck, followed by peripheral limbs. It may also occur on the vulva (vulvular intraepithelial neoplasia) or on the glans penis (erythroplasia of Queyrat). The latter is typically found in uncircumcised males. If BD is suspected, a biopsy for histological diagnosis is imperative. Nodulation or ulceration of the lesion may indicate progression to SCC. Surgical excision is the mainstay of treatment. Other treatment options include radiotherapy, photodynamic therapy and topical chemotherapy.

A Dermatology A11 – Management of malignant melanoma

1. **F – Stratum granulosum.** Breslow's thickness or depth is one of the most important prognostic indicators in malignant melanoma. It measures the depth of tumour cells invasion, which is measured from the stratum granulosum to the deepest point of tumour invasion. Of note, the epidermis is divided into five layers: the outermost stratum carneum, stratum lucidum, stratum granulosum, stratum spinosum and stratum basale, the innermost layer of the epidermis. Histopathologists depend on biopsy samples in order to measure the depth of invasion. Excisional biopsy of the tumour usually yields most accurate results.

2. **B – 80%–96%.** The approximate 5-year survival rates associated with different Breslow's thickness measurements are as shown in Table 10.

TABLE 10 Breslow's thickness and the associated 5-year survival rates

Breslow's thickness	5-year survival rates
Melanoma in situ	95%–100%
<1 mm	95%–100%
1–2 mm	80%–96%
2.1–4 mm	60%–75%
>4 mm	50%

3. **D – Level 3**. Clark's level is used for T1 MM tumours (i.e. tumours of less than 1 mm in depth) and is of little use for larger tumours. Clark's level classification is as follows:
   - Level 1 – localised to epidermis
   - Level 2 – spread to papillary dermis
   - Level 3 – spread to papillary-reticular dermis junction
   - Level 4 – spread to the reticular dermis
   - Level 5 – spread beyond dermis into subcutaneous fat.

4. **G – T3N2M0**. This staging is based on the American Joint Committee on Cancer staging system. The classification is based on a multivariate analysis of 30 946 patients with stage I–III malignant melanoma and 7972 patients with stage IV malignant melanoma.

5. **I – Wide local excision with 2 cm margin**. Various factors influence the chosen treatment option. Tumour type, stage, patient age and associated co-morbidities all influence a clinician's decision. A multidisciplinary approach is essential in the treatment of malignant melanoma and the patient must be part of the decision-making process. Surgical excision is the mainstay of treatment. The following points outline the approach to management in different stages of malignant melanoma.
   - Stage 0: this refers to melanoma in situ; here a 0.5–1 cm excision margin of the tumour is sufficient. Patients are followed up regularly to investigate for disease recurrence.
   - Stage I: 1 cm excision margin for a T1 tumour (<1 mm Breslow's thickness), 2 cm excision margin for deeper tumours. The defect created by wide local excision can be closed by the use of skin grafts, local flaps or even free flaps.
   - Stage II: this stage refers to any T2N0M0 (with ulceration) tumour or T3/4N0M0 (with or without ulceration) tumour. Wide local excision of the lesion with a 2 cm margin is recommended. There is no evidence

TABLE 11 American Joint Committee on Cancer staging system for malignant melanoma

Classification: T	Thickness	Ulceration status
T1	≤1.00	a: without ulceration b: with ulceration or mitosis
T2	1.01–2.00	a: without ulceration b: with ulceration
T3	2.01–4.00	a: without ulceration b: with ulceration
T4	>4.00	a: without ulceration b: with ulceration
Classification: N	**Metastatic nodes (n)**	**Nodal metastatic burden**
N0	0	n/a
N1	1	a: micrometastasis b: macrometastasis
N2	2–3	a: micrometastasis b: macrometastasis c: In transit metastases/satellites without metastatic nodes
N3	4+	
Classification: M	**Site**	**Serum lactate dehydrogenase**
M0	No distant metastases	n/a
M1a	Distant skin, subcutaneous or nodal metastases	Normal
M1b	Lung metastases	Normal
M1c	All other visceral metastases Any distant metastases	Normal Elevated

for using larger excision margins. If nodal metastasis is suspected, therapeutic lymphadenectomy is carried out. A sentinel lymph node biopsy is carried out in order to investigate for nodal metastasis if clinical evidence is low; however, this is controversial and there is no consensus on this practice.

- Stage III: this stage refers to any tumour with nodal metastasis, regardless of tumour depth. Wide local excision with 2 cm margins is treatment of choice. Lymph node dissection of regional lymph nodes is also indicated. There is a role for adjuvant chemotherapy in stage III disease.

- Stage IV: management of stage IV disease must take into account various factors and a patient must be an integral part of the decision-making process. Five-year survival rates are <20%. Wide local excision of the primary is offered. Depending on the site of metastasis, different treatment options are available. Surgical resection is offered for isolated symptomatic metastases. Palliative radiation has a role in symptomatic relief.

A Dermatology A12 – Infective cutaneous lesions I

1. **A – Group A streptococcal impetigo**. Impetigo is a highly contagious superficial cutaneous infection caused by *Staphylococcus aureus*, Lancefield group A *Streptococcus* (*Streptococcus pyogenes*) or a combination of both. There are two types of impetigo caused by these respective organisms; the bullous form is usually caused exclusively by *S. aureus*, and the non-bullous caused in most cases by the beta-haemolytic strains of *Streptococcus*. Both these infections frequently occur in children, particularly with pre-existing skin diseases (e.g. eczema) or when the skin's integrity has been compromised through trauma. Risk factors include humid climates, overcrowding and poor hygiene. The lesions are acute in onset and present over a few days. The boy in the scenario presents with the non-bullous form, which typically occurs in children between the ages of 2 and 5 years, affecting the face and extremities most frequently. The lesions start as thin-walled, clear vesicles on an erythematous base that may become pustular before rupturing. Rupture releases their serum, which leaves an area of exudation that dries into a honey-coloured crust – the hallmark of impetigo. Pruritis may lead to excoriations due to scratching which may exacerbate the extent of infection. There may be multiple lesions that spread locally and coalesce. There are usually no constitutional symptoms. Impetigo is usually diagnosed on clinical grounds, although culture of the skin is taken to determine antibiotic sensitivity. The finding of Gram-positive cocci in chains indicate *Streptococcus pyogenes*, while Gram-positive cocci in clusters indicate *S. aureus*. Treatment involves removal of the infected crusts using warm saline or olive oil soaks. If the infection is localised and mild, topical antibiotic therapy may be all that is necessary (e.g. mupirocin). The use of systemic antibiotics is indicated when infection is more severe, involving lymph nodes, or where there is risk of acute post-streptococcal glomerulonephritis (non-bullous impetigo). The drug preferred for streptococcus is penicillin and for staphylococcus is clindamycin.

2. **E – Recurrent herpes simplex virus type 1**. Herpes simplex virus (HSV) is an infection caused by the herpes virus hominis and is spread by close contact via mucosal surfaces. There are two types: primary HSV type 1 usually causes orofacial disease and HSV type 2 traditionally affects the anogenital mucosa via sexual interaction. However, both viruses may infect any part of the body. Subsequent infection can arise without re-exposure, as the virus has the ability to settle and replicate in the nervous system (neurovirulence) and resides dormant in sensory ganglia (latency). The location depends upon where primary infection initially occurred: HSV type 1 infection resides in the trigeminal ganglia and type 2 resides in the sacral plexus. The latent virus may reactivate; risks for reactivation include immunocompromise (including other viraemia, immunosupressive therapy, stress or disease), trauma, sunlight and menstruation. The primary infection is clinically more significant than the recurrent attacks. Despite this, many infections are subclinical. The typical primary infection presentation is a child with acute gingivostomatitis, painful vesicles and ulcers on the hard and soft palate and the lips, with a prodromal febrile illness. Although most herpes infections are spread via mucosal surfaces, herpes may also develop from direct contact, e.g. on the fingers (herpetic whitlow) or on the face (scrum pox). Recurrence of the dormant virus in the trigeminal ganglia is the manifestation of recurrent HSV type 1, as seen in this scenario. Appearance of the vesicular lesions is usually preceded by parasthesia, burning and itching of the affected area. Primary infection lasts approximately 2–3 weeks and recurrences clear within 1 week in the absence of secondary infection. When the integrity of the skin has been disrupted (e.g. eczema), herpes can spread more severely and may become life threatening (eczema herpeticum, otherwise known as Kaposi varicelliform eruption). Herpes encephalitis can occur as a complication without any cutaneous manifestation and has a recognised and somewhat predictable site of infection: the temporal lobes. Diagnosis of cutaneous HSV is usually made on the clinical picture but if there is doubt, culturing vesicle fluid is the investigation of choice. Alternatively, a Tzanck smear test can be done (histological examination of scrapings from the base of the lesion reveals Tzanck cells – degenerated epithelial cells separated from adjacent cells). The majority of HSV infections are self-limiting. Antiretroviral treatment can be used for more severe or recurrent attacks to shorten the duration of symptoms and reduce the risk of dissemination. Systemic aciclovir is the therapy of choice, although this will only be of benefit if introduced at an early stage of the infection (i.e. the tingling or early vesicular stage).

3. **K – Varicella zoster virus (chickenpox).** Chickenpox is an infection caused by the varicella zoster virus (VZV), another virus part of the herpes genome. Do not confuse this with shingles, which is a distinct clinical entity caused by reactivation of VZV. The primary infection of VZV is spread by the respiratory route. Chickenpox is mainly a paediatric disease, with most of the cases under the age of 10 years. On primary exposure to the virus, the child acquires lifelong immunity. Similarly to HSV, however, it remains dormant in the sensory dorsal root ganglion. If reactivation occurs, the clinical syndrome is known as shingles. Chickenpox consists of a characteristic rash that at any one time is in different stages of development and healing. Therefore, the diagnosis depends on distinguishing discrete crops of lesions across the body, predominating across the trunk (centripetal), varying from papules to clear vesicles and finally progressing to crusts. It is only when all the lesions have crusted over that the patient is not infectious anymore. Children may also suffer with a fever but prodromal symptoms are more commonly seen in adults. The severe pruritic stage is usually associated with the vesicular stage and excoriations from scratching may lead to a bacterial superinfection. Other complications include pneumonitis of which more than 90% occur in the adult population, and haemorrhagic complications (e.g. thrombocytopenia or purpura), which are seen more frequently in the immunocompromised. Investigations are not required but for a definitive diagnosis VZV can be cultured from vesicle fluid or a Tzanck smear test can be done. Chickenpox is usually self-limiting although calamine lotion topically may be used for the itching. In patients older than 12 years of age, immunocompromised patients or patients with severe infections, aciclovir can be used at the onset of symptoms to reduce severity and duration of disease. Varicella zoster immunoglobulin (VZIG) is additionally used for immunocompromised patients and for babies that were born to mothers who had the onset of chickenpox fewer than 5 days before delivery or within 2 days post delivery. This is necessary in this time period, as the mother's antibodies have not had sufficient time to cross the placenta, in order to provide passive immunity for her baby. If no intervention is done, severe disseminated neonatal varicella infection results, with significant mortality. It is of note that patients should not be given aspirin for the fever as it is associated with the development of Reye's syndrome in children.

4. **C – Molluscum contagiosum** is an infectious cutaneous lesion caused by the common poxvirus. Infection is spread by direct contact or shared clothing or towels (via fomites). It is more common in children (ages 1–5 years),

the sexually active and the immunocompromised. The lesions are benign, shiny pink or pearl, relatively translucent, hemispherical papules with a central punctum, which may contain a cheesy center, giving the characteristic umbilicated description. They grow slowly until they are about 5 mm in diameter. The lesions are not painful but may itch. They can occur at any site but are most commonly seen on the face and neck. In immuno-compromised individuals (e.g. AIDS), the lesions are more extensive and are spread by scratching. Diagnosis is made clinically, as the lesions have a characteristic appearance. No investigations are required; the virus cannot routinely be cultured and if confirmation of diagnosis is required then biopsy is necessary for histology. One should consider assessing HIV status in adults with extensive infection. Treatment is usually unnecessary as the infection typically clears in 6–9 months. As the condition is contagious until the lesions have disappeared, some clinicians advocate treatment. Intervention options include cryotherapy, curettage and topical imiquimod (immune response modifier). Puncturing the lesions may also be used, as this leads to inflammation and subsequent resolution.

5. **L – Varicella zoster virus (shingles).** Herpes zoster, shingles, is a cutaneous infection caused by the same virus that causes chickenpox (VZV). Shingles results from an inability of the patient's immune system to contain the latent virus replication. It is a disease of adult life; up to half of individuals living beyond 80 years will develop shingles. The virus usually lies dormant in the ganglia of the sensory spinal ganglia and the cranial sensory ganglia. This means that when reactivation occurs in a particular ganglion, characteristic sensory and cutaneous findings are felt along the respective dermatomes. Shingles usually begins with prodromal burning pain and parasthesia along a single unilateral dermatome without any skins signs. This is soon followed by erythema and grouped herpetiform vesicles in the defined dermatome. The vesicles may be clear or blood-filled initially but rapidly become purulent, rupture and crust. Local lymphadenopathy is common. The neuralgic pain may persist well beyond resolution of the cutaneous manifestations; this is known as post-herpetic neuralgia and is seen more commonly in the elderly. Of note, individuals who have not had varicella are at risk of being infected by direct contact. Other complications include secondary bacterial infections that may lead to scarring, ophthalmic involvement that may lead to blindness, geniculate ganglia involvement causing pain and blistering in the external ear (Ramsay Hunt syndrome type II), and uncommonly motor nerve involvement. Dissemination outside the affected dermatome may indicate

underlying immunosuppression or malignancy, which should be examined for. Diagnosis is usually clinical although culture of the virus from the vesicle fluid or a Tzanck smear test may be required if there is doubt. Prompt treatment at the onset of symptoms is important as this can limit the extent of disease, reduce pain and reduce incidence of post-herpetic neuralgia. Use of antiretrovirals such as aciclovir, with analgesia and calamine lotion to control symptoms is common practice. In immunocompromised individuals, administration of varicella zoster immunoglobulin is considered.

A Dermatology A13 – Infective cutaneous lesions II

1. **C – Measles** is a highly contagious infection with the myxovirus, spread via the respiratory route. Prevention is by the three-part combined vaccine against measles, mumps and rubella (MMR). Since the introduction of the MMR vaccine, the rates of measles have dropped profoundly. Despite this, because of the claims of the association between the vaccine and autism, uptake rates dropped remarkably and measles infection rose. Research supporting the connection was deemed fraudulent and there is no scientific evidence at all for such a link. It will take some time to regain the people's confidence in this vaccine again, so it is important to recognise the symptoms. The infection is usually contracted in childhood and is initially characterised by the 4-day fever and the 3 Cs: coryza, cough and conjunctivitis. This is occasionally followed by appearance of pathognomonic pale spots on an erythematous base on the buccal mucosa (Koplik's spots). The rash then develops; it is a generalised, net-like maculopapular rash that characteristically starts behind the ears and becomes blotchy and confluent. The rash develops usually 2 weeks after exposure to the virus. Complications include otitis media, encephalitis and subacute sclerosing panencephalitis. Diagnosis is made clinically: patients usually present with a fever for at least 3 days, with Koplik's spots, and/or with one of the Cs and the rash. Laboratory tests are not necessary but IgM measles antibody confers active disease. There is no treatment for measles; treatment is prevention. In this scenario, the child is only 18 months old, indicating he may not have had his first or second dose of vaccine yet (given at 12–28 months and 36 months, respectively).

2. **H – Rubella**, also known as German measles, is an infection with the togavirus that is transmitted via the respiratory route and from mother to fetus. It predominates in young children. Like measles, rubella is prevented by the MMR; however, the child in this scenario may have missed the

vaccination, as immunisation programmes are not strictly implemented in her country of origin. The presentation is usually of a fever, with a sore throat and rhinitis, but a prodrome may not always be present, particularly in children. The rash develops a few days later, typically starting on the face and spreading centrifugally down the neck and trunk. The exanthem usually lasts 4–5 days. Rarely, pinpoint red macules and papules appear in the soft palate and uvula (Forchheimer spots) prior to the rash. A tender lymphadenopathy characteristically in the suboccipital, postauricular and cervical nodes is the hallmark of this condition. The enlargement may last weeks despite the tenderness resolving. Arthralgia may also occur and may persist. The diagnosis is made based on the clinical presentation but if there is doubt, IgM rubella antibodies confer active disease. Rubella is self-limiting and there is no treatment. Like measles, prevention is key. Complications include encephalitis, peripheral neuritis and thrombocytopenia. The most severe complication is congenital rubella syndrome – rubella is acquired by the mother who is not immune and it is then vertically transmitted to the fetus in utero. If the child survives, it can develop cataracts, deafness, cardiac anomalies (commonly patent ductus arteriosus) and neurological and cognitive impairment.

3. **G – Parvovirus B19**. Erythema infectiosum, also known as fifth disease, is caused by parvovirus B19 and arises in outbreaks, particularly in the spring months. It is transmitted via the respiratory route, contaminated blood products and vertically from the mother to the fetus. There is sometimes a prodrome viraemic phase including a headache, fever and coryza. This is followed by the classical skin findings a few days later. The cutaneous rash starts off as the typical slapped-cheek erythema and within 4 days an erythematous maculopapular rash occurs largely on the extremities. Finally, the rash fades a few days later into a lace-like rash on the trunk and the limbs that can last up to 3 weeks. These cutaneous manifestations are sometimes known as the three-phased cutaneous eruption. Despite the infection being at times identified as 'slapped-cheek disease', the lacy pattern is sometimes all that is seen. Arthritic joint pain may also be a feature. Complications include infection occurring in individuals with haemolytic anaemias, e.g. sickle cell, leading to an aplastic crisis. Another complication is maternal transmission to fetus, which may lead to fetal anaemia and subsequent fetal hydrops and death. Diagnosis is usually made clinically, although a suspicion of exposure in pregnancy needs to be confirmed or excluded by serology (IgM to parvovirus B19). Erythema infectiosum is a self-limiting disease and no treatment is necessary.

4. **J –** *Streptococcus pyogenes*. Scarlet fever is a syndrome caused by *S. pyogenes*, a toxin producing group A streptococci. It is a commensal organism of the nasopharynx. This streptococcal infection manifests in three ways: direct effects cause tonsillitis/pharyngitis or cellulitis, toxin-mediated effects produce scarlet fever or toxic shock-like syndrome, and post-infectious effects lead to glomerulonephritis or rheumatic fever. Scarlet fever usually follows an upper respiratory infection, as in this scenario, but may follow a group A streptococcal infection at any other anatomical foci, and it is the erythrogenic toxin that is produced that leads to the systemic findings in scarlet fever. Infection by *S. pyogenes* to the pharynx is most common in children aged between 5 and 15 years. It is most commonly spread by the respiratory route, although it can spread via fomites. Populated vicinities like schools increase the likelihood of spread. The infection presents initially with a prodrome of fever, malaise, headache and nausea and vomiting. The typical rash is an erythematous coarse base with overlying blanching 'scarlet' macules. The exanthem appears approximately 12 hours post pyrexial onset, starting on the neck, spreading down to the trunk and the extremeties over the next day. The resolution of the rash is followed after a week by the characteristic desquamation of the skin. Pastia lines are a clinical sign of scarlet fever; confluent petechiae form hyperpigmented lines located at skin creases, particularly the antecubital fossa. Oral signs are common; the mucous membranes can become intensely red with petechiae alongside the typical tongue appearance. The tongue initially presents with a white coating, covering erythematous papillae that project through, resembling a white strawberry tongue, followed on day 5 by the red strawberry tongue when the white membrane comes away. Of note, the strawberry tongue is also seen in Kawasaki's disease and toxic shock syndrome. An additional distinguishing facial feature is a flushed face but there is perioral pallor evident. Unlike the other childhood infections with erythematous rashes in this question, scarlet fever is one where the child looks rather unwell (fever, tachycardia, lethargic, etc.). Early complications to be aware of are otitis media, pneumonia and septicaemia. Late complications include rheumatic fever and acute post-streptococcal glomerulonephritis. Investigations include a culture at the site of infection (i.e. in this scenario a throat culture) and antistreptolysin-O titres. It is important to note that streptococcus may be a commensal organism in the oropharyngeal site and thus diagnosis based on culture here must be taken in context of the clinical picture. The aim for treatment is to prevent the complications, reduce severity of the illness and shorten duration of symptoms. Antibiotics (penicillin) are the mainstay of treatment. Topical emollients may be used for

the desquamating rash, although this is self-limiting.

5. **B – Epstein–Barr virus** (EBV). Infectious mononucleosis (glandular fever) is an infection caused by EBV. EBV is usually transmitted via body secretions but also blood transfusions. It infects B immune cells and so it is spread through the reticularendothelial system, where the infection typically manifests. EBV is often asymptomatic although malaise, sore throat and fever are common. The sore throat can be either an exudative or a non-exudative pharyngitis, similar in presentation to that of group A streptococcal pharyngitis. Additionally, a third of patients with EBV have oral group A streptococcal colonisation. Confusingly, the comparable exudative pharyngitis with the positive throat culture may sometimes be mistakenly diagnosed as group A streptococcus and treated inappropriately. There may be substantial tonsillar enlargement ('kissing tonsils' is the expression used, because of the size). Patients may additionally present with a widespread faded, transient, non-pruritic maculopapular rash. It is important to recognise that this is clinically different to the rash seen when ampicillin or amoxicillin are given to an alleged streptococcal pharyngitis (which is in fact EBV) that leads to a widespread drug-induced rash. This rash is also maculopapular but itchy and longer lasting. This is not an allergic reaction, simply a rash that develops with administration of ampicillin or amoxicillin on a background of EBV infection; this is why it is so crucial to make the correct diagnosis initially despite the overlapping symptoms between the two infections. Patients may also present with features of the spread throughout the reticularendothelial system including lymphadenopathy, hepatomegaly and a tender splenomegaly; rarely splenic rupture is the first presentation. The infection does have some distinctive clinical features, including early bilateral upper lid oedema and uvular oedema. Palatal petechiae can be present – this is not seen in other viral sore throats but it is not a distinctive feature per se, as it is also seen in group A streptococcal pharyngitis. The presentation discussed thus far and in the question is that seen in the paediatric age group and the typical triad here is fever, sore throat and lymphadenopathy. An elderly individual may present with EBV with only a viral hepatitis picture, devoid of all the pharyngeal symptoms. EBV is an infection that has been shown to be related with malignancies such as Hodgkin's disease and non-Hodgkin's lymphoma, Burkitt's lymphoma and hairy leukoplakia (particularly seen in HIV patients). Diagnosis is supported by a positive Monospot test (presence of heterophil antibodies), IgM to EBV serology and atypical lymphocytes on a blood film. Transaminase will usually be mildly raised as the liver is

consistently involved, although marked elevation suggests hepatitis. No treatment is required; symptoms may last months but eventually resolve. If glandular fever is complicated with group A streptococcal co-infection, then penicillin should be used to treat the strep throat and ampicillin or amoxicillin should be completely avoided.

A **Dermatology A14 – Infective cutaneous lesions III**

1. **B – *Candida*** is an infection caused by *Candida albicans*, a yeast fungus. It is a normal commensal organism of the gastrointestinal tract (including the mouth, in 30%–60% of immunocompetent adults) and the vagina in some 13% of women. Risk factors for candidal infections include antibiotics, pregnancy and diabetes. Other factors such as maceration, moisture, high humidity, poor hygiene, obesity and perhaps the combined oral contraceptive pill also play a role. In this scenario, the patient has many risk factors, which is often the case; she is obese and has poor hygiene, which together increase the risk of moisture and maceration between the skin folds. She also complains of diabetes symptoms (loss of weight and thirst) and the recent chest infection should alarm you to her recent antibiotic use. Steroids are comparable to a growth medium for *Candida* and are sometimes applied by patients, which significantly worsens the course of disease. Asthmatics are advised to wash their mouth out after taking a puff of their inhaled steroids to avoid oral colonisation with *Candida*. Candidiasis is the term often used when referring specifically to *Candida* acting as an opportunistic infection with a preference for mucosal surfaces. Cutaneous lesions arise in skin folds where there are unusually moist conditions and/or maceration; this presents in infants as napkin candidosis and in adults as intertrigo. Intertrigo usually occurs in the axillae, the groin and the submammary folds. In both age groups, the features include a moist erythema with an irregular margin and maceration, satellite lesions and infrequent pustules. Sore fissures may develop in the folds and there may also be pruritis. Oral candidosis produces adherent white plaques on the buccal mucosa and tongue. If scraped off, there is an underlying erosive raw bleeding area. For identification of *Candida* infection, a swab is taken and analysed via light microscope with potassium hydroxide preparation; pseudohyphae and budding yeast cells will be seen. Swabs can also be taken from intact pustules for culture. It is important to also test for diabetes during investigations, as candidosis may be the first presentation. Management includes identifying the predisposing factors and eliminating them as much as possible; swabs or soaks can be used to avoid the close

contact between the opposing skin folds, aiming to keep them separated and dry. For cutaneous manifestations in immunocompetent individuals, topical nystatin and the imidazoles, such as ketoconazole, are effective. Nystatin is also available in other formulations for local application of manifestations elsewhere (e.g. oral gel, vaginal pessary). If the lesions are extensive or the patient is immunocompromised, fluconazole orally may be given. Persistent *Candida* infection should raise suspicion for an underlying immunosuppressive disease.

2. **J – Tinea corporis** is caused by dermatophytes, a type of fungi that affect the keratin in the superficial layer of skin (stratum corneum) leading to ringworm. Ringworm can produce different signs depending on the sites of infection and are thus termed accordingly; tinea corporis refers to the infection of the arms, legs and trunk. Tinea pedis affects the feet, tinea capitis affects the scalp, tinea cruris the groin area, tinea barbae the facial hair and tinea manuum affects the hands. Ringworm may be spread via contact with humans, animals and fomites. Dermatophytes thrive on warm, moist areas of the skin and thus infection typically begins in the body folds. The lesions in tinea corporis are commonly prurtic, erythematous circular plaques with raised advancing scaly edges. With central resolution, a typical ring-like pattern is seen. Inflammation is produced by the fungi metabolic products and leads to vesicles and papules, particularly at the edges. Inappropriate treatment with corticosteroids will reduce the inflammation but lead to a modified appearance known as tinea incognito. There are less scaly lesions with no distinctive raised borders that spread peripherally. Briefly, tinea pedis is the most common type of fungal infection, spread by shared showering, swimming and changing facilities. Moist interdigiting scaling and fissuring is seen, especially in the fourth toe web, with white blotting-paper skin. Tinea capitus is predominantly a condition of children. It is a fungal infection of the hair shaft that leads to well-circumscribed itchy scaling lesions with alopecia. Tinea cruris is more often seen in men. It is similar to tinea corporis although commonly itchier. Compared with candidiasis infection of the groin, the scrotum is frequently spared. Tinea barbae is similar to tinea cruris but there is often marked inflammatory reactions. Lastly, tinea manuum usually presents unilaterally with dry scaly palms, particularly evident in the creases. Diagnosis of ringworm is by microscopic examination of skin scrapings in potassium hydroxide. The sample should be taken from the scaly margin of the lesion, as this is the most active area of disease. Wood's light (black light) should be used to diagnose hair infection. Fungal culture can be done

if the diagnosis is inconclusive using microscopy. Treatment involves topical antifungals, such as allylamines and the imidazoles. Systemic therapy is indicated for extensive skin tinea corporis, hair, nail and palm infection. Griseofulvan is one of the oral agents. It is important to highlight that this is a liver-inducing drug that increases the metabolism of cytochrome P450-dependent drugs.

3. **E – Pityriasis versicolor** is a superficial skin infection caused by overgrowth of commensal yeasts. The reason why it causes disease in some individuals and not others is unknown, but there may be an element of genetic predisposition. A fifth of patients report a positive family history; these individuals have higher rates of recurrence. The condition is more prevalent in hot, humid climates and is commoner in young adults when the sebaceous glands are more active. It is also more often seen in the immunosuppressed and those with Cushing's disease. It is not infectious. Tinea versicolor is characterised by abnormally pigmented, well-marginated macules on the upper trunk, and proximal parts of the upper limbs. It can also affect the back and may become widespread. As the name implies, the macules are either darker or lighter than the adjacent skin. These patches are hyperpigmented on untanned, Caucasian skin with a fine yellow/brown scale. In tanned/darker skin, there is hypopigmentation and the macules fail to tan on sun exposure. The patches are slightly scaly and wrinkled. They are initially oval but can coalesce into irregularly shaped lesions. Seldom are the lesions itchy. They are cosmetically disturbing for the patient, despite commonly being asymptomatic. The diagnosis is usually clinical. If needed, microscopy of skin scrapings shows characteristic hyphae filaments produced by the spherical yeasts: 'the spaghetti and meatball' appearance. Topical antifungals are recommended, although recurrence is common. For widespread or persistent infection, systemic itraconazole can be used and may be curative. The lesions may take several months to resolve.

4. **D – Pityriasis rosea** is an acute self-limiting disorder of unknown cause. The increased incidence in spring and autumn and institutional outbreaks suggest an infectious source. The latest studies have indentified human herpesvirus 7 as the probable origin. It is most commonly seen in children and young adults, and in men rather than women. Stress increases the severity of clinical manifestations. Most patients develop a solitary plaque, 'the herald patch' usually seen on the trunk. This is an isolated, salmon-coloured macule that is larger, rounder, redder and scalier than the

subsequent lesions. It enlarges and develops a peripheral collarette of scale within the bounds of the well-demarcated border. Several days later, oval pink macules with peripheral scaling appear in crops mainly on the trunk, back and upper extremities. The trunk lesions are often characteristic; they have their longitudinal axes parallel to the ribs, down and out from the spine in a 'Christmas tree pattern'. In atypical cases, the lesions are not bilateral and symmetrical. Pruritis is seen in 50% of patients. The disease usually remits after 8 weeks. Pityriasis rosea-like drug-induced eruptions have been reported with commonly used drugs such as metronidazole, omeprazole and captopril. No investigations are routinely necessary. In atypical cases a biopsy may be needed to confirm diagnosis. Secondary syphilis has a very similar presentation to pityriasis rosea and there-fore serological tests for syphilis should be considered. No treatment is curative, so treatment is usually directed to symptomatic relief. Calamine lotion or a topical steroid will help with itching. Ultraviolet B light therapy relieves pruritis and hastens resolution in resistant cases.

5. **C – Common wart**. Viral warts are caused by infection with human papilloma virus. They cause benign skin and mucosal proliferation, which manifests in various forms (common, filliform, plantar and plane warts). Common warts appear as papules with a hyperkeratotic 'warty' surface, and occur most commonly in the hands. They often have red/black dots on the surface, which represent thrombosed capillaries. Spread is by direct contact, with trauma being a recognised predisposing factor. The warts may coalesce to form a plaque (mosaic warts), which occurs most com-monly on the soles. Filliform warts appear as tiny frond-like projections, commonly around the mouth. Plantar warts are rough-surfaced papules surrounded by a horny collar, and occur on the soles of feet. Unlike other types of warts, plantar warts can be very painful. Plantar warts may look similar to callus. Removing the top layer will reveal pinpoint bleeding capillaries in warts, unlike callus. Deep plantar warts usually occur at weight-bearing areas of skin. Plane warts are less common than other types of warts. They are smooth and flat-topped, skin-coloured papules that appear in areas exposed to light, most frequently the face and backs of the hands. Both common and plane warts may occur along scratch lines. Anogenital warts are usually sexually transmitted. Diagnosis of viral warts is clinical, but a biopsy may be needed to exclude other differentials (e.g. amelanocytic melanoma). Most viral warts resolve spontaneously without leaving a scar. Persistent or painful warts can be treated with topical sali-cylic acid, cryotherapy, cautery and curettage or laser therapy.

A   **Dermatology A15 – Dermatological emergencies**

1. **D – Gas gangrene**, otherwise known as myonecrosis, is a necrotising infection of the skeletal muscle caused by the toxin, gas-producing clostridium bacteria. Gas gangrene leads to rapid systemic toxicity through the exotoxins produced and can be fatal within 12 hours. The mortality rate can be up to 30% even if treated promptly. Clostridium is a partial anaerobe, indicating that the bacteria need to have low oxygen tensions in order to proliferate; high levels such as >70% inhibit their growth. The most common cause is trauma where patients have suffered injury to skin or soft tissue, such as open fractures, pressure sores and frostbite. Other causes include post-operative gas gangrene, most frequently seen in gastrointestinal surgery, and spontaneous or malignancy-related infections. Immunocompromised patients have a worse prognosis. The first symptom is sudden severe pain and tenderness disproportionate to the physical findings. As the pain worsens, there is gross oedema and overlying erythema. The wound usually has no smell or a sweet odour. The skin then changes colour from bronze to blue/black. As the disease progresses, haemorrhagic bullae are seen with a serosanguineous exudate when ruptured. Gas production ensues with crepitus palpation extending beyond the affected region. If a limb has been infected, patients often report a feeling of heaviness. Patients are usually haemodynamically shocked with respiratory distress and fever. Investigations should include a normal medical emergency work-up. A swab of the discharging wound should be taken for microscopy, culture and sensitivity. X-rays may show scanty gas bubbles within the muscles and fascia. Treatment requires immediate radical debridement of the involved tissues and continued daily exploration and further debridement if needed. If the tissue is not salvageable then an amputation is the next step. Providing a hyperbaric oxygen environment inhibits clostridial growth and is additive therapy, not an alternative to surgery.

2. **E – Staphylococcal scalded skin syndrome** (SSSS) is a widespread toxin-mediated exfoliative dermatosis. SSSS is caused by toxin-producing strains of *Staphylococcus aureus* that cause intra-epidermal splitting at the level of the granular layer. The condition most commonly affects children younger than 5 years; neonates are the most at risk, as they have a decreased renal ability to clear the toxins and a lack of advanced humoral immunity. Similarly, individuals with renal disease or immunodeficiency are at risk. Forty per cent of adults are asymptomatic nasal carriers. SSSS

starts from a focus of infection such as otitis media, conjunctivitis or nasopharyngeal infection. Patients present with a fever and a generalised rash. The rash is initially a red/orange, tender, macular erythema. At this stage a positive Nikolsky's sign can be elicited; upon mild pressure there is slippage of the superficial layer of the epithelium. This stage of the rash is also characteristically described as a tissue paper-like wrinkling of the epidermis accentuated at the flexures. After 24–48 hours this progresses to a blistering eruption where sheets of epidermis are shed. There are rapidly expanding large flaccid bullae that rupture, leaving painful erythematous raw areas. SSSS spares the mucous membranes. Despite the distressing clinical picture, superficial desquamation and healing is complete by 7 days. In adults there is a poorer prognosis; the fatality rate in children is 4% but in adults can be as high as 60%. Toxic epidermal necrolysis (TEN) may present similarly, although in TEN, splitting of the skin is deeper (at the dermo-epidermal level) and there is almost always mucosal involvement. TEN is more severe and has a higher morbidity and mortality. Skin swabs from bullae are usually negative as the lesions are toxin-mediated via haematogenous dissemination from a distant focus of infection. Culturing should therefore be taken from the remote infection site for bacteriological identification and sensitivities. Blood cultures are usually negative in children but positive in adults. Patients should be started on intravenous penicillinase-resistant anti-staphylococcal antibiotics without delay. There should be stringent attention to fluid balance. Topical wound care may be necessary in a burn centre if severe.

3. **F – Stevens–Johnson syndrome** (SJS) is a severe form of erythema multiforme involving the skin and mucous membranes. It is an immune complex mediated delayed hypersensitivity disorder that leads to cell death and subsequent separation of the epidermis from the dermis. SJS and TEN are considered by some as severity variants of the same disease, with the same symptoms and treatment. A simple classification between the two terms is as follows: SJS is where there is less than 10% of body surface area detachment, SJS overlapping with TEN is where there is 10%–30% detachment, and pure TEN is detachment of more than 30% of the body surface area. Mortality is inevitably dependent on the extent of skin involvement: rates can be as high as 5%, 35% and 50%, respectively. This scenario was quite clearly SJS. SJS is more common in male Caucasian adults. There are three main causes: drugs, infection and malignancy. Antibiotics are the most common cause of SJS. The disease usually presents with symptoms of a non-specific upper respiratory tract infection. Lesions then develop on the

skin, typically on the palms and dorsum of the hands, the soles and extensor surfaces. The lesions are nonpruritic macules with a purpuric, vesicular or necrotic centre. The lesions have a target appearance but in contrast with the typical erythema multiforme target lesions, there are only two zones of colour; the core is as described with a surrounding macular erythema. The lesions may then develop into papules or may become bullae that rupture, leaving stripped skin. Denuded skin is vulnerable to secondary infection; local worsening with fever should raise suspicion. There is concomitant mucosal involvement, which leads to erythema and swelling with ulceration, blistering and necrosis. Eye signs include conjunctivitis, corneal ulceration and visual disturbances to name but a few. The oral mucosa and lips are commonly affected but the genitourinary system and the respiratory tree may also be involved. Patients commonly present with signs of severe sepsis: febrile, tachycardic and hypotensive with an altered conscience. This is usually a clinical diagnosis but a skin biopsy is definitive, albeit rarely done. Slit lamp shows classical eye signs found in SJS. Treatment is mainly supportive and is similar to patients with extensive burns. Fundamentally, fluid resuscitation and electrolyte correction is essential. Areas of shed skin should be covered with aseptic compresses. Protein loss may be corrected by parenteral nutrition; adequate nutrition is imperative to allow healing of the lesions.

4. **A – Cellulitis** is a cutaneous infection that does not involve the fascia or muscle. It usually occurs after a break to the skin; however, occasionally cellulitis follows no evidential injury. The skin in the latter case is usually dry and cracked allowing bacterial penetration. Previous dermatological disorders such as venous insufficiency or pressure ulcers increase the risk of acquiring cellulitis. Individuals with co-morbid conditions such as diabetes mellitus, chronic liver disease, chronic kidney disease and immunodeficiency (e.g. AIDS) have an increased risk for recurrent severe cellulitis due to their altered immune response. Iatrogenic causes are common including post-operative surgical wounds or canulae sites. Most cellulitis is caused by *Streptococcus pyogenes* or *Staphylococcus aureus*. Cellulitis is more common in individuals older than 45 years. The patient presents with the four cardinal signs of inflammation: pain, erythema, swelling and warmth. Erysipelas presents similarly although cellulitis occurs at a deeper level and the cellulitic erythema is less marginated (i.e. the borders are not as elevated or clearly demarcated). In uncomplicated cases, there are usually no systemic signs of illness (such as fever, or cardiovascular responses). Complications are caused by contiguous or lymphatic spread and include

abscess, necrotising fasciitis and gangrenous cellulitis. Bacteriological swabs should be taken to identify the causative organism, although this should not delay antibiotic treatment.

5. **I – Type II necrotising fasciitis** (NF) is a severe soft tissue infection characterised by widespread necrosis of the subcutaneous tissue and fascia. NF can be classified as type I, II or III. Type I is the polymicrobial NF that usually occurs after surgery or trauma. Type II NF is that caused solely by group A beta-haemolytic streptococci. Type III NF is synonymous with gas gangrene (clostridial myenecrosis; *see* Answer 1 above). When a diagnosis is made using the term NF, it is usually referring to type II. It is important to recognise that there is no clear distinction between the causes of NF II, cellulitis and erysipelas, apart from the layer of skin that is affected – deep, middle and superficial, respectively – which dictates their presentation accordingly. Necrotising fasciitis may occur as a complication of a medical condition, such as diabetes mellitus, or surgical intervention. Any mild break in the skin such as needle puncture sites or leg ulcers can also lead to NF. All the causes of gas gangrene can cause NF; however, quite often there is no obvious cause. Infection is heralded with fever and malaise. The subsequent skin signs vary with different manifestations. A patient may begin with an erythema that is often dusky, rapidly advancing and extremely tender. Purpura with vesiculation and deep haemorrhagic bullae may appear. A necrotic eschar may develop at the periphery. Painless ulcers may also be evident. The affected area may drain a serosanguineous fluid. Occasionally there may be intact skin and the site may be difficult to differentiate from a simple cellulitis. Nevertheless, the patient's overall condition may help to discriminate between the two: the rapid progression, the severity of pain with a poor therapeutic response and the septic state. A delay in treatment has been demonstrated to increase mortality, although paucity of cutaneous signs makes early diagnosis difficult. When NF is suspected the underlying deep necrosis can then be confirmed by a deep stab incision biopsy through to the fascia. Patients are taken straight for surgery often without confirmatory investigations. Aggressive surgical debridement on a background of intravenous antibiotics is necessary to prevent spread. Tissue can be sent for microscopy, culture and sensitivity during surgery. Surgical debridement is repeated to ensure complete removal of necrotic tissue. As in gas gangrene, hyperbaric oxygen therapy can be employed, although it is not a substitute for surgery. Additionally, it is not widely available.

A Dermatology A16 – Burns

1. **B – 37% burn**. Estimating the percentage of total body surface area affected by a burn is difficult and not very accurate. There are several ways of estimating the surface area affected. A common way is known as the Wallace rule of 9s, illustrated in Figure 1.

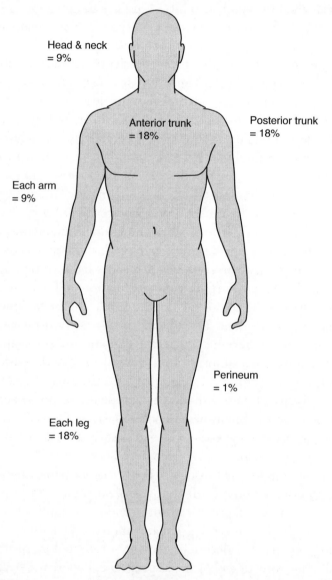

Head & neck
= 9%

Anterior trunk
= 18%

Posterior trunk
= 18%

Each arm
= 9%

Perineum
= 1%

Each leg
= 18%

FIGURE 1 Wallace rule of 9s for estimation of burns total body surface area (note: not applicable to children). Illustration by Lilas Bizrah

Moreover, the patient's palm size can be used to equate to 1% of the body surface area and this can be used to quickly estimate the size of the area affected. The most accurate method for assessment of the burns area is by use of the Lund and Browder chart. Here the areas affected can be shaded into an illustration of the body, a legend indicates the equivalent percentage body surface area affected according to the age of the patient. The total body surface area affected gives burn surgeons a quick illustration of the severity of the case, fluid requirements and the associated mortality.

2. **C – 15 000 mL**. The correct answer is 15 L. The Parkland formula refers to the total amount of fluid recommended for a burns patient over the initial 24 hours. The formula is as follows:

> Total fluid requirement in 24 hours (mL) = 4 mL × Weight (kg) × Total body surface area (%)

> In this case it would be $4 \times 78 \times 48 = 14\,976$ mL

Fifty per cent of the volume should be given in the first 8 hours from the burn injury and the remaining 50% over the course of the next 16 hours. It is imperative to mention that the Parkland formula is a guide and not an absolute protocol. The volume of fluid administered must be titrated to the patient's symptoms, urine output and vital signs. The target urine output is 0.5–1 mL/kg per hour. Of note, the amount of fluid administered should be given according to the time of injury and not admission. So if a patient is admitted to the emergency department 2 hours after the burn injury, this has to be taken into account and 50% of the fluid requirement calculated using the Parkland formula should be given over the next 6 hours. The fluid of choice varies from unit to unit and between clinicians; however, the most commonly used intravenous fluid is Hartmann's solution.

3. **F – Deep partial thickness burn**. Table 12 summarises some of the distinguishing features of different burn depths.

TABLE 12 Distinguishing features of different burn depths

Burn thickness	Appearance	Pain sensation	Scarring
Superficial	Erythematous	Painful	Minimal risk
Superficial partial thickness	Red and associated blisters (blanches with pressure)	Painful	Moderate risk
Deep partial thickness	Can vary from red to white (doesn't blanch with pressure)	Minimal to absent	Debridement and grafting needed
Full thickness	Dry texture, white or charred in colour	Absent	Severe risk of contractures

Some clinicians may use other nomenclatures when describing a burn depth such as first- or second-degree burns. 'First-degree burns' refers to superficial burns commonly caused by ultraviolet radiation exposure or limited thermal exposure when the injury is limited to the epidermis. 'Second-degree burns' refers to superficial and deep partial thickness burns. In superficial second-degree burns, a superficial part of the dermis is involved and that is commonly seen in patients after suffering a scald injury. Deep second-degree burns occur when most of the dermis is involved, usually as a result of chemical exposure or longer exposure to hot liquids or flames. 'Third-degree burns' refers to full thickness burns that involved all layers of the dermis and down to subcutaneous tissue. This usually occurs when exposure is prolonged (e.g. burnt clothes). It may also occur after exposure to high-voltage electricity or long exposure to flames or chemicals. 'Fourth-degree burns' are burns that extend down to muscle or bone.

4. **G – Escharotomy** is vital to prevent irreversible damage secondary to compartment syndrome. Circumferential burns are at high risk of developing compartment syndrome in the leg or abdomen and will affect ventilation if the burn affects the chest. Escharotomy refers to making an incision in the eschar, the inelastic burnt tissue; this can be done in the digits, across the chest wall or down the lower limb. It is vital that the incision is done longitudinally in the limbs, as this may lead to contractures if done circumferentially and hinder the patient's prospects of recovery. This will relieve the pressure in the compartments and improve perfusion. A fasciotomy may also be needed if despite initial measures tissue perfusion remains inadequate and bedside investigations such as Dopplers and compartment pressures are unsatisfactory.

Comparment syndrome refers to increased pressure in a closed facial compartment, resulting in a tissue pressure that is greater than capillary pressure. This reduces capillary perfusion, which results in muscle ischaemia, more oedema and a vicious cycle of increasing compartmental pressure and muscle ischaemia. It is vital for clinicians to be wary of the signs of compartment syndrome, which are the 6 Ps of acute limb ischaemia: **p**allor, **p**ulseless, **p**erishingly cold, **p**ain, **p**araethesia and **p**aralysis. The first of these signs are pain (bursting sensation) and reduced sensation. Use or compression of involved muscles exacerbates the pain. The presence of all the Ps indicates delayed diagnosis. Diagnosis can be confirmed by measuring compartmental pressure. However, if in doubt and unable to immediately measure compartmental pressure, seek immediate senior advice with a view to urgent fasciotomy. Muscle necrosis occurs after 4–6 hours of ischaemia!

5. **I – Split thickness skin graft**. After the initial ATLS (Advanced Trauma Life Support) approach to the management of a burn victim, both medical and surgical management must be initiated and planned. The loss of significant amounts of skin exposes the patient to hypothermia and excessive fluid loss. The initiation of intravenous fluids as already described is paramount. Moreover, warm fluids are always in abundance in a burn unit and must be used to maintain the patient's normal core body temperature. Many patients are sedated and intubated to minimise the pain and discomfort. This is essential when any inhalational injury is suspected. It is also imperative to measure carbon monoxide levels and treat if necessary with high-flow oxygen and hyperbaric oxygen therapy if required. The use of prophylactic antibiotics is debatable and usually reserved until a bacterial infection is suspected. Once the patient is stabilised, they are taken to theatre for debridement of unviable tissue. Debridement is done until viable tissue is reached; this is indicated by both appearance and bleeding from the exposed tissue. After satisfactory debridement, split-thickness autografts (from the patient's own body) are harvested to use for coverage. Alternatives such as the use of xenografts (from other species, e.g. porcine) and other temporary dressing can also be used. Autografts are meshed in order to increase the surface area they can cover and to allow for haematomas and other fluids to seep through and without jeopardising the graft. After covering the affected areas, a holistic multidisciplinary team approach to patient care is paramount. Both the patient's psychological and physiological status must be addressed. Patient education and regular monitoring for the development of complications such as contractures is essential.

A   **Dermatology A17 – Dermatological drug reactions**

Generally mild drug reactions occur within hours to 3 days post administration. However, some may develop up to 4 weeks later. Symptoms are usually benign and transient. However with a few exceptions, discussed shortly, they can be life threatening. The key to management is eliciting accurate history and a thorough examination, thereby knowing which drug was the culprit. These reactions should then be documented in the patient's medical records, with skin test follow-up if indicated. Patients should also be made aware of the reaction so they can be relayed to clinicians in the future.

1. **A – Exanthematic eruptions**. Exanthema is Greek for 'a break out'. It is a widespread rash and is the commonest cutaneous manifestation of drug intolerance. Non-steroidal anti-inflammatory medications and antibiotics, especially penicillins, are common offenders. Patients present with symmetrical maculopapular erythematous lesions that itch. Lymph node enlargement and low-grade fever (drug fever) is also a common feature as with the patient in the example given. Rarely, arthralgia may also occur. Commonly symptoms present within 3 days; however, with ampicillin it can take over 7 days. An essential differential of macular exanthemas are those caused by infectious disease such as measles. Therefore, taking a detailed history and asking about immediate contacts is imperative. Furthermore, almost all patients with previous Epstein–Barr virus (mononucleosis) infection are likely to develop exanthemas when given ampicillin or amoxicillin. Management is by withdrawal of the offending drug and systemic antihistamines.

2. **J – Type IV hypersensitivity**. This patient has had a reaction to topical medication resulting in *non*-allergic contact dermatitis or eczema. This is a delayed hypersensitivity reaction to an external allergen and is therefore a type IV reaction. Taking a thorough history is important, as the distribution of the allergen will point to a specific cause and management plan. Creams, bandages, eye drops, topical anaesthetics and antibiotics (especially aminoglycosides) are common offenders. Often one finds that the area affected may exceed the contact area. When the cause is unclear, a patch test may be indicated. This is different from scratch testing and will take about 48 hours for a delayed hypersensitivity response. Treatment is with avoidance of the identified allergen and topical steroids prior to patch testing if needed. Once the offending agent is removed, the patient should see marked and quick improvement within weeks.

3. **D – Photosensitivity**. Ultraviolet light exposure can cause dermatological reactions in the form of (a) exacerbation of underlying disease, (b) photoallergic reaction, (c) direct phototoxicity and (d) pigmentation. With photoxicity, the timeline is fast, with oedema and blistering occurring within hours, and with strict demarcation between sun-exposed areas and covered skin. In a photoallergic reaction, patients complain of initially a burning sensation, then erythema, swelling and later eczematous changes of sun-exposed areas. This patient discussed above is likely to have had a photoallergic reaction. With her recent diagnosis of rheumatoid arthritis, she was probably started on sulfasalazine, which is a known photoallergen. Other photosensitive drugs include sulphonamides, amiodarone (causing slate-grey pigmentation from melanin and lipofuscin deposition), salicylanide (in industrial cleaners) and antimalarials. Treatment here and in most cases is to remove the offending drug if possible and minimise exposure to sunlight and tanning lamps until symptoms subside. Topical steroid creams and regular sunscreen should be used.

4. **H – Type I hypersensitivity**. The patient in the example has developed urticaria and angioedema, pathognemonic of an anaphylactic reaction. Urticaria is the formation of 'wheals' post exposure to certain foods, plants or medications. Patients with a history of atopy are more susceptible. This reaction is triggered by IgE antibodies sensitising mast cells to release histamine and/or basophilic leucocytes. The result is initially pruritus or stinging, followed the development of wheals. These are oedematous plaques that can be skin-coloured or erythematous. They vary in size and shape and can be localised, regional or generalised. Urticaria usually clears up without scarring within a few hours if managed promptly. Key to examining a patient with acute urticaria is assessing for angioedema. Swelling around the eyes, of the lips and oropharynx indicate airway compromise. This is a medical emergency as it is part of a systemic anaphylactic reaction. Management is as per guidelines for anaphylaxis, however, the urticarial feature responds to parenteral H_1 antihistamines and avoidance of the offending agent. Table 13 summarises the different forms of hypersensitivities.

TABLE 13 Different types of hypersensitivity reactions

Type of hypersensitivity		Examples of associated dermatological disorders	Mediators
I	Allergy	Anaphylaxis, atopy	IgE
II	Cytotoxic	Drug-induced thrombocytopenia, haemolytic anaemia	IgM, IgG Complement
III	Immune complex dependent	Arthus reaction, systemic lupus erythematosus, erythema multiforme	IgG Complement
IV	Delayed hypersensitivity	Contact dermatitis Mantoux test	T-cells
V	Autoimmune	Hereditary epidermolysis bullosa	IgM, IgG Complement

5. **B – Nikolsky's sign** is a cardinal sign in pemphigus vulgaris and toxic epidermal necrolysis (TEN) alone. Pressure at the edge of a blister with a finger or forceps causes the epidermis to slide off, leaving erosion that heals very slowly, if at all. The question in the example described TEN occurring as an adverse drug reaction. Note the patient had been diagnosed with gout and may have recently been started on allopurinol. Also known as drug-induced Lyell's syndrome, this is a rare acute loss of large areas of necrotic epidermis. Extensive loss of epidermis results in dehydration and protein depletion. Drugs such as allopurinol, co-trimoxazole, NSAIDs, antiobiotics and phenytoin can cause TEN. Symptoms usually start with a prodrome of flu-like illness followed by a cutaneous eruption with extensive sloughing. This is very painful. Circulatory failure can result in shock and organ failure. TEN is a medical emergency and requires intensive care and supportive management similar to burn victims with withdrawal of offending drug if known; intravenous immunoglobulins; fluids and electrolyte replacement; parenteral feeding; and infection control. Steroids have not been shown to be of significant benefit. Mortality rate is about 30% in spite of this, as patients suffer from sepsis or respiratory distress due to damage of the airway. An essential differential is Stevens–Johnson syndrome (SJS). This, similar to TEN, is a mucocutaneous drug-induced or idiopathic reaction. TEN is seen as the extreme variant of SJS; and SJS a more sinister version of erythema multiforme. The skin becomes exquisitely tender with erythema of the skin and mucosa. This eventually leads to extensive exfoliation of these surfaces and can be life threatening. TEN and SJS can occur at any age – primarily over 40 years – and is of equal incidence in both sexes. Drugs as discussed earlier are the most common

triggers for both manifestations, particularly in TEN (90%). Certain associations between systemic lupus, HIV and HLA-B12 have been reported as risk factors. However, *Mycoplasma*, viral infections and chemicals have also been implicated more commonly in SJS.

A   Dermatology A18 – Dermatological investigations

1. **B – Dermoscopy** (or dermatoscopy). In this example, the patient has given you the diagnosis we are investigating. The early phase of malignant melanoma is difficult to diagnose as it shares many features with an atypical naevus. The examination stated is one of the naked eye. Dermoscopy is a non-invasive method that allows the in vivo evaluation of colours and microstructures in the epidermis, the dermo-epidermal junction and the papillary dermis, that is not visible to the naked eye (typically magnifies 10 times actual size). An experienced clinician can identify specific diagnostic patterns related to the distribution of structures and colours that can better suggest a malignant or benign lesion. A study reported that dermoscopy is more accurate at correctly diagnosing malignant melanoma with an odds ratio of 15.6 bringing the sensitivity from 74% with the naked eye to 90% with a dermascope. Dermoscopes are also used to better inspect lesions such as other skin tumours (e.g. basal cell carcinoma, squamous cell carcinoma), scabies and viral warts.

2. **J – Wood lamp examination**. The causes of alopecia are numerous, including alopecia areata, tinea capitis, psoriasis, drug reactions and trichotillomania. The diagnosis may not be a clinical one, but an examination can make us more confident with what the diagnosis is. The red papules forming a ring around the lesion are more associated with tinea capitis, and the absence of an exclamation mark sign makes it less likely to be alopecia areata. Epiluminescence microscopy is another fancy word for dermoscopy. Although dermoscopy is a logical answer to better evaluate the nature of the lesion the question has already demonstrated its use with this patient. Tinea capitis occurs mainly in children, most commonly below the age of 10 and peaking between the ages of 3 and 7 years. Tinea capitis is caused by a fungal infection from the genera *Trichophyton* and *Microsporum*. It is the most common paediatric dermatophyte worldwide. These dermatophytes are present in non-living cornified layers of skin and are sometimes capable of invading underlying living skin. Wood lamp examination is a test used since 1925 to observe fungal infections. It was discovered that when fungally infected hairs were exposed to a Wood's

lamp, the cultures would become fluourescent. In the United Kingdom and North America, *Trichophyton tonsurans* accounts for more than 90% of tinea capitis cases. Unfortunately, this particular type of tinea capitis does not turn fluorescent. However, this question specifically mentions that the family has recently arrived from Mexico, which is an area with higher prevalence of Wood's lamp positive strains.

3. **H – Skin prick test**. Asthma occurs due to a type I hypersensitivity reaction (i.e. IgE-mediated reaction). This is also the case with hay fever and eczema, which are autoimmune conditions associated with asthma. This patient has known asthma that has gotten worse due to an unidentified trigger. The best way to investigate is to induce a type I hypersensitivity reaction. The most commonly used and cost-effective method is the skin prick test. Tiny drops of allergens are dropped onto the skin (most commonly the back), then a needle is pricked through the extract into the skin. Creating point of entry for the allergen, this activates an IgE-mediated allergic cascade to cause hives where true allergens are placed. This reaction occurs in 15 minutes and up to 1 hour. If all allergens tested were negative using the skin prick test, a similar test called the intradermal allergy test can be performed. The extract is directly injected intradermally rather than just a prick on the skin. If the patient is known to have serious consequences to certain allergens such as an anaphylactic reaction, the aforementioned tests are contraindicated. However, in this example, the patient does not have any known allergies. A patch test investigates contact dermatitis, which can be due to an irritant or to an allergen. A patch test induces a type IV hypersensitivity reaction if positive. An allergen is added to a patch, which is then placed on the skin. The exact mechanism involves antigen-presenting cells engulfing the allergen and presenting it on its surface. The antigen-presenting cell travels through the lymphatic system to the lymph nodes where it brings the allergen in contact with CD4 T-helper cells. This releases cytokines and increases the numbers of T-cells that migrate to the skin lesion. This starts an immune complex cascade and causes skin inflammation, itching and irritation. This whole mechanism takes around 48 hours. Blood tests can also be used to identify certain allergens (such as the radioallergosorbent test); however, this is particularly expensive. On the other hand, the IgE quantitative blood test is very limited and only gives the clinician a better understanding whether the symptoms are secondary to an allergy or an infection. So we choose skin prick testing because, this patient has worsening asthma, which is a type I hypersensitivity reaction (patch testing investigates type IV hypersensitivity, i.e. contact dermatitis),

it is usually the first-line investigation for trigger identification as it is cheap and quick (unlike the radioallergosorbent test). If skin prick test was negative, only then do we proceed with intradermal allergy tests.

4. **I – Tzanck preparation smear**. Painful genital ulcers are most likely due to genital herpes. This is most commonly due to herpes simplex virus 1 (HSV-1). However, lesion location is not necessarily indicative of viral type. HSV-2 has been seen in orofacial regions while HSV-1 has also been observed in the genital region. Although up to 80% of infected patients remain asymptomatic, symptomatic disease causes significant morbidity to the patient. The prevalence of this disease has increased over the last decade due to the rise in immunocompromised patients, including HIV and chemotherapy patients. Hence, anyone suspected for herpes should be investigated for immunocompromise. Herpes is a lifelong disease that has latent and active phases. During active phase it manifests itself through painful ulcers. During the latent phase it lies dormant in the nerve root ganglia of the trigeminal nerve or sacral nerve (S2–5) in patients with orofacial or genital herpes. HSV is transmitted by close contact, it occurs through the inoculation of the virus into mucosal surfaces or cracks in the skin. The virus is inactivated at room temperature, so, consequently, aerosol spread is rare. Herpes simplex is best diagnosed by isolating the virus in a tissue culture. Although the results can be obtained within 48 hours, its success is operator dependent. A more rapid diagnosis can be acquired by a Tzanck smear. This can show a result within an hour by demonstrating cytological changes characteristic to HSV. Tzanck smear is done by smearing cells taken from a fresh blister or ulcer onto a microscope slide. Cells are stained in a special stain (e.g. Wright's stain) and then examined microscopically for specific changes. Herpes causes multinuclear giant cells; the shape for each nucleus appears molded to fit together to its adjacent nuclei. In the background there is a ground glass appearance containing small dark spots (inclusion bodies). Tzanck preparation can also be positive in herpes zoster patients (chickenpox or shingles).

5. **A – Allergy patch testing**. Please refer to the answer to Question 3 of Dermatology A18 – Dermatological investigations. In diagnosing allergies and skin conditions the history is crucial. From this lady's history we can reach the conclusion that her dermatitis-like picture has occurred because of use of the gloves (be it due to the latex or the chemicals in the gloves). Therefore, a conformational test can be done, which is inexpensive and takes 48 hours.

A   **Dermatology A19 – Connective tissue disorders**

1. **J – Systemic lupus erythematosus** (SLE) is a chronic autoimmune inflammatory disease commonly affecting the skin, joints, kidneys and vasculature. It is characterised by the presence of serum autoantibodies against nuclear and cell surface components, and circulating immune complex deposition. Pathogenic autoantibodies secrete B-cells that lead to the formation of immune complexes that deposit in various sites in the body. Young (aged 20–30 years) Afro-Carribean women are at increased risk. There is a female-to-male preponderance of 9:1. The cause of the disease is unknown, but multiple factors are thought to play a role in the development of the disease including genetics; there is 25% concordance between identical twins. It is more common in individuals who are HLA-B8, DR2 or DR3 positive. There is also a hormonal element (higher incidence in pre-menopausal women and Klinefelter's), immunological element (both humoral and innate) and environmental element. SLE has a variable presentation and is a relapsing and remitting condition; the triad of fever, rash and arthralgia in a woman of childbearing age should always advocate SLE investigations. There are four main dermatological manifestations in SLE:
   - Butterfly rash (malar rash): a fixed erythema over the cheeks and nasal bridge sparing the nasolabial folds. It is rarely pruritic and painful. This usually manifests in one third of individuals with SLE.
   - Discoid rash: raised rimmed erythematous plaques with keratotic scaling and follicular plugging over light-exposed regions of the skin. This progresses to scarring and pigmentation. Discoid rash occurs in 20% of SLE patients. Discoid lupus can be a benign variant of the disease whereby skin involvement is the only feature with no organ involvement (this is a distinct diagnostic entity).
   - Photosensitivity: an erythematous macular rash as a result of a reaction to sunlight. Sun exposure is an identified trigger for flare-ups.
   - Alopecia: frequently affects the temporal area.

   Other dermatological manifestations include Raynaud's phenomenon, vasculitis, urticaria, livedo reticularis (purplish mottling of the skin) and lupus panniculitis, otherwise known as lupus profundus (inflammation of subcutaneous adipose layer leading to firm, well-defined nodules). There is also commonly oral or vaginal ulceration. Palatal ulcers are more specific to SLE. Constitutional complaints are the most common presentations of SLE including fever, lethargy and weight changes. Other systemic involvements include musculoskeletal (arthralgia, myalgia, jaccoud arthropathy), renal (e.g. glomerulonephritic presentations), pulmonary (e.g. pleurisy, pleural effusions), cardiac (pericarditis), neurological (e.g. depression, headache, seizures, psychosis) and haematological (e.g. cytopenias, haemolytic anaemia, antiphospholipid syndrome). Diagnosis of SLE is made on the basis of a suggestive clinical picture in conjunction with serological evidence. Antinuclear antibodies are positive in almost all cases. Double stranded DNA (dsDNA) binding is particular for SLE but only positive in 50% of patients. Anti-Smith antibodies and antiphospholipid antibodies (anticardiolipin antibodies, lupus anticoagulant) are also commonly positive. A raised erythrocyte sedimentation rate and normal C-reactive protein levels are also common findings. Immunofluorescent stains reveal immunoglobulin complex deposits at the dermo-epidermal basement membrane. If there is renal involvement, renal biopsy may be recommended. Treatment depends on symptoms and severity of disease. NSAIDs are valuable for patients with mild disease. Patients are advised to avoid excessive sunlight. Chloroquine or hydroxychloroquine are used for cutaneous manifestations, and topical steroids can be used for discoid lupus. Systemic steroids are introduced for moderate or severe disease. Patients with renal or cerebral involvement will be given additional immunosuppressives. Targeted agents against B-cells are being developed (e.g. Rituximab) and showing promising preliminary results.

It is also important to be aware of drug-induced lupus in which dermatological and lung manifestations predominate. Drug induced lupus is commonly associated with hydralazine, isoniazid, chlorpromazine, phenytoin and procainamide. This variant remits if the triggering agent is stopped. In this variant anti-histone antibodies are seen in 100% of patients.

2. **D – Limited cutaneous scleroderma** (SS) is a multi-organ connective tissue disease characterised by excessive collagen deposition, progressive fibrosis and restricted mobility of the skin and other internal organs. Immunological and vasomotor disturbances accompany the mentioned changes. It is a disorder of unknown cause but theories suggest many factors play a role. There is an increased incidence of HLA-DR3 and HLA-B8 among individuals with SS. SS is more common in women and appears between the ages of 30 and 50 years. Patients usually present with Raynaud's phenomenon initially, prior to the development of cutaneous manifestations. Raynaud's disease must be differentiated from Raynaud's phenomenon; the former occurs with no underlying disorder and the latter is due to a secondary cause (e.g. connective tissue disease, b-blockers).

There may then be swelling of the hands and feet, leading to ulceration and subsequent gangrene. Advancing dermal fibrosis of the fingers leads to immobility with a tightened shiny appearance (sclerodactyly). The facial features are characteristic: a beaked nose, a small mouth with limitation of movement and confined opening, wrinkles radiating around the mouth and radial furrowing of the lips (rhagades). The patient's expression is often described as 'fixed'. Periungual and facial telangiectasia is common. There may be calcium deposition in the fingers manifesting as palpable subcutaneous nodules (calcinosis). There may be involvement of other organs: gastrointestinal hypomobility leads to oesohpagitis, dysphagia and aspiration, bowel changes and malabsorption. There may be fibrosis of the lungs and heart. Kidney involvement has a poor prognosis owing to malignant hypertension. A variant of SS, known as limited cutaneous scleroderma, previously known as the CREST syndrome (Calcinosis, Raynaud's phenomenon, oEsophageal involvement, Sclerodactyly and Telangiectasia) has a better prognosis. This may progress to diffuse scleroderma in subsequent years. The diagnosis is primarily based on characteristic skin findings. Serum autoantibodies are positive, particularly antinuclear antibodies (positive in 64% of cases). Anti-topoisomerase-1 [Scl70] (found in 40% of cases) and anti-RNA polymerase (found in 20% of cases) are specific for patients with diffuse disease. Anti-centromere antibodies are present in limited cutaneous disease. Radiological investigations are often required for identifying internal organ involvement: barium swallows, oesophageal manometry, X-ray of hands, CT scan of lungs. Treatment is symptomatic; vasodilators (e.g. nifedipine), immunosupressors (e.g. cyclophosphamide) and anti-fibrotics (e.g. penicillamine, intravenous prostacyclin) are used. Extracorporeal irradiation (photopheresis) is used with varying degrees of success in severe forms of the disease.

3. **A – Dermatomyositis**. Polymyositis is a rare muscle disorder characterised by inflammation and necrosis of striated skeletal muscle. When accompanied by skin manifestations it is known as dermatomyositis. There are two distinct forms, a childhood variant and the other affecting adults between 40 and 60 years. The adult variant is commonly associated with malignancy. The cause is unknown although there seems to be an autoimmune mechanism due to the presence of autoantibodies and cross-reactivity. The skin changes are characteristic: there is a heliotrope (lilac) peri-orbital discoloration and swelling, with a macular malar erythema (shawl sign – when the erythema is found on the shoulders and back). It may progress to poikiloderma, a mottled skin appearance, which are areas

of telangiectasia and skin atrophy. There are scaly streaks of erythema over the extensor aspects of the hands that may appear thickened and pale early in the disease (collodion patches). Symmetrical violaceous, flat-topped papules and plaques over the metacarpophalangeal and interphalangeal joints are also typical (Gottron's papules) and can mimic psoriasis. Skeletal muscle involvement leads to progressive symmetrical weakness and wasting. Proximal muscles of the shoulder and pelvic girdle are commonly affected, presenting as difficulty raising arms above the head or climbing stairs, respectively. Smooth muscle may rarely be involved leading to dysphagia, dysphonia and impaired intestinal motility. Extra-muscular signs include arthralgia, Raynaud's phenomenon and calcinosis. The presence of calcinosis is a good prognostic factor but responds poorly to treatment. Myocardial involvement can also be seen in the form of arrhythmias and myocarditis. Diagnosis is based upon the characteristic skin rash, muscle weakness and raised muscle enzymes (e.g. creatine kinase, alanine aminotransferase (ALT) and aldolase). Muscle biopsy is the gold-standard definitive investigation; if to be performed, electromyography can be used to identify the area of muscle involvement. Anti-Mi-2 and anti-Jo1 autoantibodies are positive. Oral steroids are the treatment of choice. Immunosuppressive therapy (e.g. azathioprine) may be of added benefit. Disease progress is monitored by obtaining regular muscle enzyme levels. The prognosis is better in adults than in children if the disease is not associated with malignancy; 50% of children die within 2 years of diagnosis.

4. **C – Henoch-Schönlein purpura** (HSP) is a generalised small-vessel vasculitis caused by deposition of IgA – dominant immune complexes in blood vessels. This condition is most commonly seen in children between 3 and 10 years of age and is more common in boys. It is often preceded by an upper respiratory tract streptococcal throat infection and peaks during the winter season. Patients typically present with a prodrome of headache, fever and malaise. The classic triad of symptoms are the '3 P' rash (painful palpable purpura), colicky abdominal pain and non-migratory arthritis. The rash is the most obvious feature and is present in all cases. It appears in crops; it may initially be urticarial pruritic papules, subsequently progressing to blanching maculopapular lesions, and finally consisting of palpable painful purpuric lesions. These are ultimately non-blanching and mainly located on the extensor surfaces of the legs and buttocks (symmetrically distributed). The torso is usually spared. The arthritis does not lead to long-term articular damage and commonly affects the knees and ankles. There is also peri-articular oedema. Renal involvement leads

to haematuria and glomerulonephritis, and gastrointestinal petechiae can lead to haematemesis, malaena and rectal bleeding. Investigations are not necessary. The disease is usually self-limiting and recovery spontaneous with bed rest and simple analgesics. Steroids may be required for severe multi-system involvement. Up to 10% of patients with renal involvement may suffer from long-term urinary abnormalities; these individuals are followed up for a year post recovery to assess their risk. Aside from the symptoms being slightly different in HSP compared with the commonly confused meningococcal septicaemia (such as tender rash, knee pain and recent throat infection), the scenario highlights the GP contacting the paediatric team rather than sending the patient immediately to the hospital with an instant dose of intramuscular benzylpenicillin.

5. **I – Reactive arthritis** is a triad of arthritis, non-gonococcal urethritis and conjunctivitis. Its cause is unknown, although it is precipitated by infectious gastroenteritis or non-specific urethritis/cervicitis. The latter is usually caused by *Chlamydia trachomatis*. Symptoms of arthritis usually occur 1–4 weeks after the infection. There is a strong association with HLA-B27 and the disease is more common in young men. Asymmetrical arthritis is the most severe element and may resemble rheumatoid arthritis. The common cutaneous manifestations are keratoderma blennorrhagica and circinate balanitis. Keratoderma blennorrhagica describes psoriasis-like red plaques and hyperkeratotic scaling papules. They are commonly on the volar surfaces of the hands and feet. The lesions may occasionally be vesicular or pustular and may extend to the extensor surfaces of the surrounding affected area (e.g. toes or fingers). Nail dystrophy may occur. Circinate balanitis is inflammation of the glans penis; there are annular erythematous scaly plaques that grow centrifugally and spread outwards across the glans penis. The lesions can become keratotic in the circumcised penis. There may be mucosal involvement with erythematous plaques and erosions in the mouth. There are no diagnostic investigations but urethral smears and stool cultures should be considered in establishing the cause of disease; although they may not be positive at onset of presentation. Erythrocyte sedimentation rate and C-reactive protein levels are both usually raised. Joint aspiration is sterile. Treatment is symptomatic and supportive. NSAIDs or local steroid injections are given for arthritis. Cutaneous lesions respond to topical psoriasis therapy. Tetracycline can be added for the urogenital symptoms.

A   **Dermatology A20 – Pharmacology in dermatology**

1. **F – Nil major known**. Emollients are the basis of managing eczema. They are available as aqueous cream or ointments and act as barriers, moisturisers and skin-softeners. They can be applied liberally without restriction or risk of major side effects. Daily emollient baths are also recommended. Other management of eczema include avoiding the precipitants or irritants of known, H_1 histamine antagonist, occlusive bandages, or antibiotics if required. Topical steroids may be mild such as 1% hydrocortisone, and may be used twice per day. More potent concentrations may be used for acute exacerbations. The face should generally be avoided when applying the latter and excessive use may cause systemic side effects as discussed shortly. Immunomodulators such as tacrolimus may be used as steroid-sparing agents in the management of eczema.

2. **D – Liver enzyme inhibitor**. *Candida albicans* affecting skin folds or mucosal surfaces of the mouth or genital tract are often managed with topical antifungals such as clotrimazole or miconazole. Nail infections, however, require systemic therapy such as with itraconazole. Itraconazole is a cytochrome P450 inhibitor; therefore, caution should be taken if the patient is on other medications, as it may serve to increase their concentrations in the body. Antimycotics are better absorbed with a fat-rich meal.

3. **E – Nappy rash**. Nappy rash is commonly caused by a prolonged exposure to urine and faeces on an occluded surface. The ammonia in urine increases pH, thus promoting faecal enzymes. The combination causes skin irritation (irritant dermatitis) and damage. Nappy rash can thereby be complicated by infections with *Candida albicans* and *Staphylococcus aureus*. Preventative measures include letting buttocks airdry and leaving the nappy off as often as possible. When applied, they must be loose and well ventilated, and changed often. Management is by using protective barriers such as paraffin ointments. *Candida* infection is treated with nystatin or clotrimazole creams and powders. Bacterial infections are treated with penicillins or macrolides.

4. **A – Dithranol**. Psoriasis can be controlled with bland emollients, calcipotriol (a vitamin D analogue) or purified coal tar when there is scalp involvement. Dithranol is highly effective in the management of psoriasis. It acts by inhibiting DNA replication, thus reducing the thickening and scaling of the skin seen in psoriasis. Dithranol can however stain skin to

a yellow-brown and stain clothing permanently. It should therefore be applied with caution only onto the affected area of skin and washed off after up to an hour with lukewarm water. When topical therapy is unsuccessful, psoralen with ultraviolet A treatment or immunosuppressants such as methotrexate may also be used.

5. **J – Urticaria**. The key to managing urticaria is identifying the cause and treating with antihistamines. The term 'antihistamines' commonly refer to the H_1-receptor blockers. They reduce the 'wheal and flare' response, by competitively binding to histamine receptors on smooth muscle, nerve, glandular and mast cells. Antihistamines are used for managing urticaria, atopy and hay fever. The sedating effect makes it highly beneficial to patients when taken at night, to enable sleep and prevent constant scratching. Non-sedating preparations such as loratidine and cetirizine are also available.

6. **I – Teratogenic**. Acne is treated by decreasing skin inflammation, sebum production and preventing bacterial infection. Topical treatments are usually first-line: keratolytics such as benzoyl peroxide, retinoid-like agents such as adapelene and antibiotics such as clindamycin and tetracycline. Second-line treatment involves low-dose antibiotics for up to 4 months, use of co-cyprindiol in women and ultraviolet B phototherapy. Retinoids are the *third* line of treatment. Examples are isotretinoin and acitretin, used in managing acne as well as psoriasis and some cancers. They are synthetic vitamin A analogues used only when all other measures have failed; there is skin scarring and/or there are severe psychological effects for the patient as a result of the acne. Side effects include thinning and drying of the skin, hair loss, and deranged liver function. Patients must have baseline blood tests prior to commencing treatment and must be closely monitored. Retinoids are teratogenic and therefore contraindicated in pregnancy. Female patients are advised to have pregnancy tests prior to commencing treatment. After the course, patients are advised to continue to take contraception for 1 month post isotretinoin. With acitretin patients are advised contraception for 3 years post treatment. In the United Kingdom, patients on acitretin are not allowed to donate blood 1 year after treatment, 2 years in the United States and 3 years in Canada, due to the risk of transfusion into a pregnant patient.

7. **G – NSAIDs**. Chronic and subacute lupus are commonly treated with oral antimalarials such as hydroxychloroquine and corticosteroids. Systemic

steroids are highly potent and used in many areas of medicine for disease and immune suppression. However, they carry multiple potential side effects, some of which are:

- acceleration of cataracts
- hypertension
- increased susceptibility to gastrointestinal ulcers
- increased susceptibility to infection
- insulin resistance
- osteoporosis
- psychological disturbance – irritability, mania, confusion
- skin thinning
- weight gain.

Oral corticosteroids have received much attention in the media and patients are increasingly wary of using them. The risks versus benefits should be discussed openly and patients should be assured that the steroids will be used only for the minimum duration and at the lowest dose necessary, with alternatives and steroid-sparing agents such as azathioprine considered. Caution should be taken with concomitant medications. Drugs such as NSAIDs are contraindicated due to increased risk of gastric and duodenal ulceration.

The key principles in dermatological pharmacology may be summarised as:

> Keep wet conditions dry,
> And dry conditions wet.
> Reduce the inflammation,
> Avoid what caused the mess!

A   **Dermatology A21 – Bullous disorders**

1. **D – Direct immunofluorescence: intercellular IgG deposits** are found in cases of pemphigus vulgaris (PV). This is an autoimmune disease targeting epidermal cells and intraepidermal units. Onset is at 40–60 years, affecting both males and females equally. IgG antibodies bind to cell surface glycoproteins – pemphigus antigens, desmogelein 1 and 3, and epithelial cadherin. This induces acantholysis (loss of cell-to-cell adhesion). PV is caused by the split and loss of adhesion within the epidermis. When these changes occur above the basal layer it is known as pemphigus

vulgaris; when they occur higher in the epidermis this is termed pemphigus foliceous. PV is more common. PV is characterised by blisters that rupture easily, and widespread erythematous lesions initially in the oral mucosa then scalp, torso, axilla and groin. Usually starts from localised to generalised acute eruptions. Lesions are randomly scattered, discrete and flaccid with serous content that rupture and bleed easily. Therefore, it is usually difficult to find intact blisters on these patients; usually extensive bleeding erosions are found instead. Nikolsky's sign is a cardinal feature of pemphigus – dislodging the epidermis with finger pressure causes erosion with lateral extension on the blister. There is no pruritus; however, there is a sensation of burning and pain and this can be very uncomfortable for patients – lesions in the mucosa cause odynophagia, leading to reduced appetite and weight loss, epistaxis, weakness and malaise. When investigating PV, biopsies should be taken of involved skin, keeping blisters intact if possible for histopathology. Samples may undergo investigation under direct immunofluorescence of tissue or indirect immunofluorescence using serum. These show IgG antibodies in the intercellular parts of the epidermis. C3 and circulating anti-epithelial antibodies may also be found. Management is by systemic high-dose steroids such as prednisolone until blisters stop and Nikolsky's sign becomes negative, followed by a maintenance dose. Concomitant treatment with steroid-sparing agents (e.g. azathioprine). Refractory disease may require cytotoxic medications such as methotrexate or cylcophosphamide. Other rare options include plasmaphareisis to reduce antibody titres, gold therapy, and intravenous immunoglobulins. Wet dressings and prophylactic antibiotics can also be of benefit. If left untreated, pemphigus can be fatal. Severe cases must be treated in hospital. Protein and fluid loss from extensive breakdown can result. Secondary infection may also occur. Toxic epidermal necrolysis also demonstrates a positive Nikolsky's sign. However, onset is quicker and usually precipitated by an identifiable drug.

2. **C – Direct immunofluorescence: basement membrane IgG deposits** are typical of bullous pemphigoid. It commonly occurs in elderly patients between the ages of 60 and 80 years with equal incidence in men and women. Auto-antibodies interact with basal keratinocytes causing activation of complement factors, neutrophils and eosinophils. The process may begin with the 'pre-pemphigoid stage' characterised by raised erythematous and pruritic areas. Bullae then form – large, tense and occasionally blood-filled. Compared with PV they are more difficult to rupture. Typical areas of involvement are the lower legs, abdomen and groin. Healing, unlike in

pemphigus, is fast. Collapsed blisters crust over with minimal scarring if any, though variants occur. Diagnosis is often clinical although biopsies can be taken for histopathology and immunofluorescence. Findings are a sub-epidermal blister (note difference with pemphigus), linear deposits of C3 along basal membranes and IgG anti-basement membrane antibodies circulating in 70% of patients. Treatment is with systemic steroids and steroid sparing agents such as azathioprine for a shorter duration than in PV. Topical steroid therapy may also be of use.

Students and clinicians sometimes find bollous pemphigoid, pemphigus, dermatitis herpetiformis, and linear IgA dermatosis difficult to distinguish clinically. They are also key differentials to be considered. Table 14 is a useful summary of the main differences.

TABLE 14 Features of different bullous disorders

Disease	Dermatitis herpetiformis	Pemphigus	Pemphigoid	Linear IgA dermatosis
Age of onset	20–60 years	40–60 years	60–80 years	Post puberty
Sex	Male > female	Male = female	Male = female	Male = female
Nature of blister	Small, firm-topped	Round, flaccid, weepy	Large, domed, tense	Grouped, symmetrical
Gluten-sensitive enteropathy?	Yes	No	No	No
Antibody deposits on fluorescence	Granular IgA deposits	Intercellular IgG deposits	Basement membrane IgG deposits	Basement membrane, linear IgA deposits
Pruritus?	Yes	No	Yes	Yes

3. **F – Hereditary epidermolysis bullosa.** This is a spectrum of rare (fewer than 20 in 1 million births) dermatoses whereby the coherence of epidermis of skin and mucosal membranes is damaged or lost (i.e. there is insufficient fixation of epidermis to dermis). This causes blister formation from minimal trauma. There are over 20 different subtypes. They are generally classified into three main groups resulting in blister above, within and below the basal lamina.

- Epidermolytic or epidermolysis bullosa simplex is usually an autosomal dominant intra-epidermal blistering mostly caused by gene mutation for keratin. Blisters, induced by trauma, are formed above the basal lamina. Epidermolysis bullosa simplex can be generalised or localised. Sites of occurrence are those most prone to trauma: elbows, knee, and feet. There is usually rapid healing and scarring is minimal.

- Junctional epidermolysis bullosa is autosomal recessive. Here there is blister formation within the lamina lucida of basement membrane. Mortality is high in the one subtype of this disease, junctional epidermolysis bullosa gravis, as skin becomes eroded. Epithelial surfaces in the respiratory, gastrointestinal and genitourinary organs are also involved.
- Dermolytic or dystrophic epidermolysis bullosa: here, blistering occurs below the basal lamina, and can result in scarring and milia formation. There are four main subtypes; however, all involve a mutation in the gene for anchoring fibril. Of note, the recessive subtype can cause syndactyly 'mitten-like' hands and feet, loss of nails, and flexion contracture, dental caries, scarring of oesophagus, urethra and anus, causing stenosis.

There is no treatment for epidermolysis bullosa. Management is supportive, with wound care, nutrition and maintaining a cool environment. Wearing soft and well-ventilated footwear can also help.

4. **H – *Staphylococcus aureus*.** Staphylococcal scalded skin syndrome or bollous impetigo occurs as a result of *Staphylococcus aureus* infection. Simply stating impetigo is non-specific and therefore it is not the right answer. Epidermolytic exotoxins A and B produced by *S. aureus* cause detachment in the epidermal layers, usually between the stratum granulosum and spinosum. The case above describes a classic history of prodromal systemic illness with respiratory tract infection, pyrexia and malaise leading to skin manifestation. Because of the history, an external chemical injury is unlikely to be the cause of her blisters and erythema. Toddlers, who have not yet developed antibodies against staphylococcal toxins, are vulnerable to staphylococcal scalded skin syndrome as are immunocompromised adults. Clinical examination reveals two key features: rapidly enlarging erythematous skin with mucous membrane sparing and bullae containing yellowish or turbid fluid. Lymphadenopathy may also be found. Diagnosis is usually clinical, however culture of the lesions usually grow group A streptococcus. Microscopy also shows Gram-positive cocci within blister fluid. Note in the example given that the young girl's thumb is swollen – this is an indication the ulceration is penetrating past the stratum corneum and into full thickness, known as ecthyma. She requires prompt treatment with systemic antibiotics such as benzylpenicillin or erythromycin as well as topical treatment with mupirocin. Healing can still occur in ecthyma,

but with scarring. In severe cases, when large areas of the skin are affected, infants should be treated at a specialised burn centre. They will require adequate fluid re-hydration as the loss of large areas of the epidermis will make the patients prone to dehydration and infection.

5. **B – Congestive cardiac failure**. This patient has dyspnoea, cough, a history of coronary heart disease and dependent oedema. Peripheral oedema in severe cardiac failure can result in the formation of bullae and vesicles on the legs due to serious water retention. This is also the most likely cause of his rapid weight gain. Underlying skin appears shiny and fluid leaks from the legs. Little can be done from a dermatological perspective for this patient. However, these patients do appear in dermatology clinics and a thorough medical clerking is essential to diagnosis. Symptoms will subside with appropriate management of heart failure including, but not limited to the use of diuretics.

   Toxic epidermal necrolysis (TEN) is a rare dermatological condition characterised by loss of the epidermal layer of skin in the entire body. In about 95% of cases this is as a result of a reaction to a pharmacological agent. Common medications implicated in TEN are NSAIDs, anticonvulsants (phenytoin, sodium valproate and carbamazepine), methotrexate, allopurinol, penicillins and sulfonamides. Mortality is around 30%. High mortality ratios are associated in patients with lung involvement and pneumonia secondary to damage of the airway linings. Treatment should be in a specialised dermatological or burns unit with Level 2 (high dependency unit) or Level 3 (intensive therapy unit) care. Patients may develop ulcerations in their mouth and necessitate nutritional support and nasogastric feeding. Intravenous immunoglobulins have a role in treatment.

A   Dermatology A22 – Pruritus

Pruritus is the experience of itching. The mechanism of production of an itch is not entirely known. Its aetiology stems from various bodily structures. Stimuli vary; most implicated are histamine and some proteinases. The sensation can be enhanced by prostaglandins and higher centres including boredom and stress. Pruritus can be categorised as localised, generalised or 'senile'. In general, definitive treatment of pruritus is by targeting the underlying cause. In general, treatment usually involves skin hydration with emollients, short-term use of topical steroids and sedating antihistamines. Hypnotics or neuroleptics may be required if pruritus causes agitation and sleeplessness. Patients with pruritus alone will respond to lower doses of neuroleptics than those required in psychiatric illnesses. It is important to take pruritus in patients seriously – not only could they be an indication of many underlying systemic diseases but they also cause intense discomfort to patients, causing insomnia and depression.

1. **A – Anogenital pruritus** refers to localised itching with two common presentations – pruritus ani, involving the perianal region, and pruritus vulvae, involving the vulva and perineum. The former is often associated with anal skin tags, fissures, haemorrhoids, foreign bodies and laxative abuse. This is because mucous or faeculent leaks cause irritation, and thereby, pruritus. Other associations are threadworm infections in children, ano-rectal carcinomas and contact dermatitis. Majority of patients are male and experience spasmodic bouts of itching, with excoriation marks evident of the intensity of the itch. Sedentary occupations are also associated with this presentation as well as patients with histories of skin disorders such as psoriasis and eczema. Clinical examination may identify peri-anal lesions, intetrigo, erythema, erosions and/or simply excoriation marks alone. Treatment involves hygiene advice, high fibre diet, local anaesthetics and antihistamines as discussed above. In the patient in this scenario, haemorrhoids are the likely underlying cause and treatment can reduce anal discharge and thus pruritus. He should be advised to keep the area cleaned regularly with soaked gauze or cotton.

2. **D – Lichen simplex**. The correct answer is lichen simplex. Constant, localised irritation leading to constant scratching can cause thickening of the skin and asymmetrical lesions. The constant itching can be habitual or triggered by stress. Plaques formed as a result of this are known as lichen simplex chronicus, sometimes referred to as 'neurodermatitis'. Nodules may also form, called prurigo. These lichenified lesions are commonly on palms and ears in both sexes; shins, ankles, scrotum and perianal area in men; forearms, nape of neck (lichen nuchae) and vulvae in women. Of note, smooth, shiny, seemingly polished fingernails are present due to constant rubbing. No clear cause of irritation is ever found, though stress is a known association. Treatment is as above for pruritus, usually with topical steroids under occlusive bandages to prevent further scratching. Tar paste can be of use. Occasionally, cognitive behavioural therapy may also be required. Pretibial myxoedema is rarely pruritic. Also, the patient in the example given had no history or clinical signs and symptoms of Graves' disease.

3. **B – Dermatitis herpetiformis**. This is an autoimmune disease most common in midlife, although it can occur from 20 to 60 years of age, associated with erythematous papules and vesicles. The key presentation is pruritus over extensor surfaces including the elbow, knees, shins, shoulders and scalp. Vesicles appear a few hours later arranging themselves in groups – hence the term herpetiformis. Symptoms can be exacerbated by gluten and iodides. Scratching will cause crusting and later hyper or hypopigmentation. Pathogenesis is unclear, however patients usually have gluten-sensitive enteropathy as with the gentleman described, whose history is likely coeliac disease. Investigation via biopsy – particularly of early papules – is preferable. It is often difficult to find intact vesicles on patients due to intense scratching. Microabscesses are found on biopsy, consisting of eosinophils and polymorphonuclear cells. In severe cases, one may have dermal infiltration. Granular IgA on immunoflurescence of peri-lesional skin (samples taken from the buttocks are best) is diagnostic. Anti-basement membrane antibodies are usually not detected in serum. Endomysial antibodies are found in most patients with concurrecnt coeliac disease and are highly sensitive. These key features from biopsied lesions are summarised shortly. Treatment involves sulphones, most commonly dapsone. Side effects include haemolysis and it is important to check G6PD level and methemoglobin levels before and during management. Sulphapyridine or sulphamethoxypyridine can also be used with careful monitoring of renal function. The patient in this example could also be started on a gluten-free diet to decrease symptoms and prevent possible progression to gut lymphoma and other malignancies. An important differential in this presentation is linear dermatosis – linear IgA deposits at dermal-epidermal junction. The key difference here is the *lack* of association with gluten diet. Linear dermatosis often occurs at puberty and can also involve the mucosa. The disease responds to dapsone and sulfapryridine and low-dose prednisolone, *not* gluten-free diet. Table 15 summarises the biopsy findings of dermatitis herpetiformis.

TABLE 15 Biopsy findings of dermatitis herpetiformis

Biopsy site	Investigation
New pink papule (preferable to blister)	Histopathology: neutophil microabcesses at dermal papillary tips at edge of vesicle
Normal skin	Immunofluorescence: granular IgA deposits in dermal papillary tips/basement membranes
Jejunum	Histopathology: villous atrophy, lymphocytic infiltration

4. **J – Wickham's striae**. The patient in this example is suffering from lichen planus (LP). LP is an acute or chronic inflammatory disease involving the skin and mucosa. *Planus* is Latin for flat. Lesions appear as a 'rash' of pink or violet, polygonal, shiny papules. Remember the Ps: purple/pink, polygonal, pruritic, papules. Lesions tend to occur in midlife and are more common in Afro-Caribbean populations and in females. Usually starting as a widespread eruption followed by coalescence into larger lesions, they can last from several weeks to years. LP occurs over the trunk and flexor aspects of the hand, shin scalp and penis. Oral mucosa can also be involved in 40%–60% of patients and are considered to be an indication of severe LP along with hypertrophy of lesions. Wickham striae are a clinical sign where white lines appear on papules when oil is dabbed on them. Some are hyperkeratotic. Examinations reveal prominent white lines in a usually reticular pattern and some erosions involving the buccal mucosa, tongue and/or gingiva. Oral LP can be precancerous and must be monitored. As lesions heal they become hyperpigmented. The cause of LP is largely idiopathic; however, drugs and minerals such as gold and mercury may trigger it as well. Treatment is aimed at reducing pruritus and reversing lesion – with topical steroids and if necessary, antihistamines. Tar-preparation can also be used. Acetretin can also be used in severe cases as an adjuvant. Erosive oral lesions may be treated with vitamin A gel. When lesions heal, areas of hyperpigmentation are left behind.

5. **G – Primary biliary cirrhosis**. Many systemic illnesses present with pruritus, therefore a systems review when clerking patients is essential. The patient above presented with primary biliary cirrhosis (PBC). This disease is a progressive destruction of intrahepatic bile ducts, leading to a build-up of bile and, over time, causing damage to hepatic tissue. PBC is thought to be an autoimmune disorder. A classical presentation of advanced PBC would be in a middle-aged woman presenting pruritus, jaundice, hepatosplenomegaly, and xanthelasma from hypercholesterolaemia. Serum blood tests will be positive for anti-mitochondrial antibodies in a majority of patients and show deranged liver function tests where alkaline phosphatase will be raised. Biopsy of the liver shows inflammation and loss of bile ducts, fibrosis and eventually cirrhosis in advanced disease. Management is with replacement of bile with ursodeoxycolic acid and reabsorption of excess bile acids with cholestyramine. Fat-soluble vitamins A, D and K need to be supplemented, as absorption is impaired. PBC in asymptomatic patients have a close to normal life expectancy if managed appropriately. However, symptomatic patients require transplantation eventually.

Table 16 summarises the causes of pruritus.

TABLE 16 Examples of causes of pruritis

Cause	Examples
Hepatic disease	Biliary disease, cholestasis in pregnancy
Infestations	Scabies, onchocerciasis, hookworm, *Candida*
Pharmaceuticals	Sensitivities to drugs, e.g. aspirin, morphine, alcohol
Malignancy	Leukaemia, multiple myeloma, lymphoma
Metabolic and endocrine	Diabetes mellitus, chronic renal failure, hyper-/hypothyroidism
Haematological disorders	Polycythemia rubra vera and iron deficiency
Psychogenic	Stress, delusions of parasitosis, neurotic excoriations
Environmental factors	Cold weather and low humidity, alkaline soaps

A Dermatology A23 – Skin infestations

1. **I – Topical antifungal and steroid cream**. Tinea pedis, commonly called athlete's foot, is a common dermatophyte infection that manifests in between toes, typically affecting young males. Predisposing factors include prolonged wearing of occlusive footwear, patients with hyperhydrosis and hot weather. It is usually transmitted in moist areas where people are barefoot such as communal showers. The patient has the risk factors of use of athletic shoes and possibly communal showers. Patients typically present with scaling, erythematous and macerating skin in the interdigital spaces. Lesions appear as annular erythematous, scaly plaques with a central clearing. Infection can spread to sites such as the hands (tinea mannum), the inguinal region (tinea cruris) and trunk (tinea corporis). Diagnosis is often clinical; however, if in doubt, the potassium hydroxide test shows the presence of hyphae confirming fungal infection. Treatment is with topical antifungals such as terbinafine, clotrimazole, econazole, ketoconazole and miconazole. Mild steroid cream can also be of benefit in this patient due to the extent of inflammation described. Contaminated socks and footwear must be washed in hot water. Patients should also be advised to keep their feet dry, wear cotton socks and use anti-mycotic powders. However, if there is nail involvement, oral treatment is necessary. It is important to treat tinea pedis, as a break in skin allows the invasion of bacteria such as *Staphylococcus aureus*.

2. **J – Topical antifungal and zinc lotion**. The patient in the example given has classic intertrigo. This is inflammation of skin surfaces in apposition. Supparative *Candida* infection of the area is common in most cases, as described in the example. Obese individuals are more succepitble to it as hot, humid areas with increased sweating worsen intertrigo. It is therefore often found in the submammary, groin and intergluteal areas. Patients with diabetes are also at risk. On examination, one would find shiny well-demarcated erythematous areas with satellite lesions of scaly foci. The scaly margins and foci are indicative of *Candida* infection. Potassium hydroxide test (potassium hydroxide) of skin scraping may be carried out to confirm fungal involvement. Treatment is with regular zinc lotion or burow (aluminium acetate) solution and topical antifungals such as miconazole or clotrimazole. Patients are also advised to dry themselves thouroghly after washing. Once healed, powders and linen gauze are advised in order to keep areas dry. Weight reduction is necessary in obese patients.

3. **B – *Cornybacterium minutissimum***. This is a Gram-positive rod part of normal skin flora responsible for erythrasma. It is a harmless, often chronic disease and an essential differential for intertrigo, discussed above. Erythrasma commonly occurs in the axillae, webspaces and inguinal region. Patients tend to be obese, elderly and/or diabetic. It presents as a red-to-brown lesion, initially smooth, that later shows fine scaling. Unlike intertrigo, erythrasma is unlikely to cause weeping or itching or satellite lesions. Diagnosis is made usually on clinical history. However, under Wood's light, lesions appear as a fluorescent coral-red. Wood's lamp is an essential tool for the dermatologist. It is simply a blacklight/ultraviolet lamp that causes certain organisms to fluoresce. Cultures from the affected area grow *Cornybacterium minutissimum*, and though rarely done, may be essential to rule out *Staphylococcus aureus* and/or 1. Treatment is with topical imidazole derivatives for Gram-positive bacteria and benzoyl peroxide. Systemic erythromycin and tetracycline are effective but not usually necessary. There are usually no known complications of this infection, though it may last from weeks to months. Patients are advised, as with intertrigo, to keep affected areas dry. Antibacterial soaps may also be of benefit.

4. **F – Scabies** is caused by infestation of the mite *Sarcoptes scabei*. Caused by skin-to-skin contact; young adults, bed-ridden patients and toddlers are most vulnerable. However, being highly infectious, it affects all social levels. *S. scabaei* thrive on and multiply in human skin only, burrowing (usually at night) into the skin as far as the stratum granulosum 2–3 mm daily. Eggs

are laid during the lifespan of the mite (4–6 weeks), laying about 50 eggs in the process. They hatch in 3–5 days. This is a major public health problem. They can remain alive in bedding and clothing for 2 days. Incubation period is 21 days. The risk of scabies in hospitals is directly proportional to age and size of the institution and inversely proportional to the ratio of beds to health care workers. Pruritis occurs as a result of sensitisation to *S. scabaei*. It is important to check household members and sexual partners. Generally patients present with persistent, intense pruritus, sparing the head and neck. On examination, lesions appear as grey or skin-coloured papules at the burrow site. These are minute elevations with a 'halo' of erythema. Later, these lesions develop weeping yellow crusts and patients complain of pain and pruritus. Burrows are usually in areas of few or no hair follicles – finger webs, wrists, feet, genitalia and buttocks. It is significant diagnostically when papules present on the shaft of the penis in men and in the mamillary region in women. Diagnosis is usually clinical. However, scrapings of burrows will demonstrate mites under microscopy. Scabies is managed by treating the individual and contacts within the last month, if possible. Scabicides/acaricides such as permethrin 5%, malathion 0.5% cream can be applied to all skin sites from the neck down. It is then washed off after 12–24 hours. Patients are advised to avoid hot baths prior to application, in order to prevent systemic absorption. The British National Formulary recommends applying scabicides twice, 1 week apart. Note that pruritus can continue for several days post treatment. Antihistamines may therefore be of use.

5. **C – Pediculus humanus capitis**, commonly called pediculosis or head lice. Lice affect the scalp, occiput and behind the ears. Lice continue to be fairly common, with outbreaks occurring from time to time in communities, particularly schools and in urban more than rural areas. These present as yellow crusty excoriations associated with pruritis. Children may also be restless and inattentive. The route of transmission is direct, head-to-head contact with a person infected with lice. Transmission can also occur indirectly with clothing, bedding and brushes. Examination with a magnifying glass shows 1 mm nits (a nit is the egg of a louse) close to the scalp and lice up to 4 mm long. Live lice are required for confirmation of diagnosis. Lifespan on non-eradicated lice is about 30 days. Lice are also found in neglected patients. Three types of lice are pathogenic in humans:
   - Pediculus humanus capitis – head lice, discussed above.
   - Pediculus humanus corporis – body lice. Associated with lower socio-economic groups, poor hygiene and crowded environments. Louse

bites provoke itching and the result is excoriation marks and papules, making skin hyper and hypopigmented. This is called 'vagabond skin'. Examination of clothing shows lice in the seams.

- Pediculus pubis – pubic lice or 'crabs', most commonly affecting the pubic areas but also other hair-bearing areas including the eyelids and axillae. PP most commonly affect young adults in close contact, such as sexual partners. As such, screening for sexually transmitted diseases may be indicated.

Preferred treatment is with the insecticide malathion. Pyrethroids such as permethrin and phenothrin, and carbaryl can also be used. Reapplication is recommended 7 days later. As described in the question, wet-combing, at least twice per week until three consecutive brushes are clear is required. Dimeticone lotion may also be used as third-line treatment. Vinegar is believed to help in the management of head lice and patients will often ask clinicians about it. Vinegar does not kill lice but may loosen nit attachment to hair, though evidence is weak. Prevention of spread is to examine contacts and treat accordingly as well as rewashing clothing and bedding.

A Dermatology A24 – Hair and nails

1. **D – Hypothyroidism with alopecia**. Alopecia is a chronic autoimmune disorder affecting hair follicles leading to hair loss. It is often associated with other autoimmune conditions such as thyroid disease and vitiligo. It can occur at any age but most commonly between 10 and 30 years. Alopecia can be categorised into scarring and non-scarring alopecia. The scarring form is irreversible and the non-scarring form may be reversible if the underlying disorder causing it is treated. There is a characteristic presentation in alopecia areata; there are round or oval areas of balding, commonly on the scalp or beard. 'Exclamation mark' hairs are pathognomonic at the edges of the bald patch; the hair is narrow and less pigmented and broken off about 4 mm from the scalp. These hairs may easily detach by mild traction. There is typically no inflammation, scarring or scaling. Spontaneous re-growth usually occurs, albeit slowly. Re-growing hairs appear in the centre of the bald patch and may be white. Conversely, the hair loss may involve the whole scalp (alopecia totalis) and the entire face and body (alopecia universalis). There can also be nail involvement in 50% of patients that may indicate extensive disease. Nails are roughened with subtle regular pitting (trachyonychia). Investigations are not usually necessary. Organ-specific antibodies may be demonstrated, although do

not alter management. Topical, intralesional and/or systemic steroids can be used but they are of limited use. Topical immunotherapy such as contact sensitisers (e.g diphencyprone), irritants and PUVA (psoralen with ultra-violet A treatment) may also help. In other localised alopecia conditions, such as traction alopecia, there may be broken hairs but not the typical 'exclamation mark' hair. Tinea captius (fungal infection of the scalp) also presents with scaling of the scalp. Telogen effluvium (thinning and shed-ding of hair due to premature entry of the hair follicle into the resting phase (telogen phase) of its growth cycle) may occur during pregnancy. There is increase in hair follicles during the pregnancy and a shedding after birth, giving rise to hair thinning.

2. **G – Polycystic ovaries**. Hirsutism is the growth of terminal hair in females that has a male-pattern distribution. These areas include the beard, the shoulders, the chest, around the nipples and in the male pattern on the abdomen and pubic region. The hairs are darker, coarser and thicker. Hirsutism is typically caused by increased androgen levels. Endocrine disorders of the pituitary, adrenals or ovaries can lead to hirsutism such as acromegaly, Cushing's and virilising tumours, respectively. The most common causes are idiopathic and polycystic ovarian syndrome (PCOS). Other causes include iatrogenic, such as androgenic drug. If the patient has a regular menstrual cycle, then an endocrine disorder will be unlikely and the patient's hirsutism is probably idiopathic. Treatment with these cases involves hair removal remedies such as waxing, shaving and laser therapy. If there is menstrual irregularity (oligomenorrhea or amenorrhoea), then a full endocrine workup should be performed (hormonal profile including testosterone, cortisol, sex hormone-binding globulin, follicle-stimulating hormone and luteinizing hormone). The patient should be referred for a transvaginal ultrasound of the ovaries and an abdominal ultrasound of the adrenals if the history deems necessary. Management depends on the cause of endocrine dysfunction. In PCOS, dianette oral contraceptive, which contains the anti-androgen cyproterone acetate, can be used if the patient does not have fertility aspirations. It must be used for at least 6 months before any improvement is seen. The patient in this scenario presented with the typical symptoms of PCOS. Patients may also present with acne. Being overweight propagates the disease but it is not a consequence of PCOS. Cushing's disease presents with hirsutism and menstrual irregu-larity, centripetal obesity and a 'moon' plethoric face, thin and easily bruised skin. Hypertrichosis refers to generalised increased growth of terminal hair and does not follow the androgen-induced pattern. This is

caused by drugs such as phenytoin, thyroid disease and the paraneoplastic syndrome.

3. **J – Tinea unguium**. Tinea unguium is a fungal infection of the nails. It is usually associated with tinea pedis or tinea of the surrounding skin. It is very common and is thus often found incidentally. The initial changes occur at the free edge of the nail, with yellow colouring, thickening and crumbling. This then spreads down the nail bed to the cuticle. Separation of the nail from its bed may follow (subungual hyperkeratosis). Microscopy and culture of nail clippings will confirm the diagnosis. Treatment involves systemic antifungal therapy; however, there are topical nail preparations such as amorolfine and tioconazole solutions that may be trialed initially. Tinea unguium is sometimes confused with psoriasis of the nails; however distinguishing features include asymmetry, tinea of surrounding skin and lack of pitting. The history of hip pathology given in the question is a red herring and depicts the way tinea unguium is commonly incidentally diagnosed.

4. **A – Alopecia with punctate leukonychia**. Leukonychia is the white discolouration of the nail and the surfacing of the nail from its nail bed. Leukonychia presentations can be subdivided into total and partial. Total leukonychia is where the whole nail is white. It can be associated with systemic diseases where it is a sign of hypoalbuminaemia. Conditions with low albumin levels include liver disease, nephrotic syndrome, chronic inflammatory disease (e.g ulcerative colitis) and sepsis. It can also be caused by a rare autosomal dominant condition: Bart–Pumphrey syndrome. This condition consists of total leukonychia, sensorineural hearing loss, knuckle pads and palmoplantar keratoderma. Partial leukonychia is commonly caused by trauma. It can be classified into three morphological variants: punctuate, transverse and longitudinal. Punctuate leukonychia is the most common form and is characterised by small white spots on the nail. It can be a completely normal finding, although can also be seen in alopecia areata and is found increasingly in nail-biting individuals. Transverse leukonychia is seen in patients with frequent manicures (transverse white lines across the nail that run parallel to the lunula) and longitudinal leukonychia is seen in Darier's disease (autosomal dominant condition characterised by dark keratotic papules that may affect in part of the skin). Notice, although this scenario is exemplifying a patient with an alcoholic addiction and possible subsequent cirrhosis, she has no other signs except leukonychia and alopecia, so there is no reason to believe at this stage that she is suffering

from liver damage without any further information (e.g blood tests, scans, and clinical signs of decompensated liver disease).

5. **I – Thyroid acropachy** describes rare hand changes seen in Graves' disease. These include clubbing, periosteal new bone formation and swelling of the fingers. Thyroid acropachy is often associated with the other typical features seen only in Graves' – namely, pretibial myxoedema and the eye signs (exopthalmos and opthalmoplegia). As is commonly seen with Graves' disease, the patient in the scenario has another autoimmune disease, pernicious anaemia.

Nail terms are as follows:
- *Paronychia* – nail infection.
- *Koilonychia* describes thin, spoon-shaped nails. This is a sign of iron deficiency anaemia. Rarely, it is congenital.
- *Onycholysis* is the distal detachment of the nail from its bed. It occurs in psoriasis and in hyperthyroidism.
- *Yellow-nail syndrome* is a rare condition affecting lymphatic drainage associated with compromised respiratory function such as bronchiectasis and pleural effusions, or lymphodema of the legs. The nails are usually thickened and yellow/green.
- *Clubbing* is associated with several medical conditions and has three key features: (1) loss of the normal angle between the nailbed and the nail fold, (2) increased curvature of the nail, and (3) softening and fluctuation of the base of the nail (increased ballotability).

An easy way to remember the causes:
A – Abscess, Asbestosis
B – Bronchiectasis, inflammatory Bowel disease
C – Cystic fibrosis, Cancer (bronchial + mesethilioma), Cirrhosis, Cyanotic Congenital heart disease
D – Drugs (e.g. laxative abuse)
E – Empyema, Endocarditis
F – Fibrosing alveolitis

A   **Dermatology A25 – Dermatological disorders II**

1. **E – Lichen sclerosis** is a chronic atrophic condition, characterised by scarring and inflammatory dermatosis, commonly of the vulva and perianal skin. Normal elastic tissue is replaced with hard collagen. The cause

is unknown but it is associated with autoimmune disease. Lichen sclerosis may coexist with morphoea (localised scleroderma characterised by thickening of skin due to excessive collagen deposition). It is more common in women and their peak incidence occurs in children and around the menopause, indicating a hormonal influence in the disease process. Patients present with white non-indurated plaques with follicular plugging, hence the alternative name of the disease, 'white spot disease'. The lesions may coalesce forming atrophic areas of skin that may become purpuric. Bullae can form and cause ulceration. The lesions may be itchy. In the most frequently affected site, the genital tissue, there may be shrinkage and architectural distortion. The genital organs can be so severely affected that in females the labia minora is lost, the clitoris is buried and the introitus is significantly restricted. In men, there is some degree of phimosis, adhesion formation between the foreskin and the glans penis, and stenosis of the urethral meatus. Extragenital affected sites are most commonly the neck and upper back. Children presenting with genital lichen sclerosis complain of discomfort and bleeding that can sometimes be misdiagnosed as childhood sexual abuse. Diagnosis is usually clinical, although a skin biopsy is indicated for unclear cases. Topical steroids may be necessary for symptomatic genital lesions and may reduce scarring. Emollients and soap substitutes are also recommended. In men, circumcision may be curative. The presence of lichen sclerosis is a risk for vulval carcinoma and can develop in up to 5%. Patients should be followed up long term for pre-malignant change. Lichen planus is sometimes confused with lichen sclerosis because of similarity in terms, but they present very differently. Lichen planus affects the skin, mucous membranes and genitalia. White lacey lines or plaques are found in the latter sites. The lesions of skin in lichen planus are violaceous, flat-topped, shiny, itchy papules. A white streak pattern can be seen on the surfaces of these papules (Wickham's striae). Lichen planus presents with either hypertrophic, hyperkeratotic plaques or erosive disease. Clobetasol diproprionate cream, a topical corticosteroid, is the mainstay of treatment and requires regular long-term application. Vulval ablation is another treatment option that relieves the sensation of itching. By menarche, 50% of children with lichen sclerosis become asymptomatic.

2. **F – Pemphigoid.** Bullous pemphigoid is a chronic autoimmune blistering disorder caused by circulating IgG autoantibodies against the dermo-epidermal junction. It is mainly a disease of the elderly. It is characterised by large tense blisters on an erythematous urticarial area.

The flexure regions of the limbs are commonly affected. The lesions are itchy rather than painful. The blisters can remain intact for several days before haemorrhaging. Nikolsky's sign is negative. Oral lesions are rare; however, there is a variant of pemphigoid, known as mucous membrane pemphigoid that specifically targets the oral mucosa, conjunctivae, and other mucous membranes of internal structures. Investigations include skin biopsy, bullous pemphigoid antigen identification (BP1 and BP2) and immunofluorescence of perilesional skin. Direct immunofluorescence demonstrates IgG and complement deposition in a linear band along the basement membrane and indirect immunofluorescence demonstrates circulating antibodies specific to this site. Pemphigoid is usually self-limiting; however, in the acute phase steroids are required. Localised disease may respond to topical steroid therapy, although widespread disease requires high-dose systemic steroids. Steroid sparing agents, such as azathioprine, may also be used with steroids or as monotherapy for severe disease. If the condition is mild, patients may respond to dapsone alone. Pemphigus is a term that is sometimes confused with pemphigoid. They are both autoimmune blistering diseases, although pemphigus blisters are more flaccid and rupture easily by pressure or friction, although unlike pemphigoid, they are not haemorrhagic. When pemphigus blisters rupture, they form widespread raw areas, erosions and crusts that are painful but not itchy. Nikolsky's sign is positive – lateral pressure on the skin causes the epidermis to glide over the dermis revealing a raw region. In contrast, mucous membranes are commonly affected. Pemphigus IF studies show intercellular epidermal IgG and complement deposits.

3. **C – Keloid scar**. A keloid is characterised by excessive collagen production and an exaggerated growth of dense connective tissue in the skin in response to injury. There is a significant genetic factor in keloid development. Keloids are more common in young adult Afro-Caribbeans and may be familial. Individuals of darker skin are more likely to be affected than individuals with lighter skin by fifteen folds. It affects males and females equally and rarely occurs in extremes of age. Injuries that typically lead to keloid in susceptible individuals include trauma, surgical wound sites and infection. Sites of predilection include upper back and trunk, shoulders, neck and ears. In at-risk patients, non-essential surgeries should be best avoided at these sites. Keloid scars are firm rubber-like fibrous, shiny growths over and beyond the original scars. They can be the same colour as the skin, or darker red or brown. Keloids may be itchy and painful. Hypertrophic scars are also raised scars, although as highlighted, keloids

extend beyond the primary site of insult compared to hypertrophic scars that remain confined to the site of initial damage. While hypertrophic scars may improve within 12 months, keloids are persistent and only occasionally fade with time. Investigations are not necessary; diagnosis is clinical. Treatment for small lesions involves compression with silicone oil or gel dressings that could sometimes be applied for 24 hours a day and up to a year. Compression dressings are another management option that has shown positive outcomes. Intralesional steroid injections have been the mainstay of treatment; they work by inhibiting collagenase inhibitors and thus reducing collagen production. Five-year recurrence rates range from 10% to 50% with steroid injections. Surgical excision may be an option, although keloids often recur unless followed by intralesional steroid injection or post-operative radiotherapy. Combined treatment in the form of surgery, steroid injections and pressure dressings has a response rate of 90%–100%.

4. **J – Strawberry haemangiomas** are benign proliferative tumours of the vascular endothelium, occurring in early infancy. They are not usually apparent at birth but appear in the first few weeks, then grow rapidly for a few months during the first year of life and then clear spontaneously over the next 3–4 years. They occur in 10% of infants and are more common in females. They most often develop on the head and neck. They may be superficial (strawberry haemangiomas), deep (cavernous haemangiomas) or mixed depending on the depth of involved blood vessels. The superficial lesions are bright red compressible swellings and the deeper lesions have a bluer shade. When spontaneous regression occurs, the surface fades and whitens centrally. In half of children, regression is complete at 5 years and 90% of children are clear by the age of 9 years. Occasionally, there is a residual area of whitened atrophy. Deeper cavernous angiomas do not shrink as completely and resolution is often not complete. Seldom they are very large and may bleed following trauma or ulcerate. Periocular haemangiomas may obstruct vision, which may lead to blindness in the affected eye. Management involves serial monitoring and observation. The larger lesions may respond to intralesional or systemic steroids. If the above measures fail and spontaneous regression has not occurred, surgery may be necessary for the larger unsightly haemangiomas. Port wine stains are sometimes confused with strawberry naevi. Unlike haemangiomas, port wine stains are caused by dilated superficial dermal capillaries and are visible at birth. They are unilateral pink or purple flat macules over the face and neck. If the port wine stain affects the trigeminal area, Sturge–Weber

syndrome may develop where there is vascular malformation of the ipsi-lateral leptomeninges. This may lead to epilepsy or hemiparesis.

5. **H – Polymorphic eruption of pregnancy** is a benign dermatosis that occurs in pregnancy in less than 1% of women. The cause is unknown but it is commoner in primips and twin pregnancies. It typically appears in the last trimester and presents with exceptionally itchy urticarial papules, plaques and small vesicles located on the abdomen and within the striae. There is sparing of the periumbilical region. Within a few days the lesions may spread to the proximal arms and legs. There is no maternal or fetal adverse consequences associated with this rash. Management includes wet soaks, emollient creams and topical steroids to relieve the pruritis. Delivery is the cure of the rash. Prurigo of pregnancy also occurs in the third trimester of pregnancy, however it usually persists after delivery for a few months. The lesions are similarly intensely pruritic papules, although they are most commonly on the extensors of the extremities and occasion-ally on the abdomen. In polymorphic eruption of pregnancy, excoriations are rarely found, unlike prurigo of pregnancy where linear abrasions and crusting is seen.

Section C

ENT EMQs

Q ENT Q1 – ENT investigations I

A. Caloric tests
B. Distraction test
C. Dix–Hallpike manoeuvre
D. Epley manoeuvre
E. Evoked response audiometry
F. Impedance audiometry
G. Pure tone audiometry
H. Speech audiometry
I. Stenger test
J. Visual reinforcement audiometry

From the list above, choose the most appropriate investigation for each of the following examples.

1. The most reliable hearing test for a 3-month-old infant.
2. Most useful test to assess the presence of a middle ear effusion.
3. Most reliable hearing test for suspected malingerers.
4. Used in conjunction with pure tone audiometry for selection of appropriate hearing aid.
5. Used to diagnose benign paroxysmal positional vertigo.

Q ENT Q2 – ENT investigations II

A. Acoustic neuroma
B. Gentamicin toxicity
C. Glue ear
D. Ménière's syndrome
E. Nasopharyngeal carcinoma
F. Noise-induced hearing loss
G. Ossicular discontinuity
H. Otosclerosis
I. Presbycusis
J. Wegner's granulomatosis

From the list above, choose the most appropriate diagnosis for each of the following examples.

1. Sensorineural hearing loss of low-frequency sounds.
2. Sensorineural hearing loss predominantly around frequencies of 3–6 kHz.
3. High-frequency sensorineural hearing loss with oscillopsia.
4. Conductive hearing loss with the Carhart's notch.
5. Type B tympanogram.

ENT Q3 – Vertigo
A. Acoustic neuroma
B. Benign paroxysmal positional vertigo
C. Cerebellar infarction
D. Labyrinthitis
E. Lateral medullary syndrome
F. Ménière's disease
G. Migraine
H. Multiple sclerosis
I. Postural hypotension
J. Vestibular neuritis

From the list above, choose the most appropriate diagnosis for each of the following examples.

1. A 43-year-old woman presents to her GP complaining of episodes of severe dizziness. These episodes last for about 3 hours at a time, during which she feels everything around her to be spinning and she subsequently vomits. She also notices a ringing in both ears. She has a past medical history of irritable bowel syndrome, and takes senna occasionally. On examination, she does not have nystagmus, abnormal middle ear signs or loss of balance. Pure tone audiometry reveals sensorineural hearing loss, predominantly of the lower frequencies.

2. A 66-year-old man presents with sudden-onset vertigo that started 12 hours ago with associated severe nausea and vomiting. His wife tells you that he is unable to pronounce words clearly. The patient has Horner's syndrome, nystagmus, facial numbness and loss of pain and temperature sensation on the right side of his face. He does not complain of any hearing loss or tinnitus. He has a past medical history of multiple sclerosis, hypercholesterolemia and hypertension, but has been non-compliant with his medications in the past.

3. A 62-year-old man presents to his GP complaining of a sensation of intense dizziness and spinning that occurred this morning while driving his car. On further questioning, he mentions that he has noticed some hearing loss in the right ear over the past 6 months, and now prefers to hold his cellphone to the left ear. He has been experiencing a pulsatile tinnitus in the left ear as well as nausea and vomiting over the past 10 days or so. He has a past medical history of hypercholestrolaemia, type 2 diabetes mellitus,

hypertension and peripheral vascular disease. On examination, he does not have nystagmus or abnormal middle ear signs. Weber's test lateralises to the left ear. Rinne's test is positive in both ears.

4. A 56-year-old woman presents to her GP complaining of episodes of severe dizziness for the past week. On further questioning, she explains that when she sits up in bed she sees the whole bedroom spinning for about a minute or two and feels very nauseous. She does not complain of any hearing loss or tinnitus. No hearing loss can be detected with Rinne's and Weber's tests. She has a past medical history of head trauma that occurred 3 weeks ago after falling off her bike. She was seen in A&E and told that her head scans are normal.

5. A 37-year-old man presents to his GP with a 3-day history of vertigo, nausea and vomiting. The vertigo started rapidly and was worse in the first day. He thought he may have caught a nasty bug, but is now worried it might something more serious. He does not complain of tinnitus or hearing loss. He is normally fit and healthy, but smokes about 30 cigarettes a day. On examination, he has a bilateral nystagmus. No hearing loss can be detected with Rinne's and Weber's tests.

ENT Q4 – Otalgia

A. Acute otitis externa
B. Drug allergy
C. Furunculosis
D. Giant cell arteritis
E. Glue ear
F. Necrotising otitis externa
G. Oropharyngeal neoplasia
H. Referred pain
I. Temporo-mandibular joint dysfunction
J. Tonsillitis

From the list above, choose the most appropriate diagnosis for each of the following examples.

1. A 15-year-old girl is brought to the GP by her mother with a right earache. She has been complaining about earache since yesterday, but there has been no discharge or a temperature. She has a past medical history of a middle ear effusion, and has had a tonsillectomy 5 days ago. On examination, the patient is afebrile, and does not appear systemically unwell. Both the external ear canal and tympanic membrane look normal.

2. A 73-year-old lady presents to her GP with a severe right earache. This pain has been intermittent for a week. She also complains of pain on mouth opening, and there is tenderness on palpation of the muscles of mastication. Her ear is not red, swollen or tender. On examination, she is afebrile, and both the external and middle ear look normal on close inspection.

3. A 32-year-old man presents to his GP with a left earache and a sore throat. This started about a month ago, and if anything is getting worse. He is otherwise fit and well, and does not smoke or drink alcohol. On examination, he is afebrile and there are no signs of systemic upset. You cannot see an abnormality at the external or middle ears. On inspection of the throat, there is unilateral tonsillar enlargement with an overlying ulcer.

4. A 42-year-old man presents to his GP with a severe left earache. The ear began itching 3 days ago, and started to become painful yesterday. He has tried paracetamol with no avail, and his pain has severely worsened today. He is normally fit and healthy, and plays tennis or swims on an almost daily basis. He does not smoke or

drink alcohol. On examination, his outer ear is erythematous, and there is significant pus in his external ear canal.

5. The 42-year-old man in the previous example comes back to the GP 2 days later with a swollen, red, shiny and tender pinna. There is no ear discharge. On examination of his ear, the pus in the external auditory canal appears to have improved, and the eardrum looks normal. He feels unwell, however, and has a fever (38.1°C).

ENT Q5 – Dysphagia

A. Achalasia
B. Benign oesophageal stricture
C. Bulbar palsy
D. Globus pharyngeus
E. Laryngeal carcinoma
F. Oesophageal carcinoma
G. Oesophageal spasm
H. Pharyngeal pouch
I. Pseudobulbar palsy
J. Vocal cord palsy

From the list above, choose the most appropriate diagnosis for each of the following examples.

1. A 67-year-old man presents to his GP with his daughter complaining of difficulty in swallowing. He first noticed it about 3 or 4 months ago but was not keen to be seen by a doctor. His daughter visited him today and noticed he has developed a hoarse voice, and insisted that he seeks a medical opinion. On further questioning, his dysphagia has been getting worse, and has unintentionally lost about 8 kg over the past 3 months. He has a past medical history of coeliac disease. He also drinks about 35 units of alcohol weekly and smokes at least 30 cigarettes a day.

2. A 61-year-old man presents to his GP with difficulty in swallowing. He has been finding it increasingly difficult to swallow both solids and liquids over the past few weeks, and sometimes gets regurgitation of liquids back into his nose. You notice that his voice is hoarse and that his speech is slightly slurred. He has lost 3 kg in weight over the past few months unintentionally. He has a past medical history of gastro-oesophageal reflux disease. On examination, his tongue looks wasted, but he does not have any signs of cranial nerve lesions or peripheral neurological signs.

3. A 69-year-old man presents to his GP with difficulty in swallowing. It started about 2 months ago, and has since been getting worse. He does not get any chest pain or heartburn, and does not have pain on swallowing. Sometimes, he gets regurgitation of undigested food back into his mouth on lying down. He has also noticed that his breath smells worse, and is shy to be in close contact with people. He has not noticed any recent

weight loss. He has a past medical history of lymphoma, which has been treated. He also smokes about 25 cigarettes a day.

4. A 66-year-old woman presents to her GP complaining of a lump in her throat. She is worried it might be a cancer, and is scared to eat because of the lump. She can swallow foods and liquids normally if she tries, although she has noticed the discomfort is worse on swallowing saliva. She does not have pain on swallowing, and does not complain of any chest pain or heartburn. Her appetite is the same, and she does not think she has lost any weight over the past few months. She has a past medical history of gastro-oesophageal reflux disease.

5. A 61-year-old woman presents to her GP with difficulty in swallowing that has been getting worse over the past few weeks. She finds that swallowing anything is difficult, regardless of whether it is solid or liquid. She has also noticed some chest pains recently, especially after eating. She has not noticed any heartburn or pain on swallowing. She has a past medical history of premature ovarian failure and osteoporosis, and is otherwise fit and healthy. A barium swallow shows a dilated oesophagus that tapers at the lower oesophageal sphincter.

Q ENT Q6 – Hearing loss

A. Bilateral conductive deafness
B. Bilateral sensorineural deafness
C. Left-sided conductive deafness
D. Left-sided sensorineural deafness
E. Mixed right-sided conductive and sensorineural deafness
F. Normal hearing
G. Right-sided conductive deafness
H. Right-sided sensorineural deafness
I. Mixed left-sided conductive and sensorineural deafness
F. None of the above

From the list above, select the type of deafness from each of the following examination findings of patients presenting with hearing loss.

1. Rinne's test is positive on the left and negative on the right. Weber's test: vibration sound is heard louder on the right side.
2. Rinne's test is negative bilaterally. Weber's test: vibration sound is heard equally bilaterally.
3. Rinne's test is negative on the left, positive on the right. Weber's test: vibration sound is heard louder on the right side.
4. Rinne's test is positive bilaterally. Weber's test: vibration sound is heard louder on the left side.
5. Rinne's test is positive bilaterally. Weber's test: vibration sound is heard equally bilaterally.

Q ENT Q7 – Management of inner ear disorders

A. Brainstem evoked auditory response
B. Dix–Hallpike manoeuvre
C. Epley manoeuvre
D. Oral aciclovir and eye care
E. Oral aciclovir, corticosteroids and eye care
F. Plasmapheresis
G. Prochlorperazine
H. Reassurance, counselling and rehabilitation
I. Stenger test
J. Tell the patient that his/her hearing is better than described

From the list above, select the next line of treatment for each of the following examples.

1. A 45-year-old lady (Jehovah's Witness) attends the ENT clinic with vertigo, hearing loss and tinnitus for 3 years. This was initially intermittent and lasted for 20 minutes per episode. She has seen her GP who has prescribed betahistine, topical and oral steroids, and prochlorperazine. This did help some of the symptoms during the attacks. However, the symptoms are now constant with a persistent hearing loss bilaterally and a residual unsteadiness. Otoscopy appears normal, horizontal nystagmus is noted, Romberg's sign is positive and audiometry reveals bilateral sensorineural hearing loss. She does not want any invasive procedures done.

2. A 40-year-old gentleman presents with a 3-day history of vertigo, and was brought in by his concerned partner after noticing that he was drooling and unable to close his right eye. On questioning he reveals that he has been having a mild sharp pain in his right ear for 2 days. On examination there is an obvious right-sided facial droop. Romberg's sign is positive, and Unterberger's test is positive with the patient rotating to the right side. Otoscopy shows small vesicles within the right external auditory canal, and a normal tympanic membrane.

3. A 69-year-old lady is brought into hospital by her daughter. The patient has been lying in bed for a week now because she is afraid that she will have an episode of vertigo and injure herself. She has been getting the feeling of the room spinning every time she turns around in bed and when she sits up. She has vomited several

times. There is no hearing loss or tinnitus. The daughter enquires about a treatment for her condition.

4. A 36-year-old recently recovered from a sore throat, for which she was given oral antibiotics (penicillin V). For the past 2 days she has been experiencing episodes of vertigo that have been reducing in intensity. She would prefer not to take any medication for these symptoms.

5. A 12-year-old girl with a 1-year history of deteriorating school performance has presented to your ENT clinic after scoring poorly on a hearing test. Her pure tone audiogram indicates normal hearing, which is out of keeping with the severity of hearing loss elicited from the examination. What do you do next?

Q **ENT Q8 – Ear infections and their complications**

A. Acute mastoiditis

B. Acute otitis externa

C. Acute otitis media

D. Brain abscess

E. Cholesteatoma

F. Chronic suppurative otitis media

G. Facial paralysis

H. Meningitis

I. Otitis media with effusion

J. Recurrent otitis media

From the list above, select the most likely diagnosis for each of the following examples.

1. A 24-year-old lady presents with a 3-day history of severe left ear pain that has not settled with paracetamol. She experienced similar symptoms a month ago that resolved with oral antibiotics. She also admits to reduced hearing from the left ear. On examination, she has conductive deafness on the left side. There is no redness or tenderness around the pinna, but the tympanic membrane is red, inflamed and swollen.

2. A 6-year-old girl is brought into hospital by her concerned parents. She has been complaining of right ear pain for the past 2–3 weeks with associated pustular discharge from the ear. She has been given oral antibiotics by her GP for a 'middle ear infection'. In the last 2 days she has been crying constantly, and she has been spiking temperatures despite taking antipyretics. On examination, the pinna is deviated down and forwards. Otoscopy reveals a right auditory canal obscured by discharge.

3. A 19-year-old swimmer presents with constant sharp pain in her right ear that is worse on chewing or on touching her ear. She has had ear pains in the past, but this episode is much worse. On examination, movement of the pinna is very tender, the concha appears cellulitis. Otoscopy reveals a swollen, red canal that is debris abundant, and an intact inflamed tympanic membrane.

4. A 32-year-old gentleman presents to A&E complaining of a suddenly worsening headache that started mild and progressed over the last 2 weeks. This originated from a left earache, which improved with oral antibiotics given by his GP. He is pyrexial, and complains of new onset photophobia. On neurological

examination he has mild left-sided weakness, bilateral optic disc swelling, and a positive Kernig's sign.

5. A 15-year-old girl attends the ENT clinic as she has suffered from recurrent pustular discharge from her right ear for 2 years. She is not in any pain but states that she thinks hearing is reduced on the affected side. On examination, there is right-sided conductive hearing loss, mucoid discharge within the external auditory canal, and a small perforation on the lower, anterior section of the eardrum.

Q ENT Q9 – Management of middle ear disorders

A. Cochlear implant
B. Intravenous antibiotics
C. Mastoid abscess drainage
D. Mastoidectomy
E. Myringotomy
F. Oral antibiotics
G. Reassurance
H. Regular ear surveillance
I. Stapedectomy
J. Topical antibiotic ear drops

From the list above, select the most likely next line of treatment for each of the following examples.

1. A 24-year-old lady is referred to your ENT clinic from her GP. She presents with a 9-month history of worsening hearing loss. Her mother has been wearing hearing aids from the age of 38. On examination, Rinne's test is negative bilaterally. Otoscopy reveals a normal-looking tympanic membrane. She would like to discuss alternative treatment options to hearing aids.

2. A 4-year-old boy presents with a 3-day history of worsening right ear pain and runny nose. His parents state that he has been constantly tugging on his right ear and hasn't slept all night. On examination, he is pyrexial at 40.5°C, otoscopic findings suggest an inflamed, bulging tympanic membrane. There is no regional lymphadenopathy.

3. A 26-year-old gentleman presents after experiencing a sharp pain in his left ear during the landing of his flight from the United States. It is now 8 hours after landing and the pain has persisted. He also complains of mild hearing loss in the left ear. He has no tinnitus, discharge from the ear, or preceding symptoms. Otoscopic examination demonstrates blood within the external auditory canal and a small perforation in the tympanic membrane. There are no signs of any infection.

4. A 30-year-old male presents with an ongoing left ear pain that began a week ago. He visited his GP who gave him amoxicillin. He has completed a 5-day course but the pain is getting exceedingly worse. He is pyrexial at 39.6°C, has no regional lymphadenopathy; however, there is mastoid tenderness on deep

pressure palpation. Otoscopy reveals an inflamed bulging yellow tympanic membrane.

5. A 55-year-old gentleman presents with a foul-smelling flaky discharge from his right ear that has progressively increased over the last 5 months. He has also noticed a significant loss in hearing on the ipsilateral side. He has a history of recurrent ear infections. On examination the ear canal was filled with flaky discharge and a perforation is noted at the superior border of the attic.

Q **ENT Q10 – External ear disorders**
A. Acute mastoiditis
B. Acute otitis media
C. Bell's palsy
D. Cellulitis
E. Contact dermatitis
F. Exostosis
G. Furunculosis
H. Malignancy of the external auditory canal (EAC)
I. Necrotising otitis externa
J. Ramsay Hunt syndrome

From the list above, select the most likely diagnosis for each of the following examples.

1. A 68-year-old gentleman with a background of hypertension, diabetes mellitus and epilepsy presents to the emergency department with severe right ear pain that has been keeping him up all night. There is no discharge, hearing loss or vertigo. On examination, he is apyrexial, with a blood pressure of 176/110 mmHg, and a blood sugar level of 21.4 mmol/L. The right pinna appears normal and there is erythema and granulations seen on the floor of the external auditory canal. There is right-sided facial palsy without sparing of the forehead, and difficulty swallowing.

2. A 30-year-old lady presents with left ear pain for the last 3 days, getting progressively worse. There is no hearing loss, tinnitus or vertigo. On examination she is apyrexial, and the pinna appears normal, however it is extremely tender on movement. A localised red tender swelling is seen on the superior aspect of the outer canal and a normal tympanic membrane. There appears to be a small tender lump over the mastoid process.

3. A 72-year-old gentleman presents to the emergency department with left ear pain, and vertigo for the last 3 days. He has also noticed partial left-sided hearing loss. On examination he has a left-sided facial droop and reduced facial power without sparing of the forehead. A vesicular rash is noted in the concha and within the external auditory canal.

4. A 23-year-old lady presents with right ear itchiness and mild ear pain that started a week ago. She was seen by her GP 5 days ago and was given ear drops for otitis externa. She claims that her

symptoms have become significantly worse. On examination pinna appears erythematous and dry. This extends into the external canal.

5. An 82-year-old gentleman presents with severe right ear pain that started initially a year ago, but has progressively become worse. He also complains of dry right eye and drooling on the right side. On examination he has right preauricular lymphadenopathy as well as localised polypoid swelling and blood within the external auditory canal.

Q ENT Q11 – Hoarse voice and dysphonia

A. Arytenoid nerve
B. Bleeding mucosa
C. Counselling
D. Injection of muscle relaxants
E. Left recurrent laryngeal nerve
F. Neck CT scan
G. Perichondritis
H. Reinke's oedema
I. Right recurrent laryngeal nerve
J. Vocal cord cancer
K. Vocal cord nodule

From the list above, choose the most appropriate answer for each of the following examples.

1. A 45-year-old news presenter presents to the voice clinic with hoarseness. She is otherwise well and has no difficulty swallowing. She admits being a smoker with a 20-pack-year history. On examination, her voice is low-pitched and husky. On nasoendoscopy it is noted that the vocal cords are fluid-filled bilaterally. There are also polypoid changes at the anterior third of the right vocal cord. What is the most likely diagnosis?

2. Lulu is a singer, busking daily at an innercity train station. She presents to the ENT clinic with changes in her voice over the past few weeks. Her range is reduced and it is occasionally painful to sing. On examination, her voice is breathy and husky. This is not normal for Lulu. Laryngoscopy shows a smooth mass on the medial and upper third of the left vocal cord. She has no significant medical history and does not smoke. This is really affecting her work and career dreams and she hopes it is not permanent. What is the most likely diagnosis?

3. Mr Wilder has been referred to the voice clinic by his GP. Excerpts of the letter are as follows:

   Dear Colleague,

   Many thanks for seeing this unfortunate gentleman who presented to my practice with hoarseness and 'breaks' in his voice. He also complains of a sensation of something in his throat . . . He has recently been discharged from hospital following a 2-week stay in the intensive therapy unit with ventilator support secondary to an anterior myocardial infarction and massive pulmonary embolism.

On examination, his voice is harsh and hoarse. A pale, unilateral granulomatous lesion is seen on laryngoscopy at the posterior aspect of the vocal fold. With the history and examination what else would one find?

4. Mr Palmer presents to the ENT clinic for routine follow-up after his hemi-thyroidectomy. Since the surgery, he has noticed that his voice has become coarser. He also finds that the more he talks the worse his voice becomes in terms of quality. He also finds he has to strain to be heard. On scoping it is noted that his left vocal cord adducts with voice production, but the right remains in place. On coughing the right vocal cord 'bows out'. Which nerve is most likely to have been damaged intra-operatively?

5. Blake is a young banker who presents to clinic with a 'strained voice'. He also complains of neck pain and the sensation of a lump in his throat, making it difficult to swallow. On examination, he has no obvious neck lump but is tender on palpation. His vocal cords also appear normal on scoping. A gentle pull of his larynx downwards causes the pain to dissipate. Other than a busy lifestyle, Blake has no significant medical history and does not smoke. What is the most appropriate next step in managing this patient?

Q ENT Q12 – Rhinitis and sinusitis

A. Acute rhinosinusitis
B. Allergic rhinitis
C. Aspirin sensitivity
D. Chronic rhinosinusitis
E. *Klebsiella ozenae*
F. Porphyria
G. *Pseudomonas aeruginosa*
H. *Staphylococcus aureus*
I. Urgent CT scan, IV antibiotics and drainage
J. Urgent IV antibiotics, steroids and CT scan

From the list above, choose the most appropriate answer for each of the following examples.

1. Martha presents to her GP with a 'cold that won't go away'. For 3 weeks her nose has been running and she is constantly sneezing. She also complains of painful cheeks, worse on leaning forward. This is the first time she has experienced such a 'cold' and she is worried that something might be wrong. She has no history of asthma, allergies or recent trauma. Martha works as a banker in a highly stressful position. She admits she has recently been relieving tension with recreational drugs. On examination, there is clear mucous discharge from both nostrils. There is no evidence of swelling, however on palpation, Martha is tender over the infraorbital region. What is the diagnosis?

2. Samuel is 12 years old and has cystic fibrosis. His mother brings him to the ENT clinic, because he has had a runny nose for close to 4 months. She thought his symptoms would improve after the summer, but they have not changed. His nose is constantly running and he complains of a sore face. Samuel's sense of smell is also impaired. On examination, Samuel is in obvious discomfort, with bilateral discharge and inflammation of the nasal mucosa. There is no foreign body in his nose. What is the diagnosis?

3. Eight-year-old Sofyan's parents bring him to A&E. He is visibly distressed, with a temperature of 38.2°C. On examination his left eyelid is oedematous. With difficulty, he lets you open his eye, which is weepy, and there is obvious proptosis and chemosis. Sofyan's vision is impaired in the affected eye. He reports seeing double with pain on moving the eye. He is only able to read four of 17 Ishihara plates correctly with the left eye, and can read all

17 plates in the right. Sofyan's mother informs you that he has been unwell recently with sinus problems. Otherwise he has no significant medical history. What would the management of this patient involve?

4. 32-year-old Mr Marshall presents regularly to the ENT clinic. His nasal polyps have returned and are causing him great discomfort. He is having difficulty smelling things and it is becoming increasingly difficult to breathe through his nose. On examination, there are bilateral pendunculated polyps. Mr Marshall has had yearly polypectomies. He also developed asthma late in life. What would the other unique feature be to Mr Marshall's condition?

5. An 18-year-old female presents to clinic for review. As she enters the examination room, one is immediately aware of a foul smell from the patient. She is embarrassed by this and very distressed. She cannot smell it, but has been told and has seen people's reactions in her presence. She reports she has always had trouble with nasal congestion and had recently experienced episodes of nosebleeds. On examination of the nasal cavities, there is extensive green crusting on the mucosa with areas of pallor. Nasal turbinates also appear eroded. Removal of the crusts causes bleeding. What is the most likely causative organism?

Q ENT Q13 – Pharyngitis, tonsillitis, laryngitis and epiglottitis I

A. Amoxicillin

B. Bacterial tonsillitis

C. Gently but quickly asses patient's airway with a tongue depressor

D. Quinsy

E. Reassurance, analgesia, bed and voice rest

F. Splenic rupture

G. Steeple sign

H. Take patient to resuscitation room and contact senior anaesthetist and ENT surgeon

I. Thumbprint sign

J. Urinary tract infections

From the list above, choose the most appropriate answer for each of the following examples.

1. You are a junior doctor in A&E. Five-year-old Kofi arrives with his mother. Kofi has been unwell today with a sore throat. His mother reports she was nursing him at home with calpol and liquids. Now he has a fever and his breathing sounds 'strained'. He also can't seem to swallow his juice anymore and dribbles more than usual. On examination, Kofi looks pale and shocked and is in obvious discomfort. He is not talking or active and is leaning forward and drooling. His head is raised and his mouth is open as he struggles to breathe particularly on inspiration. The A&E nurse describes his breathing sound as 'stridor'. There is no obvious rash and he has no known allergies. What is your next step in the management of this patient?

2. It is January, and 1-year-old Sidath presents with his parents to the paediatric emergency unit. He has been suffering from a cold over the last 2 weeks this winter and hasn't been quite his happy self. He has a temperature of 37.8°C and respiratory rate of 30, and heart rate of 140. Of note, he also has a biphasic stridor, and a loud cough that sounds like a seal's bark. He is up to date on his vaccinations. With this clinical presentation, what would an anterior-posterior neck X-ray show?

3. A 30-year-old woman presents to A&E with a 3-day history of a sore throat and a fever. She is finding it increasingly painful to swallow, and has developed foul breath and earache. A snapshot of blood results are as follows:

White cell count: 14.3 × 10⁹/L; Neutrophils: 8 × 10⁹/L; C-reactive protein: 154 nmol/L; Paul–Bunnell: negative.

On examination, she is drooling and there is cervical lymphaden-opathy. Her tonsils are enlarged and sloughy. The left side of the soft palate is more swollen and erythematous than the right. Her uvula is also displaced to the right. What is the diagnosis?

4. 18-year-old Marlon presents to A&E with a rash over his torso. He reports seeing his GP 3 days ago because of a severe sore throat and malaise and was given medication. The rash appeared today and he is anxious that he is having an allergic reaction. On examination, Marlon has a low-grade fever and cervical lymphadenopathy. His tonsils are enlarged with areas of petechial haemorrhages on the soft palate. Over his upper body, there is a widespread maculopapular rash. A snapshot of blood results are as follows:

White cell count: 11.3 × 10⁹/L; C-reactive protein: 25 nmol/L; Paul–Bunnell: positive.

From the list of options given, what was the most likely medication he was given by his GP?

5. Marlon re-presents to A&E 10 days later following a collapse. His mother reports his tonsillitis had improved and within a week Marlon was back to his normal active self. In fact, he took part in a rugby tournament the day before and did very well. He complained of some abdominal pain afterward; however, his mother took no notice of it. On examination, Marlon appears pale and disorientated. His systolic blood pressure is 85, heart rate is 119 bpm. His abdomen is generally tender and mildly distended. He is not jaundiced. Nurses report his urine dipstick is positive for blood. What condition is essential to rule out?

Q **ENT Q14 – Pharyngitis, tonsillitis, laryngitis and epiglottitis II**
A. Amoxicillin
B. Epiglottitis
C. Epstein–Barr virus
D. Foreign body
E. Group A streptococcus
F. Koplik's spots
G. Lichen planus
H. Paracetamol
I. Parapharyngeal abscess
J. Reassurance, analgesia, bed and voice rest
K. Referral to ENT outpatient clinic
L. Retropharyngeal abscess

From the list above, choose the most appropriate answer for each of the following examples.

1. 60-year-old Mr Jonathan is recovering from a terrible cough and cold and has noticed that his voice has become hoarse. It started yesterday, when he found it increasingly painful to cough and swallow. Mr Jonathan does not smoke but admits to drinking two glasses of wine per day. His diabetes is well controlled and he is otherwise well. There is no history of weight loss or haemoptysis. He has read about changes in voice being a sign of cancer and he is very anxious. On examination, his voice is notably hoarse. There is so sign of pyrexia or lymphadenopathy. How would you treat this patient?

2. Mrs Xui brings her 3-year-old son to the GP surgery. She is worried that he has an infection. His nose is running, he has a cough and has developed a temperature. He is not his usual active self, is irritable and has lost interest in food. He is otherwise a well child and is up to date with his immunisations. On examination, her son is alert, with bilateral creamy nasal discharge. There is no obvious foreign body in both nostrils and he is able to swallow. On further questioning, she admits that three other children in his play school have similar symptoms. Mrs Xui wants antibiotics for her son's infection. What would you prescribe?

3. Gary presents to his GP having developed a cough, nasal discharge and a sore throat over the past week. He is having chemotherapy for bowel cancer. You notice that his eyes are red and swollen. On examination he has whitish-grey irregular lesions

in the mucosal lining on the cheek. In view of the history and clinical examination, what are the lesions in the mouth likely to be?

4. 17-year-old Dylan presents to the surgery with a 5-day history of feeling generally unwell with muscle pains and a severe sore throat. He also reports fevers, chills and headaches. He has no cough. On examination, his tonsils are enlarged with whitish exudate. There are also purpuric eruptions on his palate. On further questioning he reluctantly admits that his girlfriend also has a sore throat. What is the causative pathogen?

5. 12-year-old Florence is brought to A&E with noisy breathing, drooling and a fever. She is visibly distressed. Her head is tilted to the left. Her father notes she has had a sore throat for a few days now. An urgent lateral neck X-ray shows soft-tissue shadowing and an air-fluid level in the pre-vertebral space. What is the diagnosis?

Q ENT Q15 – ENT epidemiology

A. Bell's palsy
B. Oral thrush
C. Parotid tumours
D. Persistent generalised lymphadenopathy
E. Pneumococcal vaccine
F. Poor dental hygiene
G. Prophylactic antibiotics
H. Rhinosinusitis
I. Stroke
J. Submandibular tumour

From the list above, choose the most appropriate answer for each of the following examples.

1. Most frequent cause of a facial nerve palsy.
2. The most common ENT manifestation of HIV.
3. Has been found to be beneficial in reducing the risk of recurrent acute otitis media.
4. The cause of most presentations to the GP with halitosis.
5. Accounts for 80% of salivary tumours.

ENT Q16 – Epistaxis

A. Acute lymphoblastic leukaemia
B. Acute myeloid leukaemia
C. Aspirin
D. Cocaine
E. Disseminated intravascular coagulation
F. Goodpasture's disease
G. Immune thrombocytopenic purpura
H. Von Willibrand's disease
I. Warfarin
J. Wegener's granulomatosis

From the list above, choose the most appropriate diagnosis for each of the following examples.

1. A 23-year-old lady comes in to hospital with severe epistaxis. She has a past medical history of systemic lupus erythematosus and menorrhagia, which was previously investigated in gynaecology outpatients. No gynaecological cause was found. She is haemodynamically stable and there are no rashes or patechiae of note. Full blood count shows haemoglobin (Hb) 12.6, mean corpuscular volume 88, white cell count (WCC) 6.0, and platelets 60.

2. A 64-year-old trader attended A&E with epistaxis. He is known to the cardiologists, with a history of hypertension, two previous myocardial infarctions and atrial fibrillation. The patient has a 30-pack-year history and he is obese. He is on several medications but he cannot recall the names. His observations are as follows: heart rate is 68 bpm and regular, blood pressure is 148/92, respiratory rate is 14 breaths per minute, saturations 97% on air and afebrile. He denies any recreational drug use.

3. A 17-year-old male presented to A&E at 5 a.m. complaining of uncontrollable bleeding from his left nostril. He had just come from a nightclub and was very distressed and nervous. He did not want his parents to be informed. He was found to be Gillick competent to make this decision.

4. A 58-year-old lady visited her GP complaining of recurrent episodes of spontaneous bleeding from her nose. She denies any trauma or nose picking to trigger it. On further questioning she has also noticed she is more tired than normal. She was admitted into hospital twice for community acquired pneumonia in the last

3 months and is just recovering from a recent pharyngitis. Bloods of relevance: Hb 7.9, platelets 98, WCC 10.2. Blood film reveals blasts and Auer rods.

5. A 46-year-old Caucasian gentleman was referred to the ENT clinic for recurrent epistaxis episodes. The patient has not noticed any exacerbating features but he also reports having oral ulcers and on examination is found to have a saddle nose deformity. Bloods of relevance: Hb 9.1, WCC 8.3, platelets 210, urea 8.9, creatinine 238, sodium 138, potassium 4.8 and normal liver function tests.

ENT Q17 – Airway obstruction I

A. Asthma
B. Croup
C. Epiglottitis
D. Haemorrhage post tongue cancer resection
E. Peritonsillar cellulitis
F. Quinsy abscess
G. Retropharyngeal abscess
H. Tonsillar haemorrhage post tonsillectomy
I. Tonsillitis
J. Tracheomalacia

From the list above, choose the most appropriate diagnosis for each of the following examples.

1. A 13-year-old boy was taken to the GP by his mother after school as his physical education teacher thought he was struggling with his breathing on the pitch. On further questioning by the GP, the child is experiencing a terrible cough that keeps him up most of the night. He feels the lack of sleep is the reason why he is struggling on the pitch.

2. A 3-year-old boy was taken to A&E by his parents as he has developed a barking cough after having a fever.

3. A 19-year-old girl was rushed into A&E as her partner found her bleeding profusely from her mouth. This was compromising her airway and she was unable to verbalise or give any history. Her partner reports that she had an operation yesterday in her mouth but he can't remember the procedure. She is otherwise fit and well.

4. A 33-year-old gentleman presents to his GP complaining of feeling generally unwell. His voice sounds muffled. He has a painful throat that is worse on the right side, and he is starting to find it difficult to swallow. There is a restricted examination as the patient has difficulty opening his mouth. With the use of a tongue depressor, the only thing that can be seen is a swollen uvula deviated to the left. The patient is febrile (38.2°C) but haemodynamically stable.

5. A 6-year-old child was brought to A&E as her parents noticed she was finding it difficult to breath. She has been quite unwell recently with a temperature, although earlier today they noticed her becoming increasingly unwell. On examination, the child

is embracing the tripod position. The child is previously fit and well and on no regular medications, although the parents do not believe in vaccination.

ENT Q18 – Airway obstruction II
   A. Abdominal thrust
   B. Bronchoscopy
   C. Encourage cough
   D. Five back blows
   E. Give 10 mg chlorphenamine IV and 200 mg hydrocortisone IV
   F. Give 10 mg chlorphenamine IV and 200 mg hydrocortisone PO
   G. Intubate and ventilate
   H. Laryngoscopy
   I. Nebulised O_2 driven bronchodilators and 100 mg hydrocortisone IV
   J. Repeat adrenaline dose (0.5 mg 1:10 000 IM)
   K. Repeat adrenaline dose (0.5 mg 1:1000 IM)

From the list above, choose the most appropriate management option for each of the following examples.
   1. A 12-year-old boy was playing football with his friends when he suddenly felt very short of breath. He initially described his chest tightening although on arrival of the paramedics he was unable to complete his sentences. On examination, he is bradycardic and there is reduced air entry bilaterally.
   2. A 12-year-old child was taken to A&E as he had acute airway compromise. The patient was on a school trip and developed immediately during lunch. On examination, he has an urticarial rash over his torso, and his lips and tongue are grossly enlarged. He has a past medical history of infantile eczema. He is on no medications and is up to date with his immunisations. In the ambulance the patient received 100% oxygen via a non-rebreathing bag. The child was given one dose of adrenaline. Upon arrival to the hospital the patient's airway condition has improved and he is able to maintain it alone.
   3. A 12-year-old child was taken to A&E as he had acute airway compromise. The patient was on a school trip and it developed immediately during lunch. On examination, he has an urticarial rash over his torso, and his lips and tongue are grossly enlarged. He has a past medical history of infantile eczema. He is on no medications and is up to date with his immunisations. In the ambulance the patient received 100% oxygen via a non-rebreathing bag. The child was given one dose of adrenaline.

Upon arrival to the hospital the patient's airway condition has not improved.

4. A 3-year-old child was rushed to A&E as his parents noticed he was finding it difficult to breathe. He has been very well and was playing with his toys when he suddenly had a bout of coughing. The child was unsupervised. On examination, he is presently able to maintain his airway, albeit struggling. When he is asked 'can you cough?' he answers 'yes' and tries to cough, although with no initial success.

5. A 3-year-old child was rushed to A&E as his parents noticed he was finding it difficult to breathe. He has been very well and was playing with his toys when he suddenly had a bout of coughing. The child was unsupervised. Since then, the child has become unable to cough effectively. On examination, he seems like he is in significant distress. When he is asked 'can you cough?' he nods, but is unable to do so.

ENT Q19 – Head and neck tumours I

A. Anaplastic thyroid carcinoma
B. Follicular thyroid adenoma
C. Follicular thyroid carcinoma
D. Hürthle cell carcinoma
E. Medullary thyroid carcinoma
F. Multiple endocrine neoplasia 1
G. Multiple endocrine neoplasia 2A
H. Multiple endocrine neoplasia 2B
I. Papillary thyroid carcinoma
J. Thyroid lymphoma

From the list above, select the most likely diagnosis for each of the following examples.

1. A 45-year-old male presents with a lump in the right lobe of the thyroid gland that has been gradually growing over the past few months. He denies any pain or difficulty in swallowing. Blood investigations reveal a normal thyroid function test and elevated calcitonin levels.
2. An 82-year-old female with known hypothyroidism attends the GP with a rapidly growing painful thyroid nodule. She has been having increasing difficulty in swallowing over the past 3 weeks. On examination the nodule is hard and irregular.
3. A 50-year-old female presents with a thyroid lump that has been increasing in size over the past 3 months. On examination, there is a left-sided thyroid nodule that is hard and non-tender on palpation. The mass moves up and down on swallowing, but does not move on tongue protrusion. Blood tests reveal normal thyroid function tests and elevated levels of thyroglobulin.
4. A 35-year-old female presents with bilateral non-tender thyroid nodules and cervical lymphadenopathy. Histological assessment of biopsies from the nodules show calcified psammoma bodies.
5. A 50-year-old male presents having noticed a unilateral thyroid mass. Blood investigations reveal raised calcitonin levels. Further screening tests reveal that the patient has elevated urinary catecholamines and parathyroid hyperplasia. On further examination there is no evidence of any cutaneous abnormalities.

Q ENT Q20 – Head and neck tumours II

A. Acinic cell carcinoma
B. Adenoid cystic carcinoma
C. Frey's syndrome
D. Mucoepidermoid carcinoma (high grade)
E. Mucoepidermoid carcinoma (low grade)
F. Pleomorphic adenoma of the superficial lobe of the parotid gland
G. Pleomorphic adenoma of the deep lobe of the parotid gland
H. Sialadenitis
I. Sialolithiasis
J. Warthin's tumour

From the list above, choose the most appropriate diagnosis for each of the following examples.

1. A 38-year-old man complains of recurrent pain and swelling in the region of the left submandibular gland for the past 2 months. The pain is exacerbated by eating and lasts for about an hour each time. The patient is afebrile and is otherwise fit and well. No lump is palpable on palpation of the submandibular and parotid glands. There are no palpable neck nodes.

2. A 45-year-old woman presents to clinic with a slow growing lump below her right ear, which she first noticed two months ago. The lump does not hurt, and she has not noticed any acute swelling on eating. On examination, the lump is situated over the angle of the right jaw. It is smooth, firm and non-tender on palpation. Examination of the mouth and oropharynx are unremarkable. There are no signs of facial weakness, and no palpable neck nodes.

3. A 55-year-old woman presents with a painful lump over the angle of the jaw. She first noticed the lump about a month ago and put it down to a viral infection. On examination, there is hard solid lump in the region of the left parotid gland. There is evidence of weakness in the muscles of facial expression. Histological assessment following a parotidectomy shows a prominent presence of epidermoid cells and a few mucous cells.

4. A 72-year-old man presents with a slowly growing lump in the parotid region. He denies any facial pain. On examination there is a smooth firm non-tender lump that seems to mainly affect the tail of the parotid gland. After a number of investigations, he is told that this condition almost never becomes malignant.

275

5. A 70-year-old man is diagnosed with a parotid gland carcinoma. He is told that his facial nerve must be sacrificed, as it is almost always involved by this type of tumour, which can lead to spread of the cancer.

Q **ENT Q21 – Congenital neck swellings**
A. Cystic hygroma
B. Dermoid cyst
C. First branchial cleft cyst
D. Infected thyroglossal cyst
E. Laryngocele
F. Plunging ranula
G. Pneumatocele
H. Second branchial cleft cyst
I. Thymic cyst
J. Thyroglossal cyst

From the list above, select the most likely diagnosis for each of the following examples.

1. An 8-year-old girl is brought to A&E by her father, as she has complained of a painful neck lump. On examination, the patient is apyrexial and haemodynamically stable. The lump is in the midline at the level of the thyroid gland. It is firm and tender on palpation. It moves superiorly on tongue protrusion. The overlying skin is non-erythematous and there is no discharge. An ultrasound scan shows a thick-walled mass with mixed echogenicity.

2. A 32-year-old male is referred by the GP to the ENT outpatients clinic. He reports a large lump on the left side of the neck. On examination, there is a soft globular lump lying lateral to the pharynx and medial to the left sternocleidomastoid muscle. The lump transilluminates. The patient denies any pain but is worried that it may be cancer.

3. A 12-year-old girl presents to the general ENT clinic with a midline neck lump that is superior to the hyoid bone. The patient denies any pain but wants it removed because her school friends have made funny remarks about the lump. On examination the lesion is well defined with a smooth surface. The lesion is not tethered to underlying skin and does not transilluminate.

4. A 2-year-old child presents with an enlarging swelling in the posterior triangle of the left neck. The patient's mother reports that it has gradually increased in size since birth.

5. A 68-year-old male with known chronic obstructive pulmonary disease presents to the ENT clinic with a peculiar neck lump that

has developed over the last few days. On examination, the swelling enlarges when asking the patient to blow while closing his nose.

Q ENT Q22 – Acquired neck swellings

A. Bacterial tonsillitis

B. Familial carotid body tumour

C. Hodgkin's lymphoma

D. Hyperplastic carotid body tumour

E. Infectious mononucleosis

F. Ludwig's angina

G. Non-Hodgkin's lymphoma

H. Sporadic carotid body tumour

I. Submandibular abscess

J. Tuberculosis

From the list above, select the most likely diagnosis for each of the following examples.

1. A 19-year-old university student presents with a 2-week history of fatigue, lethargy and fevers. He reports generalised swellings in his neck. He has recently been treated by his GP for a presumed lower respiratory tract infection with amoxicillin, which was stopped due to the development of a rash. On examination there is cervical lymphadenopathy.

2. A 48-year-old HIV-positive lady presents to A&E with bilateral swelling of the upper neck and increasing difficulty breathing. Upon questioning the patient reports having a recent dental procedure.

3. A 42-year-old man with known Eisenmenger's syndrome is referred to the ENT clinic because of a lump in the anterior triangle of the neck. The patient denies any pain. On palpation, the lump only mobilises in the transverse plain.

4. A 25-year-old man presents to his GP with generalised swelling of his lymph nodes affecting his neck and axillae. He reports unexplained weight loss, night sweats and fevers. On examination the lymph nodes are best described as being rubbery. A lymph node biopsy reveals Reed–Sternberg cells.

5. A 69-year-old male presents with bilateral enlarged lymph nodes in his posterior triangle. He does not complain of any systemic symptoms. On examination he has painless lymphadenopathy in his axilla and inguinal region. Hepatosplenomegaly is evident. Fine needle aspiration cytology is inconclusive.

Q **ENT Q23 – Sleep apnoea**

A. 10-second cessation of breathing
B. 10-second cessation of breathing with reduction of ventilation by at least 50%
C. 5-second cessation of breathing with reduction of ventilation by at least 50%
D. Advise to stop work
E. Central sleep apnoea
F. Continuous positive airway pressure
G. Home oxygen
H. Obstructive sleep apnoea
I. Sedation
J. Sleep studies

From the list above, choose the most appropriate answer for each of the following examples.
1. What is the definition of apnoea?
2. Mrs Demarco presents to the GP with her husband Carlos. She is anxious that Carlos is not getting enough sleep and very tired in the mornings. He works as a bus driver and admits to occasionally losing concentration on the job. Mrs Demarco confesses it is affecting their relationship, as she is sleeping in their guestroom because his snoring has become unbearable. He also has moments in the night where it is as though he has 'stopped breathing'.
On examination, Carlos is a middle-aged gentleman with a large neck circumference and a body mass index of $35\,kg/m^2$. He does not drink but he smokes 10 cigarettes per day on average. What should be the GP's first step in managing this patient?
3. Carlos is scheduled for sleep studies. A snapshot of his results is as follows:

> 60 episodes of apnoea . . . Observations: patient struggling to shift air during REM phase, thrashing and snoring loudly. During 10% of sleep time, oxygen saturations were below 90%. No arrhythmias seen.

What type of apnoea is he likely to have?
4. Margaret is a 60-year-old patient who presents to the emergency unit with shortness of breath and 'bloating'. She is known to have sleep apnoea, for which she had been using mandibular splints.

On examination, there are reduced breath sounds bilaterally, a displaced cardiac apex and pitting oedema to the mid-thighs. Oxygen saturation is 85% on air and blood pressure is 198/99. Margaret is diagnosed with and treated for cardiac failure secondary to sleep apnoea. Mandible splints are not enough. From the list of options given, select the most likely treatment.

5. Margaret undergoes repeat sleep studies. A snapshot of her results is as follows:

> 30 episodes of apnoea. Observations: no obvious struggle to breathe, during desaturations.

What type of sleep apnoea is described here?

Q **ENT Q24 – ENT disorders**

A. Apthous ulcer
B. Glottic laryngeal carcinoma
C. Leukoplakia
D. Lichen planus
E. Oesophageal cancer
F. Oral squamous cell carcinoma
G. Oropharyngeal cancer
H. Pharyngeal diverticulum
I. Supraglottic laryngeal carcinoma
J. Tracheo-oesophageal fistula

From the list above, select the most appropriate diagnosis for each of the following examples.

1. A 65-year-old man presents with a 1-month history of dysphagia, lethargy and weight loss. He also reports that his family have told him that his voice has changed recently. He has a past medical history of gastro-oesophageal reflux disease. He smokes 10 cigarettes a day and drinks 20 units of alcohol weekly.

2. A 45-year-old male of Chinese origin presents to his GP with pain in the right ear. He has presented to his GP several times in the past few months complaining of a painful indurated ulcer in the base of his mouth. His has a past medical history of Crohn's disease. He reports a 35-pack-year smoking history and drinking about 25 units of alcohol per week. On examination the ulcer is white and red in colour with exophytic margins.

3. A 60-year-old man presents to his GP complaining of white lines on the inside of his cheek. He noticed them after feeling a stinging sensation on eating food. He has no significant past medical history and is not on any medications. On examination there are white lines in a lace-like pattern on his left buccal mucosa. These cannot be scraped off using a spatula. On further questioning, he has a 40-pack-year smoking history and consumes a large amount of alcohol.

4. A 75-year-old male is admitted to hospital with aspiration pneumonia. The patient looks cachetic. After the patient is stabilised, he explains that he has been having difficulty swallowing and experiencing gurgling sounds in the neck for the past few weeks. A barium swallow is diagnostic for the condition.

5. A 72-year-old male presents to his GP complaining of difficulty in swallowing. He explains that he has had a persistent cough for a few weeks. More recently, he cannot seem to keep anything down, as he coughs violently on eating or drinking. He has suffered from two chest infections over the past 3 months. He has a past medical history of prostate cancer, a 20-pack-year smoking history and drinks 15 units of alcohol per week.

ENT answers

A   ENT A1 – ENT investigations I

1. **E – Evoked response audiometry** (ERA). The only reliable test for infants below the age of 6 months is ERA. This gives an objective assessment of hearing loss. Unlike pure tone audiometry, the ERA gives an objective assessment of hearing. Moreover, pure tone audiometry is only possible in children above the age of four. Skin surface or trans-tympanic electrodes are used to detect evoked potentials in the cochlea, eighth cranial nerve, brain stem or auditory cortex following auditory stimulation. One of the main advantages of this test is that it is objective. Therefore, it is useful in patients who are unable to undergo audiometry (e.g. newborn screening, mentally disabled) or for suspected non-organic hearing loss (NOHL). Measuring the latency of evoked potentials is sometimes used in patients suspected of having an acoustic neuroma (80% sensitivity, 90% specificity).

2. **F – Impedance audiometry**. The compliance (stretching ability) of the tympanic membrane (TM) varies with changing pressures. Impedance audiometry is a method of assessing the TM and middle ear via tympanometry, giving an indirect measure of the middle ear pressure. Impedance audiometry is contraindicated in children less than 6 months of age as false readings may arise because of their soft ear cartilage. A probe tone is first inserted into the sealed ear canal. The probe then measures the degree to which a sound signal is reflected back from the TM under different pressures (+200 to –400 daPa) in the ear canal. The results are recorded on a tympanogram, in which the horizontal axis represents the pressure (negative to positive), and the vertical axis represents the TM compliance. The TM is most compliant when the pressure on either side of the TM (middle ear space and external auditory canal) is equal. Impedance audiometry can also detect the acoustic reflex. The acoustic reflex occurs when the stapedius muscle contracts as a reflex to sounds that are more than 70 dB above the patient's threshold. This reflex can be lost when there is stapedius muscle dysfunction (e.g. middle ear effusion, otosclerosis,

seventh cranial nerve lesions). Figures 2–4 are examples of type A, B and C tympanograms.

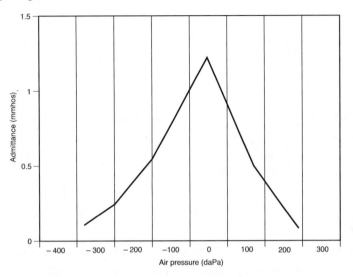

FIGURE 2 Type A tympanogram: normal ear (N.B. otosclerosis may produce a type A shape); type A can be subdivided into shallow (type As with a very low admittance peak: glue ear, otoscelorsis) and deep (type As with a very high admittance peak; disarticulation of ossicles)

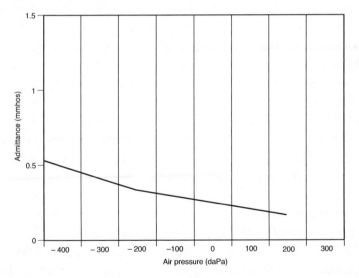

FIGURE 3 Type B tympanogram: flat trace reflects absence of compliance (a type B trace must be correlated with ear canal volume; normal volume and type B trace implies otitis media; large volume with type B trace implies a perforation; type B trace with a small canal volume implies sebum in the canal)

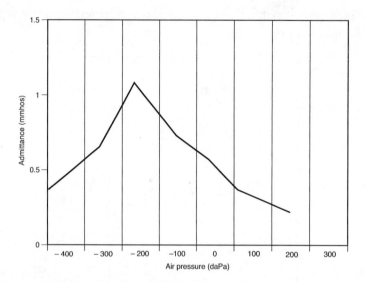

FIGURE 4 Type C tympanogram: this tracing implies negative pressure present in the middle ear; this may occur while otitis media is either developing or resolving (here usually the peak is less than −150 daPa)

3. **E – Evoked response audiometry**. The gold standard test to detect NOHL is ERA. This gives an objective assessment of hearing, unlike pure tone audiometry. Another useful but reliable test for suspected NOHL is the Stenger test – a test for psychosomatic hearing loss. This is when a 512 Hz vibrating tuning fork is placed at a 5 cm distance from each ear in turn. The patient will deny hearing in the 'bad' ear. Two tuning forks are then used; one placed 5 cm from one ear and the other placed 15 cm from the other ear, and vice versa. Patients with true unilateral hearing loss should still hear the tuning fork with the good ear at any distance. Patients with NOHL will deny hearing any sound when the tuning fork is closer to the 'bad' ear. This test is not always reliable, and some of the more 'skilled' patients can still mislead experienced examiners!

4. **H – Speech audiometry** is an important test that is being increasingly used in clinical practice to assess the degree and type of hearing loss. In essence it is used to evaluate auditory discrimination. It is not used as an alternative to pure tone audiometry, rather as cross-check of the pure tone findings. In pure tone audiometry (PTA), individuals are tested against tones; however, in speech audiometry, individuals are exposed to more realistic sounds and a mixture of tones. Speech audiometry is also important for assessment of word recognition and provision of correct hearing aids. The test consists

of presenting bisyllabic words to the patient at different sound intensities. The patient is asked to repeat the sounds. They are given a percentage score of the percentage of sounds they identified. The speech recognition threshold is then calculated. This is the lowest intensity level at which the patient can identify at least 50% of the words.

5. **C – Dix–Hallpike manoeuvre.** The Dix–Hallpike manoeuvre is a useful clinical test for the diagnosis of benign paroxysmal positional vertigo (BPPV). The patient sits up on the couch at such a position so that when he or she lies down, the head is hanging off the end of the couch. When sitting up at 90 degrees, the head is turned 30 degrees to one side. The patient is asked to keep looking at the examiner's nose, and warned that he or she will be moved down quickly. The patient is then moved to the lying position at a fast pace, with their head hanging down from the couch. It is important the patient's head is still turned 30 degrees to the side, and that the examiner moves down with the patient so that the patient maintains the eye fixation position. The patient is then carefully observed for any induced nystagmus, and asked to report any vertigo. The test is then repeated on the other side. A positive Dix–Hallpike test indicates BPPV. Over 90% of cases can be treated with the Epley manoeuvre.

Caloric tests involve irrigating each ear with cold or warm water and assessing for any difference in the nystagmus produced on irrigation of each ear. Cold water should cause nystagmus beating towards the opposite ear, while warm water should cause a nystagmus towards the irrigated ear (COWS: cold = opposite, warm = same). The caloric testing is helpful in confirming an inner ear pathology in patients presenting with loss of balance. In electronystagmography, electrodes placed in close proximity to the eyes allow a recording of electrical activity induced by eye movements. It is used to produce a record of nystagmus, and is often used to assess nystagmus in response to tests of vestibular function (e.g. Dix–Hallpike test, caloric test).

Tests used to test hearing in children also include the **distraction test** (age 6–18 months), **visual reinforcement audiometry** (6 months to 2–3 years), play audiometry (above 2.5 years), **pure tone audiometry** (above 3 years) and speech discrimination tests (school children).

Pure tune audiometry (PTA) is the most common test used to assess hearing loss in adults. The patient sits in a sound-proofed room, wears headphones and is asked to press a buzzer when they hear a noise. This gives a measure of the air conduction thresholds. To test the bone conduction threshold, a vibrating device placed on the mastoid is used instead of a headset. Pure-tone thresholds indicate the softest sound audible 50% of the time. The results are plotted on a graph (audiogram). On the audiogram, the horizontal axis represents frequency (Hz). The frequency range on the audiogram is from 250 Hz (low) to 8000 Hz (high), which is the frequency hearing level needed for understanding speech. The vertical axis represents the sound intensity (decibels, dB). Thresholds are tested in 5 dB steps. The reference range for normal hearing is –10 to 25 dB. The higher hearing threshold, the more profound the hearing loss. A value of 0 dB refers to the sound a normal person is able to hear at least 50% of the time.

TABLE 17 Hearing threshold in different degrees of hearing loss

Hearing loss	Hearing threshold (dB)
Normal range	0–20
Mild hearing loss	21–40
Moderate hearing loss	41–55
Moderately severe hearing loss	56–70
Severe hearing loss	71–90
Profound hearing loss	>90

Table 18 explains several symbols used on most audiograms.

TABLE 18 Symbols used on the audiogram

Symbol	Description
0	Right air conduction
X	Left air conduction
<	Right bone conduction
>	Left bone conduction

In a normal individual, air conduction should be better than bone conduction. In sensorineural hearing loss, there is similar air conduction and bone conduction threshold reduction (difference between air conduction and bone conduction of <10 dB). Conductive hearing loss, on the other hand, is characterised by reduced air conduction thresholds. The difference between BC thresholds and the lower AC thresholds is typically >10 dB.

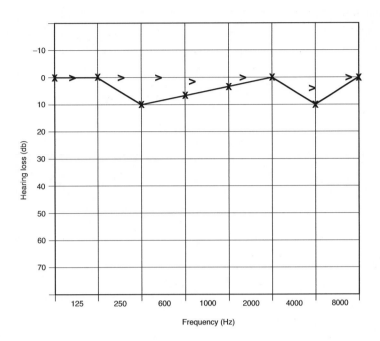

FIGURE 5 Normal audiogram of the left ear

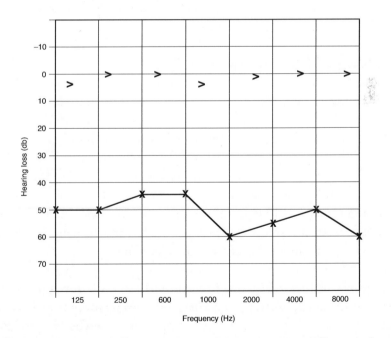

FIGURE 6 Left ear conductive hearing loss audiogram (the difference between bone conduction thresholds and the lower air conduction thresholds is typically >10 dB)

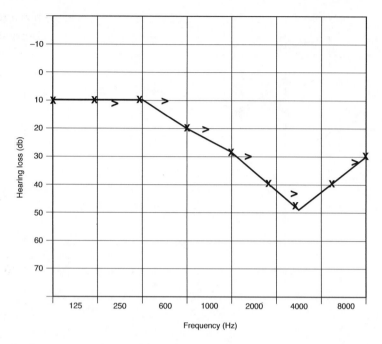

FIGURE 7 Left ear sensorineural hearing loss (SNHL) audiogram, illustrating the characteristic 4000 Hz 'dip' or 'notch' typically observed in noise-induced SNHL

A   ENT A2 – ENT investigations II

1. **D – Ménière's syndrome**. In Ménière's syndrome (also known as 'endolymphatic hydrops') there is a fluctuating sensorineural hearing loss (SNHL) often affecting the low frequencies. As the disease progresses, the SNHL becomes permanent and affects all frequencies. It is important to be aware of the tetrad of symptoms in Ménière's syndrome, which are: (1) recurrent spontaneous episodes of vertigo lasting from 20 minutes to 12 hours (most 2–4 hours), (2) unilateral or bilateral fluctuating SNHL, (3) constant or intermittent non-pulsatile tinnitus (usually preceding vertigo), and (4) feeling of fullness in the affected ear.

2. **F – Noise-induced hearing loss** most commonly develops after many years of noise exposure at the workplace (occupational). It is a bilateral sensorineural hearing loss, which stops progressing when there is no more exposure to excessive noise. The peak of SNHL is usually at 4 kHz, with the 4 kHz audiogram notch being preserved even at the most advanced SNHL stages.

3. **B – Gentamicin toxicity**. Gentamicin (an aminoglycoside) has a narrow therapeutic index, and levels must be closely monitored during therapy. It is both ototoxic and nephrotoxic. Gentamicin is a leading cause of bilateral vestibular damage. Patients present with balance problems and oscillopsia (visual blurring with head movements). Gentamicin also classically causes SNHL initially affecting the high frequencies, which can be associated with tinnitus.

4. **H – Otosclerosis** is an autosomal dominant conditioin. New bone is formed around the stapes footplate, resulting in a conductive hearing loss. It has a prevalence of 1 in 100 000 and affects females more than males. The hearing loss is bilateral in approximately 70% of cases. Patients present with an insidious onset of hearing loss. Rinne's test is negative (abnormal), and Weber's test usually lateralises to the worse affected ear. The majority of affected patients report tinnitus as well. Pure tone audiometry characteristically shows conductive hearing loss with the typical Carhart's notch. The Carhart notch is a dip in conductive hearing loss at 2 kHz, without a corresponding decrease in SNHL. It is important to note that middle ear effusions also cause a conductive hearing, which is more rarely associated with the Carhart's notch. Therefore, although it may be a useful sign to look for, it is not diagnostic. Clinically, it is also useful to look for the Schwartze's sign (detected on otoscopy), which is a flamingo pink blush of the TM that is anterior to the oval window. Otosclerosis also causes loss of the acoustic (stapedial) reflex, which is normally detected on tympanometry. Treatment can be conservative with the use of hearing-aids, medical with the use of fluoride therapy (otosclerosis had a higher prevalence in countries with low water content of fluoride – 20 mg of daily oral fluoride supplements may be used; however, the evidence is not substantial) and surgery in the form of a stapedectomy (replacement of stapes with prosthesis), stapedotomy (a hole is created in the foot of the stapes and a prosthesis is inserted) or a bone-anchored hearing aid.

5. **C – Glue ear**. The compliance (stretching ability) of the tympanic membrane varies with changing pressures. The TM is most compliant when the pressure on either side of the TM (middle ear space and external auditory canal) is equal, in which a type A (bell-shaped) waveform is obtained on tympanometry. This peak pressure is shifted to the negative side (type C tympanogram) when there is reduced middle ear pressure, due to Eustachian tube dysfunction. In the presence of a middle ear effusion (e.g. glue ear) or TM perforation, the TM becomes less stretchable

and produces a type B (flat) tympanogram. In children, glue ear usually presents as a gradual onset of bilateral hearing loss. Glue ear is an extremely common condition, affecting 80% of people at some point in childhood. Less commonly, glue ear may present as a unilateral sudden-onset hearing loss (e.g after an upper respiratory tract infection). Unlike more subjective tests (e.g. audiometry), the only compliance needed from the patient for the test is to sit still for a few minutes. This makes it especially useful for the assessment of children with glue ear. Parents are now able to use home tympanometers to monitor their children's middle ear pressure.

Presbycusis is age-related hearing loss. It is the most common cause of gradual-onset bilateral hearing loss in the elderly population. It is also the most frequent cause of high-frequency sensorineural hearing loss on audiometry.

An **acoustic neuroma** is a more rare cause of gradual onset high-frequency sensorineural hearing loss. It is normally unilateral, often associated with tinnitus and more rarely associated with vertigo.

Autoimmune conditions can cause a sudden-onset unilateral or bilateral sensorineural hearing loss. **Wegner's granulomatosis** is a necrotising granulomatous vasculitis affecting the upper respiratory tract, lungs and kidneys. Over 90% of patients are C-ANCA positive in active disease. Treatment is with cyclophosphamide. About 90% of patients have a sensorineural hearing loss, and 20% have a conductive hearing loss with effusion.

Vascular causes (e.g. labyrinthine or anterior vestibular artery occlusion) present as a sudden-onset unilateral sensorineural hearing loss with or without vertigo.

Nasopharyngeal carcinoma may present as a gradual-onset conductive hearing loss due to a middle ear effusion. This can cause a type B tympanogram, but the much more common cause is a glue ear. Other clinical features of this cancer may be present, such as epistaxis, nasal obstruction, lymphadenopathy and headaches.

Ossicular discontinuity is usually caused by head trauma, middle ear infection or a cholesteatoma. It results in a sudden-onset unilateral conductive hearing loss. Management is with a hearing aid or surgical reconstruction.

A   ENT A3 – Vertigo

Vertigo is an abnormal sensation of severe dizziness and the illusory spinning of the affected individual or surroundings. It is usually rotational, with patients describing the room to be spinning. Most patients experiencing vertigo will present to their physician complaining of dizziness. This is why it is crucial to establish exactly what the patient means by dizziness. It may be associated with sweating, nausea or vomiting. The cause of vertigo is either peripheral (inner ear), or less frequently central (vestibular nerve nuclei, brainstem or cerebellum). If the cause of vertigo is otological, the patient may experience hearing loss and/or tinnitus. It is essential to ask about the triad of vertigo, hearing loss and tinnitus in any patient presenting with any one of the three. Nystagmus is defined as an involuntary rhythmical oscillation of the eye(s), and commonly occurs with vertigo. A nystagmus usually has a fast and a slow phase. The fast phase is the direction of the nystagmus, i.e. horizontal versus vertical. A nystagmus of peripheral origin has the same direction in all positions, while a nystagmus of central origin may change direction in different gaze positions (gaze-evoked nystagmus). If the nystagmus occurs in directions other than horizontal, the cause is central rather than peripheral.

1. **F – Ménière's disease** (also known as 'endolymphatic hydrops') is named after Prosper Ménière, a French physician, who first described it in 1861. It accounts for approximately 10% of cases presenting with vertigo and has an incidence of 15/100 000 of the population. It usually starts in middle age (30–40 years of age), and is more common in females. Most cases are idiopathic (Ménière's disease). The other two leading causes are head trauma (injury and post otological surgery) and late-stage syphilis. Theories suggest that 'dark cells' in the middle ear produce abnormally high amounts of endolymph in the semicircular canals. Other experts postulate that it is a result of poor absorption of the endolymph → obstruction of the endolymphatic duct → increase in pressure eventually dislodges the obstruction → re-flow of the endolymph that causes the vertigo episode. This theory is known as the saccin theory. Essentially, it is characterised by a tetrad of symptoms: (1) recurrent spontaneous episodes of vertigo which can last from 20 minutes to 12 hours (most 2–4 hours), (2) unilateral or bilateral fluctuating SNHL, (3) non-pulsatile constant or intermittent tinnitus that usually precedes vertigo, and (4) a feeling of aural fullness in the affected ear. It is also associated with loss of balance (this may last for several days) and loudness recruitment. The latter is when the patient cannot tolerate

loud noises due to hyperacusis. Patients also usually experience symptoms such as sweating, nausea and vomiting. When the patient experiences vertigo, a horizontal or rotational (horizonto-rotatory) vertigo is always present. The attacks occur in clusters, and the patient may continue to feel unwell and have a poor balance after the attack has resolved. Frequency of Ménière's attacks is highly variable between patients. An interesting variant of the disease/syndrome is Lermoyez's syndrome – here the symptoms occur in reverse; vertigo relieves the hearing loss, tinnitus and sensation of fullness. A severe variant is termed 'crisis of Tumarkin' – this affects 2% of individuals with Ménière's. In this variant individuals experience sudden collapses without any preceding symptoms. The diagnosis of Ménière's disease is made clinically, which is why a detailed history is crucial in any patient presenting with vertigo, hearing loss or tinnitus. A pure tone audiogram may reveal a low-frequency SNHL, unlike the high-frequency SNHL characteristic of presbycusis. The hearing loss fluctuates early in the course of the disease before becoming permanent and affecting higher frequencies. An MRI scan is indicated if the symptoms are asymmetrical to exclude a more serious cause (e.g. acoustic neuroma). Glycerol dehydration test can also be used. Here administration of mannitol improves hearing due to the decrease in plasma osmolality. Acute attacks of Ménière's may resolve by the use of a vestibular sedative (e.g. cinnarizine – an antihistamine). Prophylactic management involves consumption of a low-salt diet, avoidance of caffeine and use of oral betahistine (selective weak histamine receptor H1 agonist and strong H3 anatagonist), and some patients also benefit from the addition of a thiazide diuretic. Betahistine may also reduce the frequency and severity of attacks. Counselling and reassurance is also a vital component in management of affected individuals. More invasive options include endolymphatic sac decompression (40%–70% improvement in vertigo), vestibular nerve section (symptomatic relief in approximately 90% of patients; however, associated with high rates (5%) of cerebrospinal fluid leak), surgical labyrinthectomy (80% symptomatic relief) or medical labyrinthectomy. The latter involves injection of intratympanic ototoxic agents such as gentamycin (symptomatic relief in 80% with 5% risk of complete hearing loss), and is becoming increasingly popular for the treatment of resistant Ménière's disease.

2. **E – Lateral medullary syndrome** (LMS). The patient in this scenario does not take medications, which may imply he has uncontrolled hypertension and an increased risk of multiple sclerosis relapse. His signs and symptoms are characteristic of LMS. LMS (also known as Wallenberg's syndrome or

posterior inferior cerebellar artery syndrome) is relatively common, caused by infarction of the lateral medulla and inferior surface of the cerebellum due to occlusion of a vertebral artery or the posterior inferior cerebellar artery. The structures affected are the sympathetic pathway, vestibular nuclei, inferior cerebellar peduncle and the fifth (trigeminal), ninth (glossopharyngeal) and tenth (vagus) cranial nerves. Involvement of the vestibular system causes acute vertigo with associated nausea and vomiting. On the ipsilateral side, patients present with Horner's syndrome, facial numbness, diplopia, nystagmus, cerebellar ataxia and soft palate paralysis. There is loss of pain and temperature sensation on the ipsilateral face and contralateral limbs – a distinguishing clinical finding. Other symptoms include ataxia dysphagia and dysarthria due to ninth and tenth cranial nerve lesions. Hearing loss can also occur. Limb weakness is not a feature of LMS. Treatment resembles that of a thrombotic stroke. LMS has a variable prognosis; some patients may suffer permanent debilitating symptoms and others fully recover.

3. **A – Acoustic neuroma**. The most common presenting complaint of an acoustic neuroma (also known as 'vestibular schwannoma') is progressive unilateral sensorineural hearing loss (SNHL) with or without unilateral tinnitus, which in clinical practice is assumed to be due to an acoustic neuroma until proven otherwise. Some patients, however, present with a sudden SNHL. Giddiness is common, but much less commonly patients present with vertigo or balance disturbance. In unilateral SNHL, Weber's test lateralises (i.e. sound is heard loudest) in the unaffected ear, as is the case in this scenario. Rinne's test is positive in both ears, indicating that there is no conductive deafness. Remember that an abnormal Rinne's test is negative, which can be confusing for many clinicians. An acoustic neuroma (vestibular schwannoma) is a slow-growing benign tumour arising from the Schwann cells sheath covering the vestibular (95% of cases) or cochlear (5% of cases) portion of the eighth cranial nerve (vestibulocochlear nerve). They do not infiltrate local tissues or metastasise, but can cause compression of nearby structures. These tumours account for 6% of all intracranial neoplasms, and 80% of cerebellopontine angle tumours. The other principal differential is a meningioma, accounting for most of the other 20% of cerebellopontine angle tumours. Most acoustic neuromas are sporadic (95%), but a minority can be associated with neurofibromatosis type 2, in which patients classically develop bilateral acoustic neuromas. The first structures affected by the growth of the tumour are the vestibular and cochlear nerves. Further growth of the tumour can lead to compression of

the trigeminal nerve (causing a diminished corneal reflex, facial numbness or pain), ipsilateral cerebellar signs (e.g. cerebellar ataxia) and increased intracranial pressure. It is important to know the clinical features of raised increased intracranial pressure, which include postural headaches, pulsatile tinnitus, nausea, vomiting, visual disturbance and papilloedema. The patient in this scenario has a pulsatile tinnitus with nausea and vomiting, and it is therefore important to elicit any history of headaches or visual disturbance, and look inside the eyes for optic disc swelling. The facial nerve has a great ability to stretch, and is therefore rarely affected. In general, an acoustic neuroma should be suspected in any patient presenting with asymmetrical audiovestibular symptoms. The gold standard test is a gadolinium-enhanced MRI scan of the cerebellopontine angle. Evoked response audiometry is a useful screening tool. Management options include monitoring the growth of the tumour with serial MRI scans, surgical excision of the tumour or stereotactic radiotherapy to arrest tumour growth. Factors determining the most appropriate management option include the patient's choice, his or her age and medical condition, and the size and location of the tumour. Surgical excision is the treatment of choice for tumour eradication, with tumour recurrence being rare.

Hint: A negative Rinne's test is abnormal.

4. **B – Benign paroxysmal positional vertigo** (BPPV). The main differentials in this case are benign BPPV and postural hypotension. Unlike BPPV, postural hypotension presents as dizziness or lightheadedness rather than vertigo after sitting or standing up. BPPV is the most common cause of peripheral vertigo, usually affecting people between the fourth and sixth decade of life. It is estimated to account for at least 20% of presentations of vertigo. It is defined as an abnormal sensation of motion that is triggered by certain head movements, particularly looking up. It commonly occurs while turning or sitting up in bed. The pathophysiology of BPPV is not yet clear, but it is thought to be due to stimulation of the semicircular canals (most frequently the posterior canal) by loose otoliths that have been displaced. Most cases are idiopathic, usually starting at the age of 50 years. Twenty per cent of cases occur after a head injury. Hearing loss and tinnitus are rare. The symptoms of BPPV can be elicited by the Dix–Hallpike test (essentially patients are sat up on a chair with their head rotated 30 degrees to one side. Their heads are quickly guided down the edge of the bed with the head hanging at 30 degrees. Characteristically, there is a latent period (5–10 seconds) followed by sudden-onset rotatory

geotropic nystagmus that lasts from 30 seconds to several minutes. The nystagmus is fatigable and becomes less pronounced if the test is repeated). It is associated with both vertigo and nausea. In contrast, central vestibular nystagmus (e.g. due to cerebral mass) occurs immediately, does not fatigue and is associated with minimal symptoms of vertigo and nausea. About 90% of patients with a positive Dix–Hallpike test can be cured by the Epley head manoeuvre, in which the canalith is repositioned. No medications have been found to be helpful for the management of this condition. The symptoms normally resolve in 3–6 months. An MRI scan may be done after 3 months to exclude more sinister causes.

Hint: Latent rotatory nystagmus of limited duration following the Dix–Hallpike test is pathognomonic of BPPV.

5. **D – Labyrinthitis**. Acute labyrinthitis and vestibular neuritis present as a sudden attack of severe vertigo with nystagmus, vomiting and prostration in a previously well person. The attack reaches maximum intensity within the first day, and lasts from several days to weeks. The term labyrinthitis has been used interchangeably with vestibular neuritis. It is now recommended that the former is used when both the auditory and vestibular systems are involved, while the latter should be used if the vestibular system only is involved. The patient in this scenario does not have any evidence of hearing loss or tinnitus, and is therefore more likely to have vestibular neuritis. During the attack, the patient has nystagmus. Patients also suffer from nausea and vomiting. It usually manifests as a single attack, but can be recurrent. The usual age of onset is between 30 and 40 years, with an equal male-to-female preponderance. The disorder is usually unilateral. Labyrinthitis occurs when pathogens, or their toxins, enter the labyrinth to cause inflammation. The most common form is viral labyrinthitis, which is often preceded by an upper respiratory tract infection. Commonly implicated organisms are rubella, cytomegalovirus, herpes simplex virus, mumps and influenza. Moreover, atrophy of the vestibular nerve and endoneurial fibrosis may give rise to the symptoms. If the symptoms are asymmetrical or recurrent, a brain MRI is warranted to exclude more serious causes. Otherwise, in most cases the diagnosis is made clinically. Asking about hearing loss is very important, as it occurs in labyrinthitis and Ménière's disease but not in BPPV or vestibular neuritis. Unlike the recurrent presentation of symptoms in Ménière's syndrome, symptoms do not recur in labyrinthitis once they have resolved. Acute attacks of labyrinthitis are treated with an anti-emetic such as prochlorperazine (stat dose may

be given intramuscularly followed by an oral course), bed rest and good hydration. Benzodiazepines such as diazepam are occasionally used as a vestibular suppressant. Oral steroids (prednisolone 1 mg/kg) have shown benefit especially in cases associated with SNHL. Most cases of labyrinthitis resolve spontaneously several days to weeks after onset.

TABLE 19 A summary of the causes of vertigo and their clinical features

	BPPV	Ménière's syndrome	Acute labyrinthitis	Cerebellar infarction	Migraine
Vertigo duration	Seconds to minutes	20 minutes to 12 hours	Days to weeks	Long lasting	Usually hours
Recurrence	Yes	Yes	Rarely	–	Recurs
Hearing loss	Very rare	Progressive SNHL	SNHL can occur	No	–
Tinnitus	Very rare	Yes	Yes	No	–
Other classic symptoms	Dix–Hallpike test positive	Ear fullness	Maximum intensity within 24 hours	Reaches maximum intensity at onset	Aura, throbbing unilateral headache, photophobia
Triggers	Head movement	Spontaneous	Upper respiratory tract infection	–	Sleep excess or deprivation, menstruation, stress, cheese, chocolate

A migraine is one of the most common causes of vertigo in clinical practice. Half of patients present without headache, making the presentation diagnostically challenging. The vertigo associated with a migraine can last from several minutes to several hours. The diagnosis is made by establishing symptoms of migraine (e.g. headache, photophobia or aura) in a patient with recurrent vertigo, and excluding other causes.

A **cerebellar infarction** is present in 3% of patients with vertigo. It typically causes a sudden-onset, persistent vertigo. Patients may have other signs of cerebellar infarction such as an intention tremor, dysdiadochokinesis, dysarthria, dysphagia, ataxic gait, hypotonia, etc. Most patients with cerebellar infarction and isolated vertigo will also have severe ataxia or direction changing nystagmus. Severe ataxia presents as an inability to walk unaided. A direction changing nystagmus (or gaze-evoked nystagmus) is when the nystagmus changes direction according to direction of gaze.

In **multiple sclerosis**, the vertigo is the result of brainstem demyelination, and can last from days to weeks. Patients present with other signs of brainstem demyelination such as dysarthria, ataxia and an intention tremor.

A   ENT A4 – Otalgia

1. **H – Referred pain**. Although both acute otitis media and glue ear are important differentials, there are no signs of ear pathology or a systemic infection on examination. Otalgia after tonsillectomy is very common, and typically occurs 5–7 days post-operatively. Tonsillitis itself commonly presents with otalgia due to referred pain via the glossopharyngeal nerve. Other common causes in children that should be excluded are dental disease, negative middle ear pressure and an upper respiratory tract infection.

2. **I – Temporo-mandibular joint** (TMJ) dysfunction refers to a group of disorders that affect the TMJ and muscles. It is a very common cause of referred otalgia, and is estimated to affect up to 25% of people at some point in their lives. Giant cell arteritis (GCA) should be excluded in any elderly patient (more common in females) with jaw claudication, tenderness on palpation of the temporal artery, a tender scalp, headache (especially unilateral) and visual loss. If the diagnosis of GCA is suspected, the patient's C-reactive protein levels, erythrocyte sedimentation rate and platelet counts (inflammatory markers that are raised in GCA) should be measured urgently. The diagnosis of TMJ dysfunction is much more likely in this scenario because the patient complains of otalgia rather than a headache, and does not have any of the characteristic features of GCA. TMJ dysfunction has three principal symptoms: pain, limited mouth opening and jaw noises (i.e. clicking or crepitus). The pain can occur as an earache, headache and/or in the muscles of mastication. The referred earache classically occurs just in front of the tragus. Other features include worsening of pain on jaw movements and locking of the jaw. Pain on chewing may also be due to a misaligned bite. Most patients improve over time with conservative treatment. Psychological (for pain management), orthodontic or surgical interventions may be required in some cases.

3. **G – Oropharyngeal neoplasia**. The most frequent site of an oropharyngeal tumour is the tonsils. This is followed by the tongue base, soft palate and posterior pharyngeal wall. It is most commonly due to a squamous cell carcinoma (more than 70%), with most other cases being due to lymphoma. The purpose of this question is not simply to examine your

knowledge about tonsillar cancer, rather to emphasise the importance of excluding upper airway and upper digestive tract neoplasia in any patient presenting with non-typical or suspicious otalgia. Squamous carcinoma of the tonsils has become surprisingly more common in patients under 40 years of age in recent years, with many of the patients being non-smokers and non-alcohol drinkers. This is unusual as the population usually affected are male smokers and/or heavy drinkers. The cause of this increased incidence in this age group remains unknown. Similarly to the clinical scenario, patients may present with a sore throat, otalgia (referred), an ulcerated and/or unilaterally enlarged tonsil, neck lump, dysphagia, odynophagia and dysphonia. If a diagnosis of tonsillar cancer is suspected, a panendoscopy (endoscopic examination of upper airways) is carried out to assess tumour spread and biopsy the tonsil. A CT of the chest is used to assess for distant metastasis. MRI may be used to assess primary tumour size and invasion of local structures. Staging is via the tumour, node and metastasis staging system. Treatment options include radiotherapy, chemotherapy and radical surgical excision. The second most common tonsillar cancer is a lymphoma. It is imperative to mention that half of patients with tonsillar cancer present with palpabale metastatic nodes (if palpable fine need aspiration of the neck nodes should be undertaken). Tonsillitis occurs mostly in children, with the tonsils appearing swollen, enlarged, erythematous and with an overlying exudate. This along with long history of symptoms in this patient, the tonsillar ulcer found on examination and lack of systemic signs of inflammation makes a diagnosis of tonsillar cancer more likely.

4. **A – Acute otitis externa**. This patient presents with all of the typical features of otitis externa. Otitis externa is more likely in patients who have ear canal eczema, trauma or play watersports. It often begins with an itch, followed by severe otalgia. On examination a narrowed oedematous appearance of the external auditory canal with creamy-coloured discharge is characteristic. Patients report pain on moving the pinna. It is important to investigate for any signs of a tympanic perforation, as otitis externa can be secondary to a middle ear infection. Oraganims most commonly implicated are *Staphylococcus aureus*, *Pseudomonas aeruginosa* and *Bacilus proteus*. An important differential is necrotising malignant otitis externa, which usually occurs in immunocompromised patients (e.g. elderly diabetics). This is an osteomyelitis of the temporal bone that rapidly spreads to involve the middle ear and lower cranial nerves (facial nerve is affected in ~50% of cases). Patients are usually systemically unwell and present with

severe otalgia and cranial nerve palsies. There may be granulations on the floor of the external auditory canal. Management of acute otitis externa is with aural toilet, topical aural antibiotics, topical steroids, analgesia and frequent cleaning of the ear canal. This patient in this scenario should also avoid swimming for a while. Necrotising otitis externa needs urgent hospital referral. Treatment is with local and systemic antibiotics covering both pseudomonas aeruginosa and anaerobes.

5. **B – Drug allergy**. Patients with otitis externa who do not respond to therapy may be allergic to the drops used. The patient's otitis externa symptoms seem to have improved, however, and he now seems to have predominant inflammation of the pinna. The clinical features described are most consistent with an infection of the perichondrium. This can follow an otitis externa or other local trauma (e.g. 'high' ear piercing, mastoid surgery, burns). As in the scenario, the pinna is swollen, red, shiny, thickened and tender. Severe otalgia and systemic upset are common features. Management is with broad-spectrum antibiotics (covering both pseudomonas aeruginosa and staphylococcus aureus) until culture and sensitivity results are available. If an abscess develops, urgent surgical drainage is required.

Furunculosis is a hair follicle infection in the external ear canal usually caused by a Gram-positive bacaterial infection (e.g. *S. aureus*). Patients present with a fever and a severe and often throbbing auricular pain that can radiate to the throat or neck. A classic feature of this condition is pain on movement of the cartilaginous outer structure of the ear. The abscess often spontaneously ruptures. Diagnosis is clinical, and the condition is managed with oral antibiotics, aural antibiotic/steroid drops, analgesia and application of heat. Incision and drainage may be required for a persistent abscess.

A   ENT A5 – Dysphagia

Hint: The key symptoms of an oesophageal disorder are heartburn, chest pain, dysphagia and odynophagia. If a patient presents with one of these symptoms, it is always essential to ask about the other three. It is also worth asking about what exacerbated or alleviates these symptoms (e.g. eating, type of food, posture, exertion), as this is very helpful in narrowing down the differential diagnoses.

1. **F – Oesophageal carcinoma**. The patient in this scenario has developed a progressive dysphagia with weight loss, the most common presenting complaints of oesophageal carcinoma. Hoarse voice developed a few months later, which is the result of local invasion of the recurrent laryngeal nerve. Excessive smoking, alcohol intake, gastro-oesophageal reflux disease (GORD) and coeliac disease are all predisposing factors to oesophageal cancer. Plummer–Vinson syndrome (triad of dysphagia due to an oeso-phageal web, iron deficiency anaemia and glossitis) is also a risk factor for oesophageal squamous cell carcinoma. Laryngeal cancer is an important differential, but this is unlikely to present with dysphagia as an initial symptom. Furthermore, dysphonia is an earlier finding in most cases. Another differential is a benign oesophageal stricture, but this is unlikely to present with significant weight loss. Also, it is usually associated with a history of GORD. Oesophageal cancer is the seventh leading cause of cancer death worldwide, occurring most frequently in elderly males. It can be a squam-ous cell carcinoma or an adenocarcinoma. Adenocarcinoma usually occurs in the lower third of the oesophagus, and is associated with Barrett's oeso-phagus (30–60× risk of general population). Just as a reminder, Barrett's oesophagus is the metaplasia of oesophageal epithelium from squamous to columnar cells secondary to chronic exposure to acidic contents. Barrett's oesophagus is a pre-cancerous condition in which the cells may eventu-ally develop into an adenocarcinoma. Treatment is focused on reducing GORD (conservative measures/dietary changes, proton-pump inhibitors, treatment of *Helicobacter pylori* and surgery may be done in resistant cases in the form of a fundoplication. Regular follow-up and endoscopies are essential to monitor the disease process. Squamous cell carcinomas usually occur in the middle third, and are associated with excessive alcohol intake, smoking, salted foods, achalasia and coeliac disease. The most common presenting complaint is a progressive dysphagia affecting solids and then liquids. Other symptoms include weight loss (affecting 50% of patients) and epigastric or throat pain. As with other types of cancer, the patient may develop anaemia. A barium swallow is commonly performed as an initial investigation in patients with dysphagia, and may show oesophageal narrowing in oesophageal cancer. The gold standard investigation is an endoscopy, allowing direct visualisation of the tumour and a biopsy to con-firm the diagnosis. Further imaging (e.g. CT of the chest and abdomen) may be performed to assess for local and metastatic spread. Endoscopic ultrasound is also used to accurately determine the depth of tumour pen-etration and invasion. Oesophageal cancer has a poor prognosis, and many patients are treated palliatively. The principal curative treatment is an

oesophagectomy with or without adjuvant chemotherapy or radiotherapy, but this is associated with significant morbidity and mortality. Five-year survival rates are as low as 25%.

A laryngeal carcinoma is the most common head and neck malignancy, and accounts for 3%–4% of all malignancies. About 94% of laryngeal malignancies are squamous cell carcinomas. It predominantly affects men (8:1), occurring most frequently between the sixth and seventh decades. Most patients (>95%) with laryngeal cancer are smokers. Alcohol excess is another important risk factor, and it acts synergistically with smoking to increase the risk further. The most common site of laryngeal cancer in the Western world is the glottis, followed by the supraglottic areas. The site of the cancer determines the symptoms at presentation. Cancer in the glottis, even at an early stage, causes the patient to have a hoarse voice (dysphonia). Cancers in other sites may not be symptomatic until an advanced stage in the disease. Any patient with dysphagia and 'red flag' symptoms must be investigated for a sinister cause such as laryngeal cancer. The 'red flag' symptoms include weight loss, the presence of a neck mass, haemoptysis, hoarseness, stridor, voice change, otalgia, respiratory difficulty, food/drink regurgitation and lymph node enlargement. The latter five are signs of advanced laryngeal cancer. Endoscopic laryngoscopy is carried out to assess the extent of the cancer. The diagnosis can be made clinically, but a biopsy is essential as a number of benign conditions can mimic the clinical presentation of laryngeal cancer. The tumour, node and metastasis staging of the cancer among other factors is needed to determine the most suitable treatment option. More than 90% of laryngeal cancers can be cured if treated at an early stage. Treatment is with surgery or external beam radiotherapy.

2. **C – Bulbar palsy**. This patient has a dysphagia affecting both solids and liquids, which is characteristic of a neuromuscular disorder. The other signs and symptoms which this patient presents with are most consistent with a bulbar palsy. A bulbar palsy is a lower motor neurone weakness of the muscles supplied by the ninth (glossopharyngeal), tenth (vagus) and twelfth (hypoglossal) cranial nerves. It is not a name of disease per se, but a collection of clinical signs and symptoms. It is most commonly caused by motor neurone disease and can manifest secondary to myasthenia gravis. Intracranial tumours at the level of the brainstem can also cause a bulbar palsy. It is important to mention that lesions affecting the nuclei of the aformentied cranial nerves must be bilateral, otherwise the signs and symptoms will not be clinically apparent. There is progressive dysarthria,

dysphagia, dysphonia, poor cough and nasal regurgitation. The tongue is classically weak, wasted and fasciculating, and the lips may be tremulous. There may be peripheral signs of motor neurone disease. The most serious sequel of a bulbar palsy is aspiration, which can lead to pneumonia and death. Compare this with a pseudobulbar palsy, which is a disease of the corticobulbar tracts causing an upper motor neurone weakness of the same muscles. It is most commonly caused by a stroke. It presents similarly to a bulbar palsy but there are no lower motor neurone signs. The tongue is small, spastic and non-fasiculating. The jaw jerk is exaggerated in pseudo-bulbar palsy, but may be normal or absent in bulbar palsy. Moreover, the gag reflex is absent in bulbar palsy.

3. **H – Pharyngeal pouch**. This scenario described a classic presentation of a pharyngeal pouch (also known as a Zenker's diverticulum). This is a pulsion diverticulum through the posterior pharyngeal wall through Killian's triangle, most frequently affecting the elderly with a male-to-female preponderance of 2:1. It typically causes a progressive dysphagia with regurgitation of undigested food, halitosis and gurgling noises on lying supine. There may be a lump in the neck. Food from the pouch can be aspirated into the lungs, causing aspiration pneumonia. A good history is essential for establishing the diagnosis. The past medical history and smoking history are irrelevant to the diagnosis. A pharyngeal pouch can be confirmed with a barium swallow, which will reveal the pouch in the lateral view. A rigid endoscopy can then be carried out to exclude a malignancy within the pouch. A barium swallow is done prior to endoscopy to demonstrate the pouch, as the endoscope preferentially enters the pouch, which can lead to a perforation. The treatment of choice is an endoscopic stapling of the pharyngeal pouch.

4. **D – Globus pharyngeus** is one of the most common causes of ENT referrals and regarded as a pseudo-dysphagia, affecting women more frequently than men. Patients complain of vague feelings of a lump or discomfort in the throat, usually in the midline at the level of the cricoid cartilage. Classically, this feeling is worse on swallowing saliva rather than food or water. The symptoms come and go, and get worse when the patient is stressed or tired. It can be associated with GORD. Globus pharyngeus does not cause weight loss unless patients avoid eating, and rarely causes dysphagia. It is a diagnosis of exclusion, and it is important to exclude a hypopharyngeal malignancy in these patients, which is a key differential diagnosis. All that is required for the management of patients with globus

pharyngeus is reassurance. It is important to manage a patient holistically as this may be a presenting symptom related to a background of depression; a GP must explore this further and address any concerns.

5. **A – Achalasia**. As mentioned, a difficulty in swallowing both solids and liquids is characteristic of a neuromuscular disorder. The clinical presentation and barium swallow findings in this patient are characteristic of achalasia. Achalasia is a disease of unknown aetiology in which there is disordered oesophageal peristalsis and poor relaxation of the lower oesophageal sphincter (LOS). There have been documented cases of achalasia developing secondary to degeneration of the Auerbach's plexus (the sympathetic and parasympathetic nerve network in the muscles of the gastrointestinal tract). It causes progressive difficulty in swallowing both solids and liquids, and may result in food regurgitation and weight loss. Some patients experience significant retrosternal chest pain. A chest X-ray classically shows an air/fluid level behind the heart, and a double right heart border. A barium swallow or oesophageal manometry will demonstrate a lack of LOS relaxation and aperistalsis. The barium swallow may also reveal the classic 'bird beak' or 'rat tail' appearance. An oesophago-gastro-duodenoscopy is usually performed to exclude an oesophageal cancer. The most effective treatment options are pneumatic balloon dilatation and a laparoscopic Heller's cardiomyotomy, with a success rate of about 75%. Both procedures may not be suitable for frail elderly patients, and both have a high incidence of subsequent GORD. Moreover, some patients may benefit from botox (botulinum toxin) injections into the LOS.

Oesophageal spasm may manifest in one of two forms: (1) diffuse oesophageal spasm, in which there are uncoordinated oesophageal contractions, or (2) nutcracker oesophagus, in which there are coordinated contractions with abnormally increased amplitude. The condition causes intermittent dysphagia, odynophagia and chest pain. In diffuse oesophageal spasm, a 'corkscrew oesophagus' with curling of the barium column may be seen on barium swallow. The best diagnostic test is manometry. Oesophageal spasm is a difficult condition to treat. A number of medical options exist (e.g. calcium channel blockers, nitrates), with surgical interventions (usually a myotomy) being reserved for unrelenting cases.

Vocal cord paralysis may be unilateral or bilateral, and occurs because of recurrent laryngeal nerve, superior laryngeal nerve or vagus nerve dysfunction. Patients typically present with a weak breathy hoarse voice which is associated with a poor cough, dysphagia and sensation of dyspnoea. Patients are at risk of aspiration. Bilateral vocal cord palsy may also present as a surgical emergency. Approximately one-third of vocal cord palsies are idiopathic, one-third due to neoplasia and one-third occur after surgery.

A   ENT A6 – Hearing loss

1. **G – Right-sided conductive deafness**. A positive Rinne's test is when air conduction is louder than bone conduction (normal), and a negative test is when bone conduction is louder than air conduction (abnormal). A conductive hearing loss of at least 20 dB is required before a Rinne's test becomes positive. It is important to mask the other ear (e.g. by massaging the tragus) when performing a Rinne's test. When Weber's test is performed in sensorineural hearing loss, the sound lateralises to the better side. In contrast, the sound lateralises to the affected side in conductive hearing loss. The reason for this is because the conduction problem in the middle ear of the affected side (malleus, incus, stapes, and Eustachian tube) masks the background noise of the room, while the functioning ipsilateral inner ear (cochlea) picks up the sound via the bones of the skull, thus perceiving it to be louder on the affected side. In other words, there is no external air conducted sound to cancel out the bone conducted sound from the forehead. In this case, Rinne's test is negative on the right side – this indicates conductive hearing loss; Weber's test confirms this by lateralising the sound to the affected side.

2. **A – Bilateral conductive deafness**. A negative Rinne's test indicates a conductive deafness. Since Weber's test reveals equal sounds bilaterally, this suggests bilateral equal conductive deafness.

3. **D – Left-sided sensorineural deafness**. Rinne's test is negative on the left, suggesting a conductive deafness on the left side. However, Weber's test lateralises the sound to the right side. This contradicts the pattern of conductive deafness previously described. A false negative Rinne's test is possible; this can be caused by ipsilateral severe or complete sensorineural hearing loss. The patient can hear bone conduction louder than air conduction because of the sound travelling through the bone to the contralateral cochlear; hence interpreting it as a negative Rinne's test result. A false negative Rinne's test should always be considered in any patient with severe sensorineural deafness, bilateral conductive deafness, and if Weber's test is contradictory.

4. **H – Right-sided sensorineural deafness**. This patient has bilateral positive Rinne's tests, indicating that there is no conductive deafness. Weber's test lateralises to the left side. This is indicative of a right-sided sensorineural deafness.

5. **B – Bilateral sensorineural deafness**. Bilateral positive Rinne's tests and a Weber's test equal bilaterally, suggest that the patient would have normal hearing or equal sensorineural deafness bilaterally. In this stem it has been already established that all the patients are presenting with a reduced hearing. Therefore it is more likely that the patient had bilateral sensorineural deafness than normal hearing. Pure tone audiometry is the next step in confirming this finding.

A ENT A7 – Management of inner ear disorders

1. **H – Reassurance, counselling and rehabilitation**. The patient in the first example suffers from Ménière's disease, which has been described in Question 3 (ENT section). In an acute attack, patients experience a feeling of fullness, vertigo, tinnitus and hearing loss that lasts 20 minutes to 6 hours. The vertigo may persist for several days after an attack, but there may be permanent residual unsteadiness in late stages. Vertigo may trigger patients to feel nauseous and vomit. On examination, horizontal or horizonto-rotatory nystagmus is always present. Hearing loss is sensorineural and fluctuates, usually affecting only low frequencies; however, in later stages hearing loss can become permanent and can affect high frequencies as well. There is a range of tests that can be performed, although none are diagnostic: audiometry, MRI (rule out acoustic neuroma), electrocochleography.

    There is a spontaneous remission rate in 60%–80% of cases. Medical treatments include: supportive (reassurance, counselling, hearing aid, and vestibular and tinnitus rehabilitation), vascular (betahistine improves middle ear blood flow), vestibular sedatives, electrolyte balance (dietary salt restriction, fluid restriction, diuretics), immunological (topical or oral steroids, plasmapheresis). Surgical treatments are only indicated if medical treatments fail. These can be divided into hearing preserving or non-hearing preserving procedures. Hearing preservation procedures include grommet insertion (based on the assumption that endolymph hydrops may be secondary to negative pressure within the middle ear), intratympanic gentamicin, endolymph sac decompression, vestibular nerve section and, rarely, chochleostomy, cervical sympathectomy, cochlear dialysis, vestibular ultrasonic ablation or cryosurgery. Non-hearing preserving procedure is labyrinthectomy.

In this scenario, the patient is a Jehovah's Witness, so plasmapheresis is contraindicated (Jehovah's Witnesses refuse any blood product that have been extracted from the body – this includes their own). Having said that, it is important to discuss plasmapheresis as a treatment option with the patient and to not make the assumption that the patient will definitely refuse it. She has otherwise tried all other medical treatments; therefore, she needs to fall back on supportive treatments, which are reassurance, counselling and rehabilitation.

Romberg positive means that there is loss of proprioception or vestibular sensation. Romberg's test is performed as follows: (1) the patient stands upright with his/her feet together and arms by his/her side; (2) the patient is asked to close his/her eyes while the examiner stands nearby to avoid the patient following and being harmed; (3) if the patient loses balance, then the test is positive. Cerebellar pathology does not give a positive Romberg's test, as the patient is ataxic despite visual assistance. Unterberger's test can only be used if supported by other tests. The patient is asked to walk in one place with his/her eyes closed. If the patient rotates to one side, the patient may have a vestibular lesion on the ipsilateral side.

2. **E – Oral aciclovir, corticosteroids and eye care**. This patient has Ramsay Hunt syndrome (also known as herpes zoster oticus). This is described in Question 10 (ENT section) and is essentially caused by re-activation of varicella zoster virus in the geniculate ganglion. This patient has signs of cranial nerve VII and VIII involvement. The facial nerve palsy gives him the facial droop, the drooling, and the inability to close the right eye. Vestibular division of the vestibulocochlear nerve is affected as evidenced by the vertigo. On examination the positive Romberg's sign indicates that there is either vestibular or proprioceptive pathology. Unterberger's test suggests that he has a right vestibular lesion. Involvement of the cochlear division of the VIII nerve may result in deafness. The presence of vesicles within the external auditory canal and otalgia are classic features of Ramsay Hunt syndrome. Herpetic vesicles may also erupt on the soft palate. There is a debate as to whether this condition should be treated with high dose corticosteroids and aciclovir, or corticosteroids alone to improve restoration of facial nerve function. Most patients are treated with both. In this patient it is important to address his eye, as inability to close the eyelid can lead to corneal dryness and injury. The patient should be given an eye pad, ocular lubricants (drops and ointments) and referred to an ophthalmologist.

3. **C – Epley manoeuvre**. BPPV has been explained in Question 3 (ENT section). The Dix–Hallpike manoeuvre is used to diagnose BPPV and assess which side is affected. The canalith repositioning manoeuvres (e.g. Epley manoeuvre) are used to treat BPPV. Epley manoeuvre has a >90% success rate: (1) the patient sits upright on the examination table with legs extended; (2) the examiner rotates the head to 45 degrees in one direction; (3) the examiner then helps the patient lie flat on the examination table and holds the patient's head in a 20-degree extension over the edge of the table, while maintaining the 45-degree rotation (so far the manoevre is identical to Dix–Hallpike) and this position is held for 30 seconds; (4) the head is then turned 90 degrees in the opposite direction, and held for 30 seconds; (5) hold the head and neck in a fixed position, the patient then rolls onto the shoulder in the direction they are facing (i.e. face now points towards the floor), hold it for 30 seconds; (6) finally, the patient is slowly brought into the upright sitting posture, while holding his/her head in the 45-degree rotation. Hold this position for 30 seconds.

4. **H – Reassurance, counselling and rehabilitation**. This patient has labyrinthitis, which has been discussed in Question 3 (ENT section). Her symptoms have begun resolving on their own. The patient just needs to be reassured, as she does not want any vestibular suppressants.

5. **J – Tell the patient that his/her hearing is better than described**. This patient has non-organic hearing loss, also called pseudohypacusis. There is a discrepancy between the patient's claim of deafness and pure audiometry results. It is more common in children, and in females. There is poor repeatability on audiometry, and a discrepancy between speech and pure tone audiogram. In this scenario, audiometry results indicate the patient has good hearing, which makes further hearing tests unnecessary. Malingering patients (e.g. those making litigation claims for hearing loss) may be much more challenging to investigate for non-organic hearing loss. Multiple tests are usually used for these patients, such as the Stenger test, delayed auditory feedback tests or brain-evoked auditory response (gold standard but now rarely used).

   The physician should tell the patient that his/her hearing is better than they describe, and explore reasons for the patient's claim without being confrontational. One should also be aware of psychological disorders that may be involved. It is important for the physician to bear in mind that the child's complaints may be a result of difficulties at home or school, such as neglect or bullying.

A ENT A8 – Ear infections and their complications

Otitis media is an inflammation of the middle ear. In order to better perceive the treatments of otitis media, it is important to understand its different types. Acute otitis media (AOM) is of short duration (usually 1–5 days) especially when viral; it is usually self-limiting. Recurrent otitis media (ROM) refers to three repeated short-lived episodes within a 6-month period. AOM can persist with accumulating pus behind an intact tympanic membrane. The eardrum is very sensitive and increasing pressure behind it can cause exquisite pain. If this persists for more than 3 months, this is termed otitis media with effusion. 'Chronic' implies that the tympanic membrane has perforated secondary to the high pressure within the middle ear, and the perforation has failed to heal. Chronic suppurative otitis media (CSOM) is a term used to describe the tendency for longstanding perforations to become infected and discharge. CSOM can be divided into two distinct, separate types: safe (*muscosal*) and unsafe (*bony*). The safe entity, also known as active mucosal chronic otitis media, carries no serious risks. It affects the tubotympanic mucosa (lower front part of the middle ear cleft). On the other hand, the unsafe entity, known as active chronic otitis media with cholesteatoma is associated with erosion of surrounding bone. Cholesteatoma or chronic osteitis involves the upper back part of the middle ear cleft (atticoantral). It is termed unsafe because it threatens the spread of infection intracranially.

1. **C – Acute otitis media** is very common and is frequently bilateral. Most children develop one or more episodes of AOM before they are 2 years old. However, it can occur in any age group. The most common causative organisms are *Streptococcus pneumoniae*, 35%; *Haemophilus influenzae*, 25%; and *Moraxella catarrhalis*, 15%. Group A streptococci, and *Staphylococcus aureus* may also be responsible. Patients usually present with an acute onset of ear pain, a blocked feeling within the ear, and discharge (only a symptom if the eardrum perforates; which is usually accompanied by a sudden relief of ear pain). There may be a history of a preceding upper respiratory tract infection. On examination patients are likely to be pyrexial, demonstrate a conductive hearing loss (negative Rinne's test) on the ipsilateral side, and an inflamed possibly bulging tympanic membrane. Otitis media cannot be excluded if the view of the tympanic membrane is obscured by discharge or wax. Adjacent lymph nodes are never enlarged in simple otitis media. Paracetamol and NSAIDs will usually suffice for analgesia, but avoid aspirin in children as it may lead to Reye's syndrome. Oral antibiotics

are given for one week (amoxicillin, but if suspecting b-lactamase producing organisms – co-amoxiclav is indicated). Complications of AOM include acute mastoiditis, facial paralysis, labyrinthitis, chronic tympanic membrane perforation, meningitis, and brain abscess.

With regard to the other types of otitis media, ROM is more common in children and can cause considerable distress to the child and his/her parents. It usually resolves as the child grows older. If these attacks persist, investigation of an immunodeficiency is suggested as well as, like in otitis media with effusion, grommet insertion or long-term treatment with prophylactic low dose antibiotics. Adenoidectomy is also another possible treatment if the causative factor is enlarged adenoids, but this treatment option remains controversial.

2. **A – Acute mastoiditis** is an extracranial complication of otitis media. It is the extension of AOM into the mastoid air cells, which causes a breakdown of the thin bony partitions between the air cells that then become coalescent. This process takes 2–3 weeks. In the United States, 0.004% of patients with AOM develop mastoiditis. Patients present with persistent, throbbing ear pain, persistent or increasing copious discharge, or increasing deafness. On examination you may find the patient is pyrexic, a swelling and redness postauricularly which may displace the pinna anteriorly and inferiorly, marked tenderness over the mastoid process, and either an inflamed, bulging tympanic membrane or a perforated one with associated discharge. Mastoiditis should be considered in any patient with continuous discharge from the middle ear for more than 10 days, particularly if looking continually unwell. Once diagnosed, there should be no delay in treatment. The patient should be admitted for intravenous empirical antibiotic treatment (amoxicillin and metronidazole) until the causative organism is identified. If there is no rapid or complete response to antibiotics, or if there is a subperiosteal abscess present (confirmed by imaging), surgery is indicated for pus drainage.

3. **B – Acute otitis externa**, also known as 'swimmer's ear', is an acute inflammation of the skin of the external ear canal. Ten per cent of the population will be affected by this condition at some point in their life. Risk factors include swimming, humidity and warm climates, change in ear pH (absence of cerumen), trauma from foreign bodies or hearing aids, diabetes mellitus, immunosuppression or underlying skin conditions. The causative organisms are *Pseudomonas aeruginosa*, *S. aureus* and *Bacillus proteus*. Patients present with otalgia, and pruritus especially on moving the pinna

or the jaw. They may also complain of discharge. Examination may show an inflamed external canal rich with debris with an inflamed, imperforated eardrum. There may be spreading cellulitis. Treatment is with regular aural toilet and possible insertion of an ear wick, and antibiotic/steroid ear drops. Systemic antibiotics are indicated for extending cellulitis.

4. **D – Brain abscess** is caused by infectious intracranial inflammation with subsequent abscess formation. The infection reaches the brain by direct spread via bone and meninges or haematogenous spread. The overall rate of brain abscesses has increased markedly since the emergence of acquired immune deficiency syndrome (AIDS). Antibiotics and the availability of imaging has significantly reduced mortality from up to 80% to less than 5%–15%. Frequency of neurological sequelae depends on how quickly the diagnosis is made and treatment administered. They occur most frequently in the first four decades of life. The clinical course can range from indolent to fulminant. The causative organisms are predominantly *S. aureus*. Most symptoms are a result of the size and location of the space-occupying lesion: headache, nausea and vomiting. A suddenly worsening headache, followed by meningism is associated with rupture of the abscess. The signs on examination are pyrexia, drowsiness, confusion, seizures, focal neurological deficit, neck stiffness and papilloedema (bilateral optic disc swelling due to raised intracranial pressure). Investigations include routine blood tests (full blood count and inflammatory markers), blood cultures, lumbar puncture (may be dangerous due to the risk of coning) and CT or MRI to determine the location and size of the brain abscess. Brain abscesses can rapidly result in death, which is why rapid surgical drainage is crucial. This is drained through a burr hole or excised via a craniotomy. Mastoidectomy should be performed with the same anaesthetic. Post-operative antibiotics are essential. If left untreated, death occurs from pressure coning, rupturing into a ventricle or spreading encephalitis. In this clinical scenario, the patient is likely to have an abscess which has ruptured and irritated the meninges.

5. **F – Chronic suppurative otitis media**. This case is a classic 'safe', mucosal CSOM. This is a common condition. The patient's main complaint is of an inconvenient, recurrent, mucoid discharge from the affected ear arising from the inflamed and secreting mucosa of the middle ear giving rise to associated conductive hearing loss. Classically the perforations in the safe group are 'central'. What this means is that there is membrane surrounding the perforation. In CSOM mucosal disease, the main aim is

to eliminate discharge and improve hearing deficit. *Drying* of the ear is achieved by treating the infection. This involves regular aural toilet (using microsuction) to remove infected material and antibiotic/steroid combination ear drops to treat the infection and reduce inflammation. Once dry, this becomes an 'inactive chronic otitis media'. Recurrent discharge can be prevented by protecting the ear from water, promptly treating upper respiratory tract infections, or closing the defect of the eardrum surgically (myringoplasty). Hearing defects can be assisted with hearing aids or a tympanoplasty.

A   ENT A9 – Management of middle ear disorders

1. **I – Stapedectomy**. Otosclerosis is an autosomal dominant disorder that is more common in young females, and there is usually therefore a positive family history. It affects 10% of the white population and has been decreasing in incidence since the use of the measles vaccine (aetiology is unknown; however, measles RNA is found in otosclerotic foci). The disorder is characterised by abnormal bone formation around the stapes footplate in the middle ear, resulting in slowly progressive conductive hearing loss, usually starting at low frequencies. This is bilateral in 70% of cases. Rinne test is performed as an investigation of hearing loss. The examiner uses a 512 Hz tuning fork, strikes it and places it over the mastoid process (bone conduction) followed by placing it by the ear (air conduction). The patient then states which one sounds louder. In conductive hearing loss bone conduction is louder than air conduction (Negative Rinne's test). In normal hearing and sensorineural hearing loss air conduction is louder than bone conduction. Other signs to look for are Schwartze's sign (on otoscopy), conductive hearing loss with a Carhart's notch (pure tone audiometry) and the absence of a stapedial reflex. Very rarely, otosclerosis can present as sensorineural hearing loss, if the bone of the cochlea is involved. Treatment of otosclerosis can be conservative or surgical. Hearing aids can be used to improve quality of life, and surgical intervention can be used to improve and reduce progression of hearing loss. These include total or partial stapedectomy, or stapedotomy. There is, however, a risk of complete sensorineural hearing loss with surgical intervention, which must be emphasised to the patient.

2. **F – Oral antibiotics**. This child has acute otitis media, which is treated with oral antibiotics and analgesia. The treatment of acute otitis media is discussed in Question 8 (ENT section).

3. **H – Regular ear surveillance**. This patient has suffered a tympanic perforation. These can be traumatic or infective. Traumatic perforations are divided into direct and indirect causes. Direct trauma includes poking with sharp instruments, usually in an attempt to clean the ear. Indirect trauma includes a slap with an open hand, sudden changes in atmospheric pressure or from a blast injury. Temporal bone fracture in a severe head injury and welding spark burns can also cause indirect traumatic tympanic perforation. A tympanic membrane perforation may also occur due to infection, secondary to a growing effusion within the middle ear. Patients present complaining of a pain at the time of rupture that is usually transient but may persist. Deafness is not usually severe, tinnitus may be persistent in cochlear injury (if the stapes is driven into the inner ear) and vertigo is rare. Patients can also present with a whistling sound on valsalva manoeuvres (sneezing, and blowing nose). This is due to high-velocity air travelling from the mouth through the Eustachian tube and then through a small perforation in the eardrum. Signs on examination include: bleeding from or blood clot in the ear, conductive hearing loss, and a hole/tear in the tympanic membrane. Treatment is to *leave it alone*. Thus, *do not* clean it, *do not* put drops in it, *do not* syringe it. Oral antibiotics are only indicated if there is any evidence of infection. Patients undergo regular ear surveillance until hearing has returned to normal.

4. **E – Myringotomy**. This is another case of AOM; however, in this example the patient has already had a trial of oral antibiotics that has failed. The treatment for this is a myringotomy – an incision into the tympanic membrane to release indwelling pus. However, this is a procedure that is rarely needed in the acute phase. Myringotomy may be followed by grommet insertion in ROM. The patient in this example has demonstrated mastoid tenderness on deep pressure palpation. This is a finding in AOM that may lead to clinicians suspecting mastoiditis. In acute mastoiditis, mastoid tenderness is marked even on light palpation.

5. **D – Mastoidectomy**. Cholesteatoma consists of squamous keratinising epithelium that is trapped within the skull base. It can be trapped within the temporal bone, middle ear or mastoid and can only expand at the expense of bone surrounding it. It can cause injury to adjacent structures within the nervous system and neck. Cholesteatoma can be congenital, primary acquired or secondary acquired. Congenital arises from squamous epithelium within the temporal bone during embryogenesis. Primary acquired is due to progressively deeper medial retraction of the tympanic

membrane. Secondary acquired is the result of injury to the tympanic membrane, which is the case in this example, as the patient is likely to have sustained a perforation due to recurrent otitis media. Patients usually present with painless otorrhoea that is foul-smelling and flaky. When infected it is very difficult to eliminate, as cholesteatomas do not have a blood supply. Conductive hearing loss is another common presentation, unlike vertigo, an uncommon symptom. Rarely, they present as an abscess in the neck or with symptoms of central nervous system complications such as sigmoid sinus thrombosis, epidural abscess or meningitis. Examination shows an ear canal filled with flaky discharge and a perforation or granulation tissue in the atticoantral region. Exposed bone may be seen. The only treatment that will stop expansion of the cholesteatoma is surgery. Patients who refuse surgical intervention will need regular cleaning to help control infection and slow growth. Surgical treatment of cholesteatoma includes radical mastoidectomy or a combined approach tympanoplasty, the former of which has a lower cholesteatoma recurrence rate. Patients should be warned that repeated operations may be required before complete elimination of a cholesteatoma.

A   ENT A10 – External ear disorders

1. **I – Necrotising otitis externa**. Also known as malignant otitis externa (MOE). MOE is a misnomer; it is a rare *non-neoplastic*, progressive infection of the external auditory canal that progresses into an osteomyelitis of the temporal bone. Spread beyond the external auditory canal takes place through the fissures of Santorini and the osseocartilaginous junction. It is more common in males than females, in those over 60 years of age (although it affects people in all age groups), and is found almost exclusively in diabetics and/or immunosuppressed. It is almost solely caused by *Pseudomona* species. Rarely, *Staphylococcus*, *Aspergillus* and *Proteus* are the causative organisms. Common symptoms are severe otalgia (disproportionate to external auditory canal appearance), purulent otorrhoea and temporal headaches. Further spread of infection and involvement of the jugular foramen and hypoglossal canal can cause cranial nerve palsies (seventh, ninth, tenth, eleventh, twelfth); however, these can appear in an almost normal-looking ear canal. Symptoms may include facial palsy, dysphagia and hoarseness. More rarely, the petrous apex can get involved resulting in sixth (Gradenigo's syndrome), as well as fifth nerve palsy. On examination there is marked tenderness between the mandibular ramus and mastoid process. Fever is uncommon in MOE. Otoscopic examination reveals granulation of

the floor of the external auditory canal particularly at the osseocartilaginous junction (pathognomic examination sign), and exposed bone may also be seen. As with the case in this scenario, patients may be systemically unwell (e.g. fever, malaise) and hyperglycaemic. Cranial nerves V–XII should be examined as well as mental state, as an altered mental state may indicate intracranial involvement. Isotope bone scanning, high-resolution CT or MRI scans of the head are used to confirm skull base erosion or intracranial pathology. MOE is a serious condition that can lead to lateral and cavernous sinus thrombosis, meningitis, and death if treatment is delayed. Treatment involves admission, blood sugar control, anti-pseudomonal systemic and topical antibiotics (e.g. ciprofloxacin) for 6–12 weeks, and regular aural toilet and strong analgesia. If no improvement is seen, surgical debridement may be indicated, where a histological specimen can be taken to exclude malignancy (e.g. squamous cell carcinoma).

Hint: Always consider necrotising otitis externa in diabetics with otitis externa.

2. **G – Furunculosis**. Otitis externa can be either diffuse or less commonly localised. Localised otitis externa (furunculosis) is merely an infection of a hair follicle of the external auditory canal caused by Gram-positive bacteria – usually *Staphylococcus aureus*. A furuncle is a very tender swelling or boil that is always located in the outer ear canal, as there are no hair follicles within the inner bony meatus. As in all cases of otitis externa, patients present with severe pain (most prominent symptom in furunculosis) particularly on movement of the pinna or pressure on the tragus, making examination of the ear canal challenging. Hearing loss is only experienced if the furuncle or discharge completely occludes the external auditory canal. Fevers do not occur unless infection spreads to the front of the ear as cellulitis or erysipelas. Tender lymphadenopathy may be palpable pre- or post-auricularly (hence, over the mastoid process in this patient). Post-auricular swelling may resemble a subperiosteal mastoid abscess. However, in this case, the patient only has a history of pain for 3 days, and a normal-looking eardrum (in mastoiditis this process takes 2–3 weeks to occur, with persistent increasingly copious discharge through a perforation in the tympanic membrane). Treatment is with aural toilet, oral antistaphylococcal antibiotics (e.g. amoxicillin), analgesia and possibly incision and drainage of the furuncle (under local anaesthesia) and/or insertion of a ribbon gauze or pope wick soaked in anitibiotic-steroid drops or 10% glycerine-ichthammol solution (the later is a combination of antiseptic and hygroscopic dehydrating agent).

3. **J – Ramsay Hunt syndrome** (RHS), also known as herpes zoster oticus, is an acute peripheral facial neuropathy caused by reactivation of varicella zoster virus lying dormant in the geniculate ganglion. Although it most commonly affects the facial nerve, it may rarely spread to involve the glossopharyngeal, vagus, trigeminal, abducens or hypoglossal. RHS is the cause of 16%–18% of all facial palsies. Twenty per cent of RHS cases are misdiagnosised as Bell's palsy. It is important to understand that a Bell's palsy in which the facial paralysis does not recover is not a Bell's palsy. RHS is more common in the elderly and immunosuppressed population. Patients with HIV have a significantly higher incidence of RHS than the normal population. It is not usually associated with mortality and its primary morbidity is facial weakness (resulting from neuritis), but, unlike Bell's palsy, the full recovery rate is less than 50% (more than 90% is Bell's palsy), and only 10% if left untreated. The most prominent presenting complaint is moderate to severe pain around and within the ear. They later develop facial palsy, which may be accompanied by vestibulocochlear symptoms (hearing loss, tinnitus and vertigo). Loss of taste on the anterior two-thirds of the tongue is a common symptom. Vesicles appear 2–3 days later in the concha (the shell-shaped part of the ear), and rarely the ipsilateral soft palate and anterior two-thirds of the tongue. Early treatment is essential, with high dose aciclovir and corticosteroids.

   Hint: Always examine the ears of a patient presenting with partial or complete facial paralysis.

4. **E – Contact dermatitis**. This is a delayed type hypersensitivity reaction of the skin of the pinna secondary to contact with an allergen, such as earrings, cosmetics, hair products, antiseptics, antibiotic drops (especially neomycin and chloramphenicol), as well as extension of a meatus infection in otitis externa. Note that contact dermatitis may be due to contact with an irritant substance (irritant contact dermatitis) or, as in this scenario, a substance to which an individual has a genuine allergy to (allergic contact dermatitis). In the acute phase the skin is erythematous, oedematous, and pruritic. Small vesicles may develop and lesions begin to weep and crust over. If this develops into a chronic problem, skin can begin to thicken as a result of rubbing and scratching, resulting in lichenification and hyper-pigmentation. A patch test may be helpful in establishing the causative allergen. Treatment involves stopping the causative agent (antibiotic in this case), adequate aural toilet and topical application of a steroid-based ointment.

5. **H – Malignancy of the external auditory canal** can be either localised or spread to the temporal bone. It is a rather rare type of tumour, but very aggressive. Carcinoma of the temporal bone accounts for fewer than 0.2% of all head and neck tumours, and most of them arise from the lateral concha and pinna as they are more sun exposed and spread medially to the external auditory canal (soft tissue has minimal resistance to tumour spread) and ultimately the temporal bone; tumour spread can also extend through the tympanic membrane into the middle ear or posteriorly to the mastoid cavity. It is an important differential diagnosis for otitis externa that is chronic and/or unresponsive to treatment. The majority are squamous cell carcinomas (squamous to basal cell carcinoma ratio 4:1; however, there are other, rarer types). Patients present with severe otalgia, otorrhoea (debris and/or blood), deafness, and cranial nerve palsies. On examination, tenderness, regional lymphadenopathy (nodal metastasis is seen in 10%–20% of advanced disease), blood and polypoid mass within the ear, and cranial nerve pathology may be elicited. If there is inadequate evidence to demonstrate tumour invasion, then a deep tissue biopsy is indicated. CT and MRI can be used to assess the extent of spread. Treatments can be curative or palliative, usually in the form of combined radiotherapy and surgery. All patients who are fit for surgical intervention should undergo excision of the tumour. Different options include local canal resection, extended mastoidectomy, lateral temporal bone resection, and subtotal or total petrosectomy. Malignancy of the external auditory canal has a poor prognosis, with a 2- to 3-year survival rate of 50%.

Exostoses – these are bony overgrowths or small osteomata of the external auditory canal that are quite common and usually multiple and bilateral. It happens more commonly in those who swim regularly, particularly in cold water. The reason is unknown. There are usually tumours arising in the bony meatus that are hard, sessile, smooth, covered by thin skin and very sensitive when probed. Its rate of growth is very slow and may be asymptomatic. If the patient is symptomatic, surgical removal of exostoses may be indicated.

A   ENT A11 – Hoarse voice and dysphonia

Voice change is often referred to as hoarseness. Clinically, the terms aphonia and dysphonia are preferred, the former meaning no voice or simply a whisper and the latter meaning alteration in the quality.

There are three crucial aspects to determining the cause of voice change: a thorough history, examination and knowledge of neuroanatomy.

The questions in this stem highlight these nuances and will help you distinguish a benign and self-limiting problem from one requiring urgent clinical attention. Key points in the history are:

- onset and duration of symptoms
- determining whether the change in voice is constant or variable
- associated or preceding symptoms such as pain, otalgia and a sore throat
- occupation and working environment (e.g. teaching, working in areas of poor acoustics, irritants in the atmosphere)
- smoking history – the main risk factor for laryngeal cancer
- medical history – chest disease, neck trauma, hypothyroidism
- surgical history – thyroid, cardiothoracic surgery.

Vibration of the vocal cords produces sound and the mouth and tongue provide articulation. Examining the vocal cords enables the clinician to demonstrate if there is a lesion, structural abnormality, or immobility in one or both cords. The vocal cords are usually visualised with nasal-endoscopy or video stroboscopy. Key to examining the vocal cords are the following: general appearance, abduction during coughing, and apposition/adduction during sound production. The vocal cords are innervated by the recurrent laryngeal nerve for both abduction and adduction. Most important, listen: the patient's voice may be breathy, rough, weak (termed asthenia) or strained.

1. **H – Reinke's oedema**. The vocal cord consists of three layers:
   - epithelium
   - lamina propria – subdivided into superficial (known as Reinke's space), intermediate and deep
   - vocalis or thyroarytenoid muscle.

Vocal cord oedema is a benign condition characterised by symmetrical bilateral oedema throughout the length of vocal cords. Fluid collects in the superficial layer of the lamina propria, also known as the sub-epithelial space of Reinke. The patient discussed here has two risk factors – occupational (where she uses her voice constantly) and smoking. Other causes include reflux disease and hypothyroidism. Patients present with a deep, hoarse voice. As with the patient in this example, there may also be localised oedema usually in the anterior third of the vocal cord. This causes polyp formation. Dysphonia may persist unless the polyp is surgically removed. This has the additional benefit of ruling out malignancy. Key to management is advice on smoking cessation and speech therapy. Further management of severe forms of Reinke's oedema is microsurgery, involving a cordotomy and drainage of fluid. There are several other benign vocal cord lesions including singer's nodules and contact ulcers, both caused by voice abuse. Occasionally, human papilloma virus may cause vocal cord and laryngeal papillomas. These may (rarely) become large and obstruct the airway or become malignant. Surgical intervention is therefore required. Recurrent papillomas may require intralesional antiviral treatment such as cidofovir.

2. **K – Vocal cord nodule**. It typically presents in adult females and young males. From the history of presenting complaint, we know that she most likely sings in areas of poor acoustics, requiring her to vocalise aggressively. Hence, the other term for this condition, singer's nodule. Vocal cord nodules are benign and usually occur at the junction of the anterior medial third of the vocal cord. This is the area most traumatised by high-pitched noises such as screaming. Patients sound breathy and their pitch is lower because the presence of the mass means the vocal cords cannot appose adequately. Management is with voice therapy and to retrain patients on appropriate sound production and reducing strain. Patients, on rare occasions, may require surgery.

3. **G – Perichondritis**. This patient has a vocal cord granuloma. Key to answering the question correctly is his history of intensive therapy unit admission. It is suggestive of trauma to the larynx as a result of intubation resulting in chronic inflammation of the exposed cartilage (perichondritis). Chronic inflammation can lead to the formation of localised, rounded, pedunculated granulomas. In the vocal cords, these arise from the posterior aspect. Patients may present with dysphonia, noisy breathing and a sensation of 'something' in their throat. Management is by removing the granuloma with a carbon dioxide laser. The surgeon must be careful not to remove too much as to expose the cartilage or too little, leaving granuloma behind to re-proliferate. As with all unilateral lesions, malignancy must be excluded. Any history of reflux is important to treat to minimise inflammation. Perichondritis can lead to necrosis of the cartilage of patients intubated for long periods of time.

4. **I – Right recurrent laryngeal nerve**. This patient has a right vocal cord palsy – the immobility of the true vocal cord. This is secondary to injury of the right (unilateral) recurrent laryngeal nerve following thyroid surgery. The causes, in roughly equal incidence are iatrogenic, neoplastic

and idiopathic. Patients present with weak, breathy voices and a history of voice fatigue. They may also have a poor cough or swallow and are therefore at risk of aspiration. Note that unilateral vocal cord paralysis does not cause loss of ability to speak, but a change in quality of sound produced. On scoping, one would find unilateral muscle atrophy and poor apposition due to the immobility of the damaged cord. Management of unilateral cord palsy includes conservative measures – whereby the contralateral cord compensates till the patient is asymptomatic. If this is unsuccessful, the palsied cord is medialised surgically to allow the mobile cord to fully adduct and appose with the palsied cord. When paralysis is bilateral for the abductors, phonation is good, however inspiration is poor. The most important and first step is maintaining the airway preferably with a tracheostomy. In bilateral adductor paralysis, the opposite happens where the airway is maintained but phonation is impaired. The first step here is still to maintain an airway and prevent aspiration. The case above describes a neurological cause of dysphonia. Neurological causes may be divided into central and peripheral, whereby lesions in the nervous system can precipitate voice change. Peripheral lesions affect the vagus and/or recurrent laryngeal nerve. The left recurrent laryngeal nerve is more vulnerable to injury, as it travels a longer course. These causes are summarised in Table 20.

TABLE 20 Central and peripheral causes of dysphonia

Central neurological lesions	Peripheral neurological lesions
Guillain–Barré syndrome	Nasopharyngeal cancers
Myaesthenia gravis	Carotid surgery
Multiple sclerosis	Thyroid surgery
Motor neurone disease	Bronchial carcinoma
	Aortic arch aneurysm

5. **D – Injection of muscle relaxants**. Musculoskeletal tension disorders tend to occur in patients, like that described above, with problems of stress and overwork. Excessive tension in the intrinsic and extrinsic laryngeal muscles during times of stress may lead to voice changes. Increase in their tone results in voice changes. Patients present with a change in voice and throat pain that is exquisitely tender on palpation. Occasionally there may also be a sensation of a lump in the throat. Gently pulling down the larynx eases these symptoms. Sometimes patients also report the voice change disappears when they are on holiday (i.e. less stressful situations). Musculoskeletal

tension disorder is part of the family of psychogenic dysphonia. This is a voice disorder in the absence of laryngeal disease. Further probing may elicit a history of depression, stress, anxiety, personality disorders and psychoneuroses. Other forms of psychogenic dysphonia include ventricular dysphonia, conversion disorders and mutational falsetto. Sudden-onset aphonia should prompt investigations into a psychogenic cause.

Other important differentials for dysphonia are, briefly:
- Foreign bodies.
- Hypothyroidism can cause chronic oedema of the vocal cords and thereby dysphonia.
- Laryngeal cancer: patients present with hoarsness, dysphagia, occasionally otalgia and a history of heavy smoking. On examination there may be a palpable neck lump. Endoscopy may also reveal a unilateral lesion of the vocal cord and larynx. Cervical lymphadenopathy may be present. Systemic features of malignancy may also feature, including unintentional weight loss.
- Laryngitis: patients present with a history of sore throat and voice change. Patients respond to fluid, analgesia, voice and bed rest.
- Reflux disease – patients are advised to stop smoking and reduce alcohol and caffeine intake; adequate hydration. Non-surgical interventions may also include dietary advice and voice exercises.

A   ENT A12 – Rhinitis and sinusitis

1. **A – Acute rhinosinusitis**. Rhinosinusitis can be acute or chronic. It is an inflammatory process involving the mucous membranes of the paranasal sinuses and the nose. Fluid build-up within the cavities results in facial pain and pressure. Acute inflammation can last up to 4 weeks, subacute up to 12 weeks and chronic more than 12 weeks. Patients are said to have recurrent sinusitis if symptoms occur more than four times a year. There are multiple causes of rhinosinusitis. These can be allergic or non-allergic. Patients with allergies, genetic predispositions and anatomical variations are prone to rhinosinusitis. Infection (*Haemophilus influenzae*, *Moraxella catarrhalis*, rhinovirus, respiratory syncytial virus, pneumococcus, among others), autonomic involvement, vasomotor, trauma and iatrogenic causes must also be considered. A history of trauma will prompt the clinician to rule out cerebrospinal fluid leakage as an important differential. Patients should be asked about activities such as diving – which can force contaminated water into the sinuses – smoking, foreign bodies in the nostril and

dental procedures. There may also be a history of inhalation of irritants like cocaine in the case of this patient. Patients with rhinitis typically present with a nasal congestion, sneezing and rhinorrhea. Obstruction and congestion also occur and patients also complain about altered sense of smell, and a post-nasal drip. Sinusitis adds a symptom of facial pain worse on bending forward. Investigations are not usually necessary, but plain sinus X-rays may show fluid levels in the sinuses. CT scans will also show thickening of the sinus mucosa. Treatment is with broad-spectrum antibiotics, e.g. co-amoxiclav, analgesia and decongestants, e.g. xylometazoline (an alpha-1 agonist causing vasoconstriction in the blood vessels in the nasal cavity and hence reducing inflammation and congestion) and/or Betnesol drops (corticosteroids leading to reduced inflammation of the lining of the nasal cavity and sinuses) into the nostrils. Steam inhalation is also of benefit. In refractive cases, packing the nasal cavity with 10% medical cocaine-soaked gauze can provide immediate relief. Cocaine is an uptake-1 inhibitor and potentiates neurotransmission at the synaptic cleft, and hence acts as a sympathomimetic leading to vasoconstriction and immediate relief of the congestion and drainage of the sinuses. Furthermore, functional endoscopic sinus surgery is usually the treatment of choice in severe cases. Table 21 summarises the classification of rhinosinusitis.

TABLE 21 Classification of rhinosinusitis

Type	Duration
Acute	Less than 4 weeks in duration
Sub-acute	Lasting for more than 4 weeks but less than 12
Recurrent	More than or equal to four episodes per year
Chronic	Lasting more than 12 weeks

2. **D – Chronic rhinosinusitis** usually lasts over 12 weeks. Symptoms are as described above under acute rhinosinusitis, however patients also suffer from anosmia and may also have nasal polyps. Unlike patients with acute rhinosinusitis, investigations are necessary in this case as there is usually underlying pathology. This is most commonly bacterial in aetiology and the common pathogens are anaerobes and Gram-negative bacteria such as *Staphylococcus aureus*, coagulase-negative staphylococci. Investigations should include allergy testing, ACE, erythrocyte sedimentation rate and anti-neutrophil cytoplasmic antibodies to exclude granulomatous disease. Also, patients with a medical history of cystic fibrosis, Kartagener's syndrome, and bronchiectasis have a predisposition to chronic rhinosinusitis

because of the impairment of ciliary clearance. This is the case for young Samuel in the example. The extent of disease can be examined with anterior rhinoscopy. This reveals an inflamed nasal mucosa and discharge on the cavity and oropharynx. Rigid endoscopy allows exploration of the middle meatus and any discharge into the postnasal space. A CT scan of the sinuses will show an air-fluid level and thickened mucosa. Imaging is essential in also ruling out nasopharyngeal and skull base malignancy in cases of chronic sinusitis. Treatment is as discussed, with analgesia (particularly NSAIDs) and topical steroids. However, it is prolonged and patients with chronic disease may also require oral steroids. Antihistamines and macrolides may be indicated if allergy test is positive and in the presence of mucopus respectively. As mentioned, in resistant cases pledgets of cotton soaked in cocaine may be of benefit. Surgical intervention may be required in the form of functional endoscopic sinus surgery.

3. **I – Urgent CT scan, IV antibiotics and drainage**. This patient has an orbital abscess. This question discusses a crucial complication of sinusitis, where inflammation may spread beyond the sinus cavity, increasing morbidity and mortality. The most common point of extension of the infection is the ethmoid sinus. Patients typically present as ill, pyrexial children, with chemosis (oedema of the conjutiva), diplopia and proptosis, most likely due to underlying abscess formation. Colour vision is impaired (test with an Ishihara plate) and there may be a relative afferent pupillary defect (RAPD). Funduscopy may reveal an enlarged optic disc and engorgement of the retinal veins. Common pathogens include *Streptococcus*, *S. aureus*, *Haemophilus influenzae* type B, *Pseudomonas* and *Klebsiella*. Management is via CT imaging to check for orbital abscesses, intravenous antibiotics, and steroids to reduce inflammation. This patient will need urgent surgical drainage to prevent permanent visual loss. If optic nerve decompression is not done within two hours, this will lead to irreversible nerve damage. Orbital complications of sinusitis are classified into five main categories – Chandler's Classification:
   - Class 1: Preseptal cellulitis (cellulitis that is superficial to the tarsal plate in the eye)
   - Class 2: Orbital cellulitis
   - Class 3: Subperiosteal abscess
   - Class 4: Orbital abscess
   - Class 5: Cavernous sinus thrombosis.

   Table 22 summarises the complications of rhinosinusitis.

TABLE 22 Complications of rhinosinusitis

Sites of possible invasion	Complications
Orbital	Orbital cellulitis
Dental	Mucocoeles
Intracranial	Intracranial abscesses, otitis media, cavernous sinus thrombosis
Airways	Pharyngitis, bronchiectasis
Haematogenous – leading to sepitcaemia	Toxic shock syndrome
Lymphatic	Tonsillitis
Other	Meningitis

4. **C – Aspirin sensitivity**. The case in this example describes a genetic cause of nasal polyps. Samter's triad comprises of late onset asthma, recurrent polyps and aspirin intolerance. Nasal polyps are considered to be on the spectrum of rhinosinusitis, whereby polyps result from chronic inflammation of the mucosa. They are essentially a prolapse of the sino-nasal mucosa secondary to chronic inflammation. The underlying cause of polyps is unclear. Other contributing factors include:

   - Allergies (e.g. to mites).
   - Infection – viral or bacterial. Nasal polyps may be considered as part of the clinical spectrum of rhinosinusitis. This is because continuous inflammation of the sinus and nasal lining causes it to become thicker and later pedunculated into the cavity.
   - Note that polyps are rare in children. Their presence should prompt the investigation for coeliac disease and cystic fibrosis.
   - Vasculitis – Churg–Strauss syndrome, Wegener's granulomatosis.

   Patients with nasal polyps tell a story of gradual onset nasal obstruction, postnasal drip and hyposmia or anosmia. Occasionally facial pain can be a symptom, for example in cases of chronic sinusitis. Patients often snore or have obstructive sleep. On examination, benign polyps appear as mobile, translucent and pedunculated grape-like structures. Patients should not feel pain on probing. If they do, you are probably touching the inferior turbinate! Patients with large chronic nasal polyps can experience a widening of nasal bones and bridge. Of note, the clinician should assess whether the polyp(s) is unilateral or bilateral. Unilateral polyps should be managed as neoplastic until otherwise proven. Malignant polyps may be solid and haemorrhagic. Polyps may be investigated with CT or MRI imaging. Polyps can be managed medically or surgically. Patients may be given a course of betnosol nasal drops and short-term steroid spray. Antihistamines and nasal douche with saline also help. Patient with larger polyps may be given a short course of high dose prednisolone. Patient with Samter's triad usually require long-term topical steroids and montelukast. Management of this condition also includes low salicylate diet which means avoiding fizzy drinks, potatoes and apples. Surgical treatment includes microdebridement and functional endoscopic sinus surgery.

5. **E – Klebsiella ozenae**. This patient presents a history of atrophic rhinitis or ozaena (meaning 'the stench'). In terms of pathophysiology, there is suqamous metaplasia followed by atrophy of the sinusoids, seromucinous glands and nerves. Causes include malnutrition, hereditary factors, and chronic bacterial rhinitis commonly from *Klebsiella ozenae*. In Western countries it usually occurs as the after-effects of nasal surgery. Typically affecting females more than males, patients are usually anosmic and are unfortunately unaware of the foul smelling discharge associated with it. This can have effects on their social interactions. On examination there is crusting of the nasal cavities and atrophy of mucosa to bone. Dislodging of crusts causes epistaxis. Management of this condition is by three to four times daily alkaline nasal toilet with a water toothpick or Higginson syringe. Steam inhalation and nasal drops containing glucose and glycerine are also of benefit. Surgical intervention may be required. This involves narrowing the nasal cavity or completely closing the nostril to be reopened after a few weeks. The aim of treatment is to allow time for regeneration of normal epithelium.

A **ENT A13 – Pharyngitis, tonsillitis, laryngitis and epiglottitis I**

As doctors, particularly in the fields of general practice and paediatrics, a large volume of patients will present with coughs, colds, throat pains and general malaise. The questions ENT Q13 and ENT Q14 (Pharyngitis, tonsillitis, laryngitis and epiglottitis I and II) are designed to help you distinguish between upper airway emergencies and day-to-day complaints. In all cases, however, it is essential to take a thorough history and then examine if indicated and safe.

1. **H – Take patient to resuscitation room and contact senior anaesthetist and ENT surgeon**. This patient has acute epiglottitis. The history and presentation (duration of symptoms, history of upper respiratory tract infection and lack of rash) is not consistent with an anaphylactic reaction.

The most common pathogen for epiglottitis is *Haemophilus influenzae* B (Hib). However, since the introduction of the Hib vaccine, incidence has reduced and other pathogens such as *Candida* and *Staphylococcus* have emerged. A typical presentation is as in the example given, with a young, usually male toddler (2–7 years) with a history of sore throat, looking pale, very unwell, complaining of odynophagia, inability to tolerate liquids and drooling. The patient also demonstrates the 'tripod sign' where leaning forward with outstretched arms improves breathing. Stridor is indicative of airway compromise. Essential to the management is *not* to touch the patient and *not* to give sedation. As a junior doctor, your role will be important to keep the patient and his mother calm and to take the patient to a 'place of safety'. This can be theatre, anaesthetic room or resuscitation room and then to urgently contact a senior anaesthetist and ENT surgeon for assessment and management. A place of safety must have facilities for intubation. Humidified oxygen, nebulised adrenaline and intravenous steroids may then be considered. Intravenous third-generation cephalosporins are usually given until blood cultures reveal sensitivities. In adults, there is a similar presentation. Laryngoscopy (the gold standard for diagnosing epiglottitis) may be performed in the presence of a senior ENT surgeon, as instrumentation can cause airway spasm. A lateral X-ray of the cervical spine is no longer often done as it delays management and increases the risk of airway compromise. However, it will show a 'thumbprint' sign caused by thickening of the epiglottis. Key to initiating this plan of action is knowing the sound of stridor. It is high-pitched noisy breathing that indicates airway restriction. Inspiratory stridor is caused by narrowing of the larynx and trachea; and expiratory stridor, narrowing of the bronchi. Causes include epiglottitis as described earlier, foreign bodies, croup, retropharyngeal abscess, bilateral vocal cord palsy and malignancy. In neonates, also suspect webs, subglottic stenosis and laryngomalacia. It is essential to take a quick history, assess vital signs (particularly oxygen saturations and respiratory rates) and most importantly, to keep yourself and the patient calm. Complications of epiglottitis include pharyngeal abscesses, meningitis and (rarely) pneumo-mediastinitis.

2. **G – Steeple sign**. Laryngotracheobronchitis, otherwise known as croup, typically manifests in infants aged 6–36 months. Patients present with a barking cough that is painful, pyrexia and inspiratory stridor progressing to become biphasic. Croup typically presents in the winter time, as with the patient in the example and is usually caused by *parainfluenza*, respiratory syncytial virus or *influenza* A or B. It is more common in males with

a history of a recent upper respiratory tract infection. It is important to note the difference between croup and epiglottitis and this is explained in Table 23. In view of the causes of stridor described, an X-ray of a stable patient is indicated to rule out other differentials for stridor such as foreign bodies. An anteroposterior X-ray in a patient with croup will show a narrowing of the supraglottis known as the steeple sign. The thumbprint sign is indicative of epiglottitis and not croup. It is caused by thickening of the epiglottis and is seen on lateral X-rays of the cervical spine. Management is usually conservative – patients are admitted for observation and humidified oxygen. It is essential to exclude epiglottitis and foreign body inhalation as differentials for stridor. They may also require intravenous dexamethasone and nebulised adrenaline. Symptoms usually settle within a week. However, if croup recurs patients may require microlaryngobronchoscopy to assess for anatomical problems.

TABLE 23 Comparison between epiglottitis and laryngotracheobronchitis

Variable	Epiglottitis	Laryngotracheobronchitis (croup)
Causative pathogen	*Haemophilus influenzae* B	Parainfluenza, RSV
Age	2–7 years	6–36 months
Clinical presentation	Rapid onset of symptoms	Gradual onset of symptoms
	Pyrexia	Low-grade fever
	No cough	Barking cough
	Drooling	No drooling
	Patient generally quiet	Patient more active and distressed
	Dyspnoea ++	Variable dyspnoea
Cervical X-ray	Thumbprint sign on lateral view	Steeple sign on AP view

RSV, respiratory syncytial virus; AP, anteroposterior.

3. **D – Quinsy.** The patient in the example has tonsillitis with peritonsillar abscess, known as quinsy. This is a complication of tonsillitis. Tonsillitis is very common and should be familiarised by students and clinicians. With bacterial tonsillitis, patients present with a history of sore throat, general malaise and pyrexia. On examination, one would find enlarged tonsils with or without exudate (the term 'slough' was used in the example). With quinsy the patient is very unwell, drooling and with fetor. On examination, there will be unilateral swelling of the soft palate to the site of the abscess and contralateral deviation of the uvula. In the case of the patient in this example, she has a left-sided peritonsillar abscess. Crucial to

assessment to is to check the extent of dysphagia and airway compromise if any. Blood tests will indicate bacteraemia. The Paul–Bunnell test is an antibody test used to assess for glandular fever, using red cells of sheep in heterophile antibodies. Another is the Monospot test. This uses horse red cells, exposed to heterophile antibodies. Either will confirm infection due to Epstein–Barr virus. The patient in this example has a bacterial cause and therefore requires needle aspiration of the abscess with or without incision to drain and intravenous antibiotics. Penicillin is the antibiotic of choice. The most likely pathogens in this case are group A beta-haemolytic *Streptococcus*, *Pneumococcus*, *Haemophilus influenzae* and *Staphylococcus*. Other complications of tonsillitis include parapharyngeal abcess, chronic tonsillar hypertrophy and airway obstruction. Patients with recurrent tonsillitis or who suffer from quinsy are often offered elective tonsillectomies.

4. **A – Amoxicillin**. This patient has glandular fever or infectious mononucleosis caused by the Epstein–Barr virus (EBV). EBV also causes pharyngitis. It most commonly affects patients between the ages of 15 and 25 years and has an incubation period of 1–2 months. Transmission is via coughing, sneezing, sharing utensils or oral contact, hence the term 'kissing disease'. Here, the symptoms are similar to that of tonsillitis, but the temperature rise is mild, duration of illness is longer and there is likely a history of oral contact. On examination, there is cervical lymphadenopathy, petechial haemorrhages on the palate, and slough on the tonsils. There may also be hepatosplenomegaly. Glandular fever is usually self-limiting. Patients are managed with intravenous or oral fluids, analgesia and short-term steroid therapy. Antibiotics including amoxicillin and ampicillin are unnecessary and must be avoided in patients with glandular fever. Like the patient in the example, an extensive pruritic maculopapular rash will develop. EBV is also associated with Burkitt's and B-cell lymohoma, nasopharyngeal cancer and Duncan's syndrome. These should be kept in the clinician's mind when assessing or reassessing the patient. In general, patients presenting with the above symptoms but with *negative* Paul–Bunnell tests, the differentials include cytomegalovirus, rubella, HIV, herpes simplex and toxoplasma infection.

5. **F – Splenic rupture**. Marlon played rugby 10 days after EBV tonsillitis. A rare but important complication of this condition is hepatosplenomegaly. It is likely that he was not told patients with glandular fever must avoid contact sports for 6 weeks. This is because of the risk (and in this case the occurrence) of splenic rupture. This is a failure of patient care. If suspected,

patients must be promptly resuscitated, scanned and urgently referred to the surgical team. Other complications of EBV include those for tonsillitis – airway compromise if enlarged as well as myocarditis, haemolytic anaemia, nephritis and meningitis. However, these are very rare. Jaundice occurs in few cases of hepatosplenomegaly. In general, all patients must be advised of the following if they are suspected of having infectious mononucleosis:

- avoid contact sports for 6 weeks
- avoid alcohol during illness
- avoid amoxicillin and ampicillin.

Paracetamol and/or ibuprofen helps alleviate pain and reduce fevers.

A   ENT A14 – Pharyngitis, tonsillitis, laryngitis and epiglottitis II

1. **J – Reassurance, analgesia, bed and voice rest**. This patient has acute laryngitis. It usually presents, as with the patient in the example, as part of an upper respiratory tract infection. Patients experience a sore throat with dysphonia. Symptoms also include malaise, pain on coughing and dysphagia. On examination there may be mild pyrexia. Endoscopy, if used, will show inflammation and oedema of the larynx and vocal cords. Patients may have laryngitis following streptococcal and staphylococcal infection. Most patients with the symptoms given in this example either self-medicate or see a GP. Analgesia, steam inhalation, cough linctus and, rarely, penicillin, may be administered. Key to resolving laryngitis, however, is voice rest. This is particularly necessary for patients whose careers are voice dependent. Laryngitis can cause haemorrhage into the vocal cords causing permanent changes in voice. The following are risk factors for chronic laryngitis:

- smoking
- alcohol
- patients with chronic lung disease, sinusitis, reflux disease
- workers or residents in areas of environmental pollution
- voice overuse.

Here, constant irritation of the stratified squamous epithelium causes an increase in the presence of macrophages and lymphocytes. The epithelium of the larynx and vocal cords eventually becomes keratinised and oedematous. Patients present with the symptoms described above, as well as constant coughing, throat clearing and globus. Vocal cords will appear thickened, inflamed and erythematous. Management of chronic laryngitis includes voice rest, speech therapy and smoking cessation. Management of reflux is also important. If symptoms persist for over four weeks, ENT referral, microlaryngoscopy and/or biopsy may be required.

2. **H – Paracetamol**. Mrs Xui's son has simple coryza or the common cold, for which antibiotics are not indicated. Transmitted via airborne infected droplets or direct contact, it is likely that he contracted it in his play school. It is essential in managing patients to have a good rapport, understand their concerns and to explain that antibiotics will not alleviate their symptoms. Openly discuss these anxieties and ensure that patients are better educated and prevent unnecessary visits to the doctor in the future. This is a common written and clinical examination scenario. Key facts to note are as follows:
   - there are no drugs proven to treat the common cold
   - colds are self-limiting of up to 2 weeks
   - mild pyrexia is expected and common in infants and can be managed with paracetamol or ibuprofen
   - encourage plenty of fluids
   - cough linctus and vapour rubs may be used to keep patients more comfortable.

   As with the child in this example, it is good practice to examine the patient and rule out foreign bodies in the nose. The discharge in the latter case is more likely to be unilateral, foul smelling or blood stained. The red flags are inability to swallow, drooling and shortness of breath.

3. **F – Koplik's spots**. The patient in this example has measles and from the history he is at the highly infectious (also called the catarrhal) stage. He has prodromal symptoms of coryza, conjunctivitis and cough and his medical history (chemotherapy) suggests immuno-compromise. Koplik's spots appear as grey-white on an erythematous base in the buccal mucosa. The catarrhal stage will be followed by the morbilliform (measles-like) stage. This is a maculopapular rash, starting on the face and neck and spreading across the body. Measles is caused by droplet transmission of the RNA paramyxovirus. Measles is self-limiting; however, 1 in 10 cases may require hospitalisation and can be complicated by pneumonia, gastroenteritis, myocarditis and panencephalitis. Following the MMR scare, the incidence of measles has risen, although herd immunity prevails.

4. **E – Group A streptococcus**. This patient is suffering from streptococcal pharyngitis and tonsillitis. In the history he presents with classic symptoms of general malaise, fever, headaches and inflamed throat and tonsils. Palatal petechiae and cervical lymphadenopathy aid in the differential diagnosis of 'strep throat' as it is commonly called. Definitive diagnosis is with throat culture. This organism is highly contagious and incidences of streptococcal pharyngitis are often found in schools and other close environments. Most sore throats are self-limiting and patients are advised rest, hydration and analgesia. Treatment with penicillin V or amoxicillin can be used to prevent complications such as rheumatic fever and retropharyngeal peritonsillar abscesses. Strep throat is often misdiagnosed as infectious mononucleosis caused by the Epstein–Barr virus. Note that up to 70% of sore throats are caused by viral infections. The Centor criteria may be used to predict patients at high risk of group A streptococcal infection. The criteria are:

- history of fever
- absence of cough
- tender cervical lymph nodes
- tonsillar exudate.

However, in the case given in this example, we know that the patient scores at least 3, which implies a 40%–60% likelihood of infection with group A streptococcus.

5. **L – Retropharyngeal abscess**. This is a complication of pharyngitis. Upper respiratory tract infections can cause adenitis. If the retropharyngeal nodes are involved, abscesses – normally unilateral – may form. This is termed retropharyngeal abscess (RPA). B-haemolytic streptococci, *Staphylococcus aureus* and *Bacteroides* are the common pathogens usually from a history of tonsillitis, adenoids, infected teeth or foreign bodies. As with the case given here, RPAs are more common in children. Patients present with sore throat, fever, stridor, dysphagia, drooling or cough. In adults neck stiffness and cervical adenopathy may be additional physical signs. RPAs are distinguishable from epiglotitis in terms of lateral X-ray findings – in the former, one would note increased soft tissue density and an air fluid level in pre-vertebral space, and in the latter, a more focal swelling or 'thumbprint' at the site of the epiglottis. CT imaging with intravenous contrast can help differentiate if available and appropriate. These patients should also have a chest X-ray to monitor for aspiration pneumonia and mediastinitis, which are known complications of RPAs. Management is by keeping a

patent airway and high-dose intravenous antibiotics such as cefuroxime, clindamycin, or co-amoxiclav, with metronidazole. ENT surgeons must be informed as oral (tonsillectomy approach) incision and drainage is often required. Intravenous steroids may help reduce swelling. There are also cases of chronic retro-pharyngeal abscesses. These can be caused by spinal tuberculosis.

A   **ENT A15 – ENT epidemiology**

1. **A – Bell's palsy** is the most common cause of facial paralysis, and accounts for approximately 75% of acute facial palsies. It is a lower motor neurone type of facial paralysis, resulting in full paralysis in about two-thirds of patients. The cause is unknown (likely viral), and most patients start to recover within 4–6 weeks. It has an incidence of 20 cases per 100000 and affecting males and females equally. Bell's palsy is a diagnosis of exclusion. A comprehensive history is imperative to establish the cause of facial paralysis. This must include enquiring about any recent trauma or surgery. One must not assume that the patient will volunteer this information. The facial palsy in Bell's palsy and Ramsay Hunt syndrome (RHS) is frequently preceded by aching pain in the mastoid. Other signs of Bell's palsy include hearing impairment, taste impairment, eye dryness and hyperacusis. A chronically discharging ear with facial paralysis is most likely due to cholesteatoma. A thorough examination of the head and neck is also vital. Upper motor neurone lesions do not cause a paralysis of the upper (forehead) muscle due to bilateral nerve innervations, a sign referred to as forehead sparring. A stroke must be excluded in these patients. Lower motor neurone lesions result in paralysis of upper and lower facial muscle. The presence of a parotid swelling or a tonsillar deviation with facial paralysis may indicate a parotid malignancy. The ears should be examined for herpetic vesicles (RHS) and a cholesteatoma. RHS is a lower motor neurone-type facial palsy caused by reactivation of the dormant herpes zoster virus. It accounts for less than 10% of all facial palsies, but it has major complications (e.g. post-herpetic neuralgia). In addition to the aforementioned clinical features, patients may have a sensorineural hearing loss, vertigo and tinnitus. Mainstay of treatment of RHS is with oral antivirals (e.g. aciclovir) and steroids. There is no good evidence for the use of antivirals or steroids in Bell's palsy; however, it is common practice to offer oral aciclovir if a patient presents within 48 hours of the initial symptoms. Full recovery occurs spontaneously in more than 90% of patients; however, it may take up to a year for symptoms to resolve. Studies

have shown that symptoms are recurrent in 10% of affected individuals. Other causes of facial nerve palsies include trauma (facial lacerations and fractures of the temporal bone), bacterial (Lyme disease, acute otitis media), viral (HIV), tumours (e.g. acoustic neuromas, parotid tumours, meningiomas), acquired disorders (e.g. myotonic dystrophy), congenital (e.g. mobius syndrome: sixth and seventh cranial nerve palsy – can be unilateral or bilateral). Moreover, facial nerve palsy can be a manifestation of a systemic disease process such as multiple sclerosis, Guillain–Barré syndrome and sarcoidosis.

2. **H – Rhinosinusitis**. About 40% of HIV patients will present with an ENT disease. Rhinosinusitis is the most common manifestation of HIV infection, affecting up to 68% of patients. Patients present with nasal congestion, facial pain, headache, post nasal drip and fevers. Management is with antibiotics, but draining of the sinuses may be required in resistant cases. HIV may manifest in many different forms in the head and neck area, and may be the first sign or symptom of AIDS. It is important, therefore, to be aware of the common clinical presentation. The most common ear manifestations of AIDS are otitis media and aural polyps. Common skin presentations include molluscum contagiosum, seborrhoeic dermatitis and Kaposi's sarcoma. Cervical adenopathy is present in up to 45% of patients with HIV. Early in the course of HIV, 'persistent generalised lymphadenopathy' is a common finding. This is multisite lymphadenopathy of unidentifiable cause. The cervical lymph nodes are the most commonly affected. Bilateral parotid swelling (usually multicystic) in young individuals may be the initial presentation of HIV. Oral manifestations of AIDS include oral candidiasis (oral thrush), hairy leukoplakia, tonsillar hypertrophy and Kaposi's sarcoma. The latter is a very common cause of oral lesions in AIDS patients, with the majority of cases affecting the palate.

3. **E – Pneumococcal vaccine**. *Streptococcus pneumoniae* is the most common cause of acute otitis media (AOM) in children of all age groups. *Haemophilus influenzae* is the second most frequently isolated pathogen in AOM. AOM is a self-limiting condition, and most patients recover without the use of antibiotics. Although many advocate a conservative 'watch and wait' approach for AOM rather than using antibiotics, this is possibly associated with an increased rate of mastoiditis. Some children suffer from a recurrent AOM. In children at high risk of recurrent AOM, prophylactic antibiotics have been shown to decrease the risk. The average incidence has been found to decrease from 3 to 1.5 episodes of AOM per

year. Pneumococcal vaccine, on the other hand, has not been found to be successful in reducing the incidence of AOM.

4. **F – Poor dental hygiene**. Halitosis affects about 2.4% of adults. The most common cause of halitosis is poor dental or oral hygiene. Other common causes include chronic sinusitis, tonsillitis, dentures and poor diet. In immunocompromised and elderly patients, oral thrush (candidiasis) is a relatively common cause of halitosis and dysphagia. Patients with asthma or bronchitis who use steroid inhalers are also at increased risk if they do not wash their mouth after using the inhalers. Another important and obvious cause of bad breath is smoking, but patients do not present complaining of bad breath, as they usually know both the cause and the solution!

5. **C – Parotid tumours**. The salivary glands are made up of the parotid, mandibular and sublingual glands. Eighty per cent of all salivary tumours occur in the parotid gland, of which 80% are pleomorphic adenomas (also known as benign mixed tumours). The second most common benign parotid tumour is a Warthin's tumour (also known as an adenolymphoma). Pleomorphic adenomas also represent 90% of submandibular gland tumours. They occur more commonly in females, and tend to affect the 30- to 60-year age group. They typically present as a progressively enlarging painless lump behind the angle of the mandible. It is rare for a pleomorphic adenoma to become malignant, and this occurs in patients who have had the condition for a long time. If a pleomorphic adenoma starts to grow rapidly, becomes painful or the facial nerve is affected, a malignancy should be suspected. Imaging is usually not necessary for a pleomorphic adenoma if there is no clinical evidence of deep lobe extension. A fine needle aspiration is helpful (95% sensitivity), but some specialists prefer to go straight for a superficial parotidectomy. The latter is the treatment of choice for pleomorphic adenoma, involving a complete surgical excision of the adenoma with uninvolved margins. Recurrence after excision is rare (<4%). Frey's syndrome (gustatory sweating and facial flushing most commonly due to iatrogenic damage to the auriculotemporal nerve during surgery. The nerve heals and attaches to the sweat glands rather than the salivary glands. Therefore, sweating occurs instead of salivation) occurs in up to 40% of patients who have undergone parotid gland surgery. Diagnosis is clinical (sweating over surgical site), but can be confirmed by the starch iodine test (iodine applied to the face is mixed with starch. A food stimulus is presented to the patient hence causing them to sweat and rendering the iodine and starch mixture dark).

A   ENT A16 – Epistaxis

The nose has a very rich blood supply and the patient's presentation depends on from where the bleed is arising. When handling epistaxis, the site of the bleed needs to be grossly identified: either an anterior or a posterior bleed. More than 90% of epistaxis occurs anteriorly, from Little's area (Kiesselbach's plexus). This is an anastomotic network of blood vessels at the anterior cartilaginous septum, where blood supply from the internal carotid artery (anterior and posterior ethmoid arteries) and the external carotid artery (sphenopalatine and branches of the internal maxillary arteries) meet. Bleeding posteriorly is more profuse and frequently arterial in origin. Therefore, they are more serious, as they are more difficult to control and they pose a greater risk of aspiration of blood and airway compromise. Causes of epistaxis can be divided into three groups: local causes, systemic causes and idiopathic causes. The latter group is the most common cause of epistaxis. Local causes include trauma, septal abnormality (congenital or nasal fracture), mucosal irritation such as nose picking or cocaine abuse, inflammatory conditions such as rhinitis, local tumours and iatrogenic causes such as intranasal steroids or surgery. Systemic causes include hereditary telangiectasia, haematological malignancy such as leukaemias and lymphomas, coagulative abnormalities such as haemophilia, von Willibrand's disease, immune thrombocytopenic purpura (ITP) and other thrombocytopenias, and antiplatelet or anticoagulation drugs. Hypertension is not an independent cause of epistaxis but it may precipitate the problem. The patient population is bimodal, with peaks in children aged between 2 and 10 years, and older individuals aged between 50 and 80 years. Cocaine use should be considered in an adolescent presentation. The immediate treatment for epistaxis is the same regardless of the cause. Subsequent treatment depends upon the cause and will be discussed in the scenarios. When a patient presents with uncontrollable epistaxis, direct firm digital pressure on the lower nose (cartilaginous area) for 10 minutes compresses the vessels on the septum and arrests bleeding from Little's area. The patient should sit leaning forward and breathe through his/her mouth. Suction can be used to remove excess blood and clots. If the bleeding persists, then cautery may be used. First, cotton wool or ribbon gauze soaked in lidocaine and adrenaline is left in at the site of the bleed for about 5 minutes. Cautery can then be applied using a silver nitrate impregnated stick. If these measures fail to control the bleed, the nose may need to be packed using a ribbon gauze or a self-expanding pack (e.g. a nasal tampon). If the bleed is posterior, then a post-nasal pack can be used when the patient is under general anaesthetic or a Foley catheter can be inserted until it is visible in the oropharynx – the balloon can be inflated then and pulled back to occlude any bleeding vessel, and the catheter is secured so that the balloon remains in place. If bleeding continues despite adequate packing then the patient may require surgical intervention.

1. **G – Immune thrombocytopenic purpura** (ITP) occurs as a result of immune destruction of platelets with splenic sequestration. There is isolated thrombocytopenia, no other haematological abnormalities and typically a normal bone marrow (occasional megakaryocytes). There are two clinical presentations of ITP: the acute syndrome that presents in children and the chronic syndrome that presents in adults. Children affected are more commonly boys aged between 1 and 6 years who present with an abrupt onset of purpura, following a viral infection. Investigations are unnecessary and the disease is self-limiting in the majority of children, lasting approximately 2 months. Chronic ITP usually affects young adult women and is the commonest cause of thrombocytopenia. It usually presents gradually and persists longer than 6 months. The cause is most commonly idiopathic; however, it may present with other autoimmune diseases, such as thyroid disease and systemic lupus erythematosus, or viral infections, such as Epstein–Barr virus and HIV. Drugs such as methyldopa may also cause ITP. Patients present with manifestations of bleeding: easy bruising, gingival bleeding, menorrhagia and epistaxis. Splenomegaly is not a feature of ITP. Blood results show thrombocytopenia, normal thrombin time, partial thrombin and coagulation time. Platelet associated IgG is 95% sensitive and 50% specific. ITP is a diagnosis of exclusion; there are no laboratory results that prove the diagnosis. A platelet count above 50 does not usually require treatment; levels between 20 and 50 are treated according to clinical condition; levels below 20 are treated with high-dose intravenous steroids and intravenous immunoglobulins. Patients may require platelet transfusion although similar immune destruction of the transfused platelets may occur. A level below 10 is a medical emergency. If medical measures have failed, a splenectomy may be necessary. Dapsone is a novel therapy that has proved efficacious in recovering platelet levels. It is often difficult to differentiate clinically between ITP and other bleeding disorders such as von Willebrand's disease; clues in the question will direct you to the correct diagnosis. In this scenario the patient also has systemic lupus erythematosus and all other haematological results are normal. In von Willebrand's disease the bleeding time and activated partial thromboplastin time is prolonged and there are low levels

of VIII:C and VIII:vWF. Additionally, von Willebrand's disease is the most common inherited bleeding disorder (autosomal dominant), so the question would usually include a family history of bleeding. If the patient had disseminated intravascular coagulation (DIC) they would be very unwell and septic. The blood test results in DIC characteristically reveal a triad of: (1) thrombocytopenia, (2) prolonged prothrombin time and activated partial thromboplastin time, and (3) decreased fibrinogen. Blood film reveals schistocytes (broken blood cells).

2. **C – Aspirin**. There are a number of clues in this question; the risk factors of this typical arteriopath are male, type A personality being a trader, hypertension, history of myocardial infarctions and atrial fibrillation. The additional comment regarding the patient's medication is there for a reason: it has been left ambiguous so you can assume the examiner wants you to consider a drug cause. This patient has a CHADS2 score of 1. The CHADS2 score is a clinical prediction assessment for estimating the risk of stroke in patients with atrial fibrillation. CHADS stands for **c**ongestive heart failure, **h**ypertension, **a**ge >65, **d**iabetes mellitus and **s**troke. Each gives a score of 1, stroke gives a score of 2 alone. This scoring system is used to determine whether the patient should be treated with anticoagulation therapy or antiplatelet therapy. A score of 2 and above indicates the patient is at a higher risk of stroke and will therefore be started on warfarin. Alternatively, patients with a score less than 2 will be started on aspirin. This patient was therefore on aspirin. It is extremely important to take a full medical history in a patient with epistaxis. Importantly, hypertension is not an independent cause of epistaxis; however, it worsens the condition and propagates the complications.

3. **D – Cocaine**. This is another example of reading between the lines in a question; it is merely fashioning a stereotypical individual that would require further enquiry into recent recreational drug abuse. He is a young lad attending A&E in the early hours, returning from a nightclub. The anxiety is not an effect of cocaine; it is another hint suggesting the patient being genuinely afraid of the consequences of his illicit drug use, by either parents or police finding out.

4. **B – Acute myeloid leukaemia** (AML) is classified as acute and chronic on the basis of the speed of evolution of disease. This patient presented with AML, which is seen more frequently than acute lymphoid leukaemia (ALL), predominately a disease of childhood, in adults. There is

uncontrolled growth of leukaemic cells in the bone marrow and the peripheral blood with consequential reduction in red cells, neutrophils and platelets. The acute leukaemias present similarly as a result of the failing bone marrow; patients present with shortness of breath/palpitations/lethargy, increased risk of infection and increased bleeding tendencies. Patients may also present with unexplained irritability and gum hypertrophy. There may also be lymphadenopathy and hepatosplenomegaly. There may be testicular enlargement in ALL. Bone marrow aspirate is the most diagnostic investigation, although peripheral blood films are very informative; both these tests identify blast cells (of lymphoid origin in ALL and myeloid origin in AML). Auer rods within blast cells are pathognomonic of AML. Blood tests show anaemia, neutropenia, thrombocytopenia and usually raised white cell counts, but not always! Correction of blood counts and infection, and prevention of acute tumour lysis syndrome, by hydration and allopurinol, is important. Treatment can be curative with chemotherapy. Chronic leukaemias have different presentations and have a more insidious onset. Chronic myeloid leukaemia (CML) presents with weight loss, fever and anaemia. Massive splenomagaly is characteristic. Philadelphia chromosome is found in 95% of CML patients. The tyrosine kinase inhibitor, imatinib, is the treatment for CML and can be continued indefinitely with greater than 90% success rates. Chronic lymphoid leukaemia is the most common leukaemia of the elderly. This leukaemia is commonly asymptomatic and patients are found to have incidental lymphocytosis on blood studies. Occasionally, patients present with symptoms of bone marrow failure, painless lymphadenopathy or hepatosplenamegaly in advanced disease. Blood films show 'smear cells'. Chronic lymphoid leukaemia is incurable and management is usually palliative.

5. **J – Wegener's granulomatosis**, or its recently refined name granulomatosis with polyangiitis, is a rare multisystem vasculitis of unknown aetiology. It is one of three vasculitides that is associated with anti-neutrophil cytoplasmic antibodies (ANCA), distinctively C-ANCA; the other two include Churg–Strauss syndrome and microscopic polyangitis, which are specifically associated with P-ANCA. It occurs more commonly in men aged between 35 and 55 years, and 90% of the patient population are white. Wegener's granulomatosis has a predilection for the upper and lower respiratory tracts and the kidneys. Chronic sinusitis is the most common presenting complaint. Other common ENT symptoms include epistaxis and rhinitis. Saddle nose deformity is typical because of collapse of the nasal septum. Oral ulcers are common. Lower respiratory symptoms

include cough, haemoptysis and pleuritic chest pain. Pulmonary infiltrates and nodular reticular shadowing with cavitation is seen on imaging. Kidney lesions are present in 20% of patients; renal histological changes show focal segmental (crescentic) necrotising glomerulonephritis. Central nervous system involvement leads to polyneuropathy, mononeuritis multiplex and cranial nerve palsies. Treatment is with cyclophosphamide and steroids. Goodpasture's syndrome (anti-glioblastoma multiforme) only presents with haemoptysis (lung haemorrhage) and glomerulonephritis but *not* epistaxis.

A ENT A17 – Airway obstruction I

1. **A – Asthma** is a chronic inflammatory condition of the lungs that leads to variable airway narrowing. It is characterised by mucosal oedema, hypersecretion, bronchospasm and hyper-responsiveness. Asthma may be diagnosed clinically by recognising a constellation of episodic symptoms. Patients may complain of a cough, dyspnoea, wheeze and chest tightness. These symptoms are frequent and recurrent, typically worse at night or early in the morning, and respond favourably to bronchodilators. Triggers include exercise, animal contact, cold air, smoke and exaggerated emotions. Patients often have a substantial relevant atopic personal and family history; the atopic chain includes a history of allergies to food or drugs, eczema and hay fever. If patients have typical symptoms they can be started on therapy immediately. The treatment will be reviewed after a short period to assess the response (the trial of treatment); the aim is to identify variable airflow limitation by demonstrating a change in the peak expiratory flow rate (PEFR). This may be evident from innate diurnal variability, from responses to bronchodilators or from changes induced by exercise. The PEFRs can be recorded by the patient in a diary. Further testing can be reserved for those with poor response to therapy, although there is still no single diagnostic test. Histamine or methacholine bronchial hyper-reactive challenge demonstrates a fall in the FEV_1 (forced expiratory volume in 1 second), and allergy skin testing (radioallergosorbent test) identifies atopy. A trial of steroids may be used in those with severe airway limitation; an improvement demonstrates reversibility.

    Management aims to control the disease process; this means the patient should not experience any exacerbations, should not experience night or daytime symptoms, should not need rescue therapy, and should not have any limitation on sport activity. Their FEV_1 and PEFR should be normal for their age and height. To ensure all these targets are met, patients should be started on the management step that is most appropriate to their initial severity using the British Thoracic Society guidelines in the stepwise management of asthma.

- Step 1 (for mild intermittent asthma): short-acting β_2-agonist as required (e.g. salbutamol inhalers). If needed more than three times a week or if symptoms wake up the individual from sleep $\rightarrow$ move to Step 2.
- Step 2 (for regular prevention): the addition of an inhaled steroid, e.g. fluticasone 50–100 mcg twice a day or beclometasone 200 mcg twice a day. If symptoms still present and reliever inhaler used regularly $\rightarrow$ move to Step 3.
- Step 3 (initial add-on therapy for patients not controlled on Step 2): addition of inhaled long-acting β_2-agonist (e.g. salmeterol inhaler 50 mcg twice a day), increasing the dose of inhaled steroid used in Step 2. The benefit of the long-acting β_2-agonist is assessed and the management changed accordingly. It is imperative to recheck inhaler technique, compliance and avoidance of triggering agents. If poor control still persists $\rightarrow$ move to Step 4.
- Step 4 (for persistent poor control): the dose of the inhaled steroid may be increased gradually up to 2000 mcg per day, addition of slow-released theophylline (e.g. Slo-Phyllin 6 mg/kg twice a day orally) or a leukotriene receptor antagonist (e.g. montelukast) may be considered. If poor control still persists $\rightarrow$ move to Step 5.
- Step 5: use of oral steroid while maintaining a high dose of inhaled steroid. Referral to specialist is advised.

General notes to consider:
- Monitoring of growth is essential because of the use of steroids. Moreover, it is imperative to advise the patient and guardian to rinse their mouths after use of steroid inhalers.
- Spacers can be used in children to enhance the delivery of the medication.

Note the following changes to the aforementioned regimen in children aged between 5 and 12 years:
- Step 2: 200 mcg/day is an appropriate starting dose.
- Step 3: increase dose to 400 mcg/day.
- Step 4: increase up to 800 mcg/day.
- Step 5: maintain high dose at 800 mcg/day; refer to respiratory paediatrician.

Once control is adequately achieved, it needs to be maintained. This may involve stepping up or down accordingly, titrated against clinical response. Patients should be reviewed every 3 months by their GP. It is imperative that before a new medication is introduced compliance is checked, triggers are recognised and removed, and inhaler technique is assessed. Patients should have appropriate training of their asthma control including a written action plan advising how to act early during exacerbations.

2. **B – Croup** is a type of laryngotracheal infection characterised by mucosal inflammation and swelling. There can also be oedema of the subglottic area, which can lead to life-threatening airway obstruction. The commonest causes of croup are the parainfluenza viruses and there is a high incidence during the autumn season. It most frequently occurs at the age of 2 years, although it can occur any time between the ages of 6 months and 6 years. The typical symptoms are harsh stridor (a rasping sound heard on inspiration), barking cough, hoarseness (due to vocal-cord inflammation) and variable degrees of dyspnoea. These features are usually preceded by coryza and fever that is worse at night. No investigations are necessary. If the child has mild symptoms that only occur on exertion, then they can be managed at home; parents should be able and have confidence to recognise signs of deterioration. Nebulised steroids or oral steroids can be used to limit the duration and severity of the infection. If the child has a compromised airway, adrenaline provides benefit. It is important to recognise the difference clinically between croup and epiglottis; croup presents over days, whereas epiglottis presents within hours. Patients with epiglottitis are reluctant to speak, cough or swallow. They also appear significantly more toxic.

3. **H – Tonsillar haemorrhage post tonsillectomy**. The indications for a tonsillectomy are:
   - gross enlargement of tonsils causing airway obstruction, dysphagia or sleep disturbance (obstructive sleep apnoea)
   - recurrent tonsillitis (more than three infections per year despite treatment)
   - peritonsillar abscess (quinsy) unresponsive to medical treatment and incision and drainage.

The most common complication of tonsillectomy is haemorrhage: 1 in 30 patients suffer from this complication. Haemorrhage is grouped into primary or reactionary haemorrhage (within first 24 hours) and secondary haemorrhage (occurring between 24 hours and the first 10 days). The treatment of primary haemorrhage must be imminent as it can be catastrophic with acute airway obstruction. Superficial pressure can be initially attempted with a sponge on a long clamp to the bleeding tonsil fossa. Topical adrenaline or thrombin powder may be of benefit. If these immediate measures fail, the patient should have emergency surgical intervention; cauterising the tonsillar bed or further use of topical haemostatic agents should be trialed, and if this fails then ligation of the ipsilateral carotid artery is done. Secondary haemorrhage is usually due to an underlying infection of the tonsillar bed. Patients are often reluctant to eat postoperatively and so the lack of movement of the throat promotes the slough to become infected; bleeding occurs when the slough separates from the tonsillar base. Usually adequate analgesia and antibiotics are sufficient to control the bleeding. Rarely, patients are taken back to theatre. The patient in this scenario is more likely to have tonsillar haemorrhage post tonsillectomy rather than haemorrhage post tongue cancer removal, as this history highlights that she is otherwise well, and she is only 19 years old.

4. **F – Quinsy abscess**. A quinsy is a peritonsillar abscess presenting as an acute complication of tonsillitis. It is a collection of pus outside the tonsillar capsule that can extend into the soft palate. The abscess usually presents unilaterally (3% present bilaterally). The affected tonsil may be pushed medially because of suppuration and may obstruct the patient's airway. It is thought to occur from direct spread of an inadequately treated bacterial tonsillitis, which then progresses to a peritonsillar cellulitis before it advances to form an abscess. It is important to recognise the difference as peritonsillar cellulitis does not require surgical drainage nor a tonsillectomy. A quinsy is the most common abscess of the head and neck. It is more common in male adults in the third and fourth decades (unlike simple tonsillitis). The patient usually presents following a presumed recovered tonsillitis with recurrence on one side and worsening of symptoms. The patient looks unwell and has a high temperature and rigors. There is pain in the throat leading to dysphagia and referred otalgia. The difficulty in swallowing can be so severe that patients have pooling of saliva and are found drooling. On examination, there is trismus; however, if an adequate view is achieved the quinsy is seen to be superior and lateral to the affected tonsil, pushing it down and medially. The palate is congested and the uvula is oedematous and deviated to the contralateral side. The buccal mucosa is erythematous and may be furred. There is tender cervical and tonsillar lymphadenopathy. Patients are also reported to have a muffled 'hot-potato'

voice. Complications are rare, but a bleeding quinsy, caused by erosion of the abscess into an adjacent vessel (i.e. internal carotid artery) is important, as it may be catastrophic. Pus obtained from needle aspiration (or swabs) should be sent for microscopy, culture and sensitivity. Bacterial growth is frequently polymicrobial of oral flora origin. Treatment includes analgesia, antibiotics plus or minus surgical drainage. Patients will ultimately have a tonsillectomy, whether immediate or after the acute phase has passed. Some authorities advise to start intravenous penicillin and observe; if after 48 hours the patient has improved, they should finish the course of antibiotics and return back for an interval tonsillectomy (4–6 weeks later). If there is no relief with antibiotics alone during this trial period, then the abscess is subsequently drained. Others advocate some form of immediate drainage: needle aspiration, incision and drainage or tonsillectomy if other techniques have failed, in addition to intravenous antibiotics.

Note, it is often difficult to differentiate between peritonsillar cellulitis and quinsy; drooling and trismus are more commonly seen with an abscess. If diagnosis is uncertain, an ultrasound scan or CT may be performed for differentiation. Retropharyngeal abscesses present with more respiratory complications, such as stridor, and neck stiffness. These cases often progress to airway obstruction and attention to the airway is imperative.

5. **C – Epiglottitis** is a medical emergency characterised by localised infection of the supraglottic structures, obstructing the laryngeal inlet. It is typically caused by *Haemophilus influenzae* type B (Hib). Epiglottitis is commoner in children aged between 2 and 4 years. Since the introduction of the Hib vaccine, it has become very rare in children in the United Kingdom; nonetheless, the incidence in adults has remained the same. Epiglottitis is characterised by a rapid onset and progression of severe symptoms that may lead to death in a few hours. The patient usually presents with a high temperature, followed by difficulty breathing (air hunger). The patient embraces the typical 'tripod position' to ease her airway and maximise air entry; sitting up on hands, body leaning forward and chin hyper-extended. Sore throat, muffled hoarse voice and dysphagia are common. The mouth is frequently open with the tongue protruding; drooling occurs in 80% of patients. There may be a cough. Stridor is a late sign and indicates advancing airway obstruction. On examination the patient appears toxic! They are irritable and extremely anxious. The patient may rapidly become shocked and hypoxic. The patient's throat should *not* be examined, as it may cause spasm and worsen obstruction. Similarly radiographic evaluation is not required. In acute epiglottitis, a lateral neck radiograph

classically shows the 'thumb sign', in which the epiglottis appears enlarged and oedematous. Laryngoscopy is preferred for confirming diagnosis; again, this should only be attempted if there is no risk to the airway. Most patients are managed by endo-tracheal intubation. Mortality rates are 10% for patients whose airways are not protected compared to 1% when early intubation is performed. Few patients may require a cricothyrotomy. Patients should be managed in the intensive therapy unit. Blood cultures should be taken once patient is stable. Antibiotics (e.g. ceftriaxone) are the mainstay of treatment once the airway is secured. All close contacts should receive prophylactic antibiotics. Pneumonia and otitis media are the most common complications. Quinsy may present similarly, although the patient is not as toxic and the airway is not as compromised. Patients with quinsy additionally often have a recent history of tonsillitis. Croup can also present alike, although it usually occurs in younger children and there is more commonly a prodrome. The barking cough if present is typical and infants rarely appear as toxic.

A ENT A18 – Airway obstruction II

1. **I – Nebulised O_2 driven bronchodilators and 100 mg hydrocortisone IV**. Patients coming to hospital with exacerbations of their asthma need to be thoroughly reviewed to assess at which stage of disease they are presenting. It is important to recognise the criteria to diagnose the degree of exacerbation, as detailed in Table 24. In general, the following is the approach a clinician must take in the management of a patient after stabilisation from an asthmatic attack:
   - ABCDE approach
   - maintain oxygen saturations between 94%–98%
   - PEFR every 30 minutes to monitor response to treatment
   - urea and electrolytes daily – salbutamol and steroids may derange (hypokalaemia)
   - before the patient is discharged, the cause of the exacerbation must be identified
   - the patient needs a personalised written action plan – self-management improves outcome
   - patients with acute exacerbation need an appointment with a specialist within 30 days
   - if patient admitted with severe asthma, he/she should be under respiratory team for at least 1 year

- patients who have brittle asthma or who have experienced a near-fatal episode should be under specialist management indefinitely
- Note, NSAIDs and beta blockers are contraindicated in asthmatic patients.

TABLE 24 Clinical features and management of different severities of asthma

Variable	Asthma			
	Moderate	**Severe**	**Life threatening**	**Near fatal**
PEFR	>50%–75% of best or predicted	33%–50% best or predicted	<33% best or predicted	
RR	Normal	≥25 breaths per minute	Poor respiratory effort	
HR	Normal	≥110 bpm	Bradycardia plus or minus arrhythmia	
Features	No clinical features of severe asthma	Inability to complete sentences in one breath	Silent chest, cyanosis, exhaustion, altered conscious level	
ABG	ABG not required	ABG not required	SpO$_2$ <92% PaO$_2$ <8 kPa normal PaCO$_2$ (4.6–6.0 kPa)	With raised PaCO$_2$
Management	Bronchodilators: two puffs (up to 10 can be used) Supplementary oxygen (maintain SpO$_2$ level of 94–98%) High dose inhaled β$_2$ agonists as early as possible	Salbutamol 5 mg or terbutaline 10 mg via O$_2$ driven nebuliser Hydrocortisone 100 mg IV or prednisolone 60 mg PO	Repeat or continuous β$_2$ agonist nebulization (oxygen-driven) Hydrocortisone 100 mg IV (6 hourly) Add nebulised ipratropium bromide 0.5 mg (4 hourly) Magnesium sulphate 1.2–2 g IV infusion (over 20 minutes)	Admission to ITU and need for intubation and mechanical ventilation

PEFR, peak expiratory flow rate; RR, respiratory rate; HR, heart rate; ABG, arterial blood gas; IV, intravenous; PO, by mouth; ITU, intensive therapy unit.

2. **E – 10 mg chlorphenamine IV and 200 mg hydrocortisone IV**

3. **K – Repeat adrenaline dose (0.5 mg 1:1000 IM)**. Anaphylaxis is a severe, potentially life-threatening medical emergency caused by a generalised hypersensitivity reaction. It is a clinical diagnosis characterised by rapidly developing airway (A) and/or breathing (B) and/or circulatory (C) complications with cutaneous and mucosal changes. There is usually a history of acute exposure to an allergen causing rapid release of chemical mediators. The classic form of anaphylaxis is IgE-mediated, where there is prior sensitisation to an offending agent in a susceptible individual. It is upon re-exposure that the patient experiences the clinical symptoms through an immunological response. The most common triggers are foods (e.g. nuts, fish, shellfish, milk and eggs), drugs (e.g. antibiotics, NSAIDs, anaesthetic muscle relaxants and intravenous contrast agents) and venom. Food triggers are most common in children and drugs are more common causative agents in the older generations. Anaphylaxis should always be suspected in patients who were exposed to an allergen and then suddenly developed progressive compromising symptoms. Be aware that often the patient cannot recall exposure to a trigger. Anaphylactic reactions usually begin with the patient expressing a sense of impending doom. Symptoms can develop over hours or more acutely over a few minutes. Cutaneous manifestations are common and occur in over 80% of patients. These include urticaria (red, raised, irregular lesions) that may be intensely itchy, signs of inflammation (swelling, erythema and warmth) and angioedema. Concurrently, the patient may develop A and/or B and/or C complications. Airway compromise manifests as a hoarse voice, stridor, dyspnoea and dysphagia. Breathing compromise manifests as wheezing, shortness of breath and cyanosis. Angioedema of the larynx may be so severely obstructing airflow that hypoxia and subsequent confusion develops. Respiratory arrest may ensue and ultimately death if treatment is not instigated imminently. Patients with a background of asthma have an increased risk of death. Circulatory involvement leads to clinical signs of shock (pale and clammy) tachycardia expressed as palpitations and hypotension expressed as dizziness and syncope. Cardiovascular collapse may ensue in severe cases. Patients may also have gastrointestinal symptoms including abdominal pain, vomiting and diarrhoea. Anaphylaxis is recognised upon clinical judgement and a thorough history allows determination of the cause. With life-threatening conditions it is important to use the ABCDE systematic approach. Advanced Life Support guidelines advise that anaphylaxis is likely if all three of the following criteria are met:

- sudden onset, rapid progression
- life-threatening A, B or C problems
- skin or mucosal changes (although these can be subtle or absent in 20% of patients).

Treatment of anaphylaxis: as implied by the guidelines, although skin changes may be profound and concerning; if they are not seen in conjunction with Airway, Breathing and Circulation complications then it is not diagnosed as anaphylaxis.

Treatment must be immediate and without delay. Doses are for those aged >12 years:

- omit the offending agent (e.g. stop drug infusion)
- establish an airway* and give high-flow oxygen
- 0.5 mg intramuscular adrenaline 1:1000 into the lateral thigh – this can be repeated in 5 minutes if no response
- intravenous access and intravenous fluids
- 10 mg intravenous chlorphenamine
- 200 mg of intravenous hydrocortisone.**

*Once an airway is established it must be maintained and ventilator assistance may be needed. This may be in the form of a bag and mask. If this is not adequate, a nasopharyngeal airway may be necessary and is better tolerated than an oropharyngeal airway in the awake patient. Continuous positive airway pressure (CPAP) may also be trialled prior to advanced airways. If hypoxia persists and the above measures have failed then a supraglottic airway device (such as layrngeal mask airway) should be considered early. If there is an anaesthetist present then endotracheal intubation may be attempted (again early, avoiding delay). Nevertheless, even in skilled hands, intubation may become impossible and attempts may be catastrophic leading to worsening laryngeal oedema. Surgical airways may be the only option; cricothyrotomy rather than emergency tracheostomies as it is easier and quicker to perform.

**Option F from the list of options given is incorrect, as hydrocortisone is never given by mouth – prednisolone is the oral steroid given at the high dose of 60 mg. Even if prednisolone was the option, this would still not be the right answer because in anaphylaxis, intravenous steroids and intravenous antihistamines are recommended because of the severity of the condition.

Once the patient is stabilised, mast cell tryptase can be measured to confirm the diagnosis. Three timed samples should be taken (1) as soon as possible after resuscitation is complete, (2) 1–2 hours after start of symptoms and (3) at 24 hours. Patients should be offered an EpiPen with clear directions of its use. They should be made aware of the causative agent and advised to stay clear of its ingestion and contact. They should be referred to an allergy clinic to identify any other susceptible allergens. Patients should be monitored depending on the severity of the anaphylaxis for fear of the resumption of symptoms after the effects of the medications given wear off.

4. **C – Encourage cough**

5. **D – Five back blows**. The aspiration of a foreign body has bimodal presentations, peaking in childhood and in the elderly. In children, the highest incidence is during infancy and up to 4 years of age. It is between these years that children are curious and explore through hand-to-mouth interaction. Elderly patients are at risk when they have neurological disorders or have conditions that depress the central nervous system. Aspiration of a foreign body can have many different presentations, ranging from no signs to respiratory arrest, although greater than 90% present with choking or coughing. If there is upper airway compromise patients may present with an inspiratory stridor. However, aspirated foreign bodies more commonly settle in the right main stem bronchus. If the foreign body has lodged in the right lower lobe, patients may present a few days after the aspiration incident with a prolonged expiratory wheeze, collapse, pneumonia or pulmonary oedema. Alternatively, a ball-valve obstructive presentation may result, leading to hyperinflation of the obstructed lobe; this can be seen on inspiration–expiration films. Patients may also present in respiratory distress. If the patient is stable, chest films are useful, although CTs are more conclusive.

Foreign bodies may lead to either mild or severe airway obstruction. The degrees of airway obstruction can be differentiated by signs and symptoms and management is according to presentation.

TABLE 25 Clinical signs and management of different degrees of airway obstruction

	Mild airway obstruction	Severe airway obstruction
Signs	Able to respond to the question 'are you choking?' with yes Effective cough Able to breathe despite choking Conscious	Unable to speak and answer question but may respond by nodding Ineffective cough Unable to breathe (stridor, wheezy) May be unconscious
Pre-hospital management	Encourage patient to cough Check for relieved obstruction Check for any deterioration – if cough becomes ineffective, patient has *severe airway obstruction*	If patient is *conscious*, give up to five back blows (check if each has relieved obstruction) If five back blows have failed, give up to five abdominal thrusts (Heimlich manoeuvre) If obstruction not relieved, then alternate between five back blows and five abdominal thrusts and call ambulance If the patient becomes unconscious – (respiratory arrest) start CPR until an experienced individual is present
Hospital management	Laryngoscopy can be attempted using Magill's forceps (below the cords but above the cricoid ring) If stridor present: adrenaline via a nebuliser until bronchoscopy If unstable: rapid sequence induction until bronchoscopy If foreign body obstructing trachea below level of vocal cords: may attempt intubation to push the object down the right main-stem bronchus to relieve complete airway blockage until bronchoscopy Bronchoscopy: definitive treatment	

The prognosis is very good if the foreign body is not occlusive or is in the right main-stem bronchus. If there is complete tracheal obstruction then immediate actions need to be taken otherwise this can be a rapidly fatal event. The overall mortality rate is 1%.

Note, a sudden onset of stridor in an otherwise well child, who was unsupervised while eating or playing with toys, is a foreign body aspiration unless proven otherwise!

A   **ENT A19 – Head and neck tumours I**

Thyroid cancer accounts for 1.5% of all cancers, and 92% of endocrine cancers. As a general rule, all solitary thyroid lumps must be investigated to exclude malignancy. An enlarged cervical lymph node is the only presenting feature in 5% of cases of thyroid cancer. Patients with thyroid cancer typically have normal thyroid function tests, and never hyperthyroidism. Fine needle aspiration (FNA) is initial diagnostic test of choice in the investigation of solitary lumps. Radionuclide (scintillation) scanning is used to determine if the nodule is functioning or non-functioning. Functioning nodules are almost never malignant. Ultrasonography helps differentiate thyroid cysts from solid nodules. In general, thyroid cancer is either well differentiated (which is associated with a good prognosis) or poorly differentiated (poor prognosis). A laryngoscopy allows the clinician to visualise any vocal cord paralysis, which can be caused by invasive thyroid tumours. A partial or complete thyroidectomy is the mainstay of treatment for most thyroid malignancies. Complications include hypoparathyroidism, recurrent laryngeal nerve palsy, neck haematoma and thyroid storm (rare). It is important to document the calcium levels and vocal cord function before a thyroidectomy.

1. **E – Medullary thyroid carcinoma** (MTC) is the only thyroid cancer that causes an elevated serum calcitonin level. This type of cancer may be referred to as medullary C-cell carcinoma, as the cancerous cells originate from the calcitonin-producing parafollicular (C-cells) of the thyroid gland. Medullary carcinoma represents about 5%–10% of all thyroid carcinomas, and it is a poorly differentiated tumour. Males and females are equally affected. Patients usually present with a solitary painless nodule affecting the thyroid gland. Regional lymph nodes are involved in 50% of cases. Patients with advanced disease may present with dysphagia and hoarseness of voice secondary to invasion of surrounding structures. Raised serum calcitonin levels are characteristic, and the diagnosis is confirmed by FNA. It is imperative to mention the genetic element found in medullary thyroid carcinoma. About 75% of cases occur sporadically, and 25% are familial. Medullary carcinoma is a part of the multiple endocrine neoplasia (MEN) 2A and MEN 2B syndromes. It can also be of the non-multiple endocrine neoplasia familial type, termed familial medullary thyroid carcinoma. Mutations have been identified in MEN 2A/2B and familial medullary thyroid carcinoma. Genetic screening is offered to the children of patients with the above conditions. Prophylactic thyroidectomise is being offered

routinely; alternatively, some opt for close monitoring of calcitonin levels and performing surgery when levels rise. In general the prognosis for patients with medullary thyroid cancer is worse than patients with a well-differentiated thyroid carcinoma. Ten-year survival rates are at about 70%. The treatment of choice for both familial and sporadic causes is a total thyroidectomy with central neck dissection. Surgery is the only effective intervention, and there is no role for radioiodine treatment in medullary thyroid carcinoma. External beam radiotherapy may be considered to reduce regional recurrence. Of note when medullary carcinoma is suspected, one must exclude the concomitant presence of pheochromocytoma (free catecholamines and metanephrine in plasma or 24-hour urine collection), as it is part of the MEN syndrome.

2. **A – Anaplastic thyroid carcinoma** (ATC). Both the age of the patient and the rapid onset of symptoms point towards ATC. The main differential is thyroid lymphoma. ATC is the least common type of thyroid carcinomas and has a peak incidence in the seventh decade of life. It is an undifferentiated thyroid carcinoma, affecting females more than males (2–3:1). ATC may be associated with pre-existing thyroid disease, as is the case in this scenario. It is a rapidly growing tumour that is often painful, and hence patients present with rapidly evolving symptoms. It is locally invasive and metastasises both regionally and distantly. Occasionally, patients may present with airway obstruction. It is imperative to differentiate between a thyroid lymphoma and ATC by tissue diagnosis by an FNA or an open biopsy if necessary. The differentiation is important as lymphoma is a much more treatable condition. The prognosis for ATC is very poor, with an approximate 2-year survival of around 10%. The management of ATC is usually palliative, with great care taken to ensure airway protection. Management plans are conducted after careful consideration of patient wishes, co-morbidities, age and size of tumour. Total or subtotal thyroidectomy with or without adjuvant radiotherapy may be offered if the individual situation permits, but the response to treatment is often poor.

3. **C – Follicular thyroid carcinoma**. The main diagnostic hint in this scenario is the rapid growing nodule and the presence of elevated levels of thyroglobulin. Adenomas usually have a slower increase in size. The neoplastic cells in follicular thyroid carcinoma (FTC) are thyroid-stimulating hormone (TSH) sensitive. They vigorously convert iodine into thyroglobulin. Both the uptake of iodine and production of thyroglobulin are of diagnostic and post-operative monitoring value. FTC is one of the

well-differentiated types of thyroid carcinoma, accounting for approximately 20% of thyroid malignancies. It affects women three times more than men, with a peak incidence in the fifth decade of life. Of note, the prevalence of FTC is higher in areas with low intake of iodine. Tissue biopsy is important in order to distinguish between a follicular adenoma and a carcinoma. Histologically, vascular or capsular invasion indicates follicular carcinoma (as opposed to adenoma). Metastases usually occur via the blood. Up to 30% of patients with FTC will have distant metastases on presentation; the most common sites being the lungs and bones. Treatment for FTC is surgical excision. Total thyroidectomy is offered to patients with FTC but, because of the major aforementioned complications involved in such a procedure, many advocate a subtotal thyroidectomy. Radioiodine scanning is conducted post-operatively to investigate for metastasis and residual tissue. As mentioned before, the cancerous cells have a high uptake of iodine and this can be demonstrated with radioiodine scanning. Diagnostic doses are used for scanning and higher therapeutic doses are used for radioablation of residual and metastatic disease. Scanning is done routinely for monitoring after treatment. Patients need lifelong thyroxine replacement therapy, and the aim of treatment is to suppress TSH secretion due to the TSH-sensitive nature of the cancerous cells. Prognosis is good with 10-year survival rates of about 85%.

4. **I – Papillary thyroid carcinoma** is the most common thyroid malignancy, accounting for approximately 75% of all thyroid cancers. It usually affects patients in the third to fourth decades of life, with a 3:1 female-to-male ratio. It is strongly associated with a history of exposure to radiation. Papillary thyroid carcinoma is a slow-growing tumour that spreads via lymphatics after several years. Bilateral disease occurs in 30%–75% of cases, and the neck nodes are involved in 60%. The key word in this scenario is the presence of calcified psammoma bodies, which is a characteristic feature seen in histology. Investigations and treatment are similar to that of FTC. Surgery is the mainstay of treatment, but larger tumours also need adjuvant radiotherapy. If the neck nodes are involved, patients will also need neck dissection. The prognosis is even better than FTC, with a 20-year survival of 95% if there is no local invasion on diagnosis.

5. **G – Multiple endocrine neoplasia 2A**. MEN is a syndrome characterised by the presence of multiple tumours affecting the endocrine glands. All the variants of MEN are inherited in an autosomal dominant manner. Table 26 summarises the associated tumours in each subtype.

TABLE 26 Tumours associated with different types of multiple endocrine neoplasia (MEN)

MEN 1	Tumours affecting at least two out of the three main endocrine glands: 1. parathyroid hyperplasia/adenoma 2. pituitary adenoma 3. pancreatic endocrine tumours Also known as Wermer's syndrome In addition to tumours in these glands, patients may present with cutaneous tumours (e.g. angiofibromas and lipomas)
MEN 2A	**Medullary thyroid carcinoma**, pheochromocytoma and parathyroid hyperplasia Also known as Sipple's syndrome
MEN 2B	**Medullary thyroid carcinoma (more virulent form)**, pheochromocytoma and neuromas No parathyroid hyperplasia Also known as Williams' syndrome

Thyroid lymphoma represents about 1%–5% of all thyroid cancers (most are non-Hodgkin's lymphoma). It is eight times more common in women, especially with a past medical history of Hashimoto's thyroiditis. It occurs most frequently in the elderly. The presentation can be very similar to anaplastic thyroid cancer, as patients present with a rapidly growing thyroid mass causing local symptoms such as difficulty swallowing and hoarseness. FNA or an open biopsy is needed to confirm the diagnosis. Treatment of choice for thyroid lymphoma is combined chemotherapy and radiotherapy.

Hürthle cell carcinoma (also known as follicular carcinoma, oxyphilic type) is thought to be a more aggressive variant of follicular carcinoma. It has a higher incidence of metastasis than other well-differentiated thyroid carcinomas. FNA enables a diagnosis of a Hürthle cell neoplasia to be made, but does not enable differentiating a Hürthle cell adenoma from a carcinoma. Treatment is with total thyroidectomy.

A ENT A20 – Head and neck tumours II

1. **I – Sialolithiasis.** The scenario is a typical presentation of salivary gland stones (sialolithiasis). Sialolithiasis is common, and can occur in both the submandibular (~85%) and the parotid gland (~15%). It most frequently occurs in middle-aged men. The submandibular gland (beneath the jawbone) is more prone to developing stones because of the viscous nature of the secretions and the length of the submandibular duct. The stones are

largely composed of calcium phosphate and hydroxyapatite. The symptoms are thought to occur because of increased salivation prior to and during the consumption of food. The contraction of the smooth muscles of the glands and the ducts will exacerbate the symptoms. Patients typically present with recurrent pain and tense swelling of the affected gland immediately before, during or after meals. On examination, a stone may be visible in the floor of the mouth, or palpable in the submandibular duct. History and examination are usually sufficient for a diagnosis to be made. The salivary stones are easily seen on plain X-ray because of their radio-opaque nature. A sialogram (serial X-rays of the duct system with contrast) detects 80% of salivary stones. Conservative measures such as hydration, massaging the affected area to dislodge the impacted stone or sialologues (e.g. lemon drops) have been described. Definitive treatment is in the form of a sialotomy (cannulation of the duct) or sialoendoscopically assisted sialolithectomy of stone. Untreated, the patient may develop an infection of the affected gland, known as obstructive sialadenitis. The patient in this scenario is unlikely to have sialadenitis, as he does not show any systemic signs of infection (e.g. pyrexia), and his symptoms are precipitated by eating rather than being constant. Sialadenitis (non-obstructive) may also occur because of reduced saliva production or other causes of salivary stasis. Patients present with the affected gland being erythematous, swollen, firm and tender. The most common causative organism is *Staphylococcus aureus*. Antibiotics are required for the management of this condition. Drainage may be required if an abscess is present.

2. **F – Pleomorphic adenoma of the superficial lobe of the parotid gland.** Most salivary gland tumours occur in the parotid gland (~80%), most of which are benign (~80%). Pleomorphic adenomas (PAs) are the most common benign parotid gland tumour (~80%), also called 'benign mixed tumour'. They usually occur in the superficial lobe of the parotid gland. It occurs most frequently in the 30- to 70-year age group, affecting females more than males. Patients present with an asymptomatic slowly growing lump behing the angle of the mandible. Weakness of the facial nerve muscles or pain are red flags for malignancy. PAs are initially investigated by FNA, but this is not always accurate in differentiating a benign PA from a malignant one. Superficial parotidectomies are the mainstay of treatment for PA and enable a definitive diagnosis to be made. About 5%–10% of PAs will become malignant if not removed. Malignant lesions may require adjuvant radiotherapy. Careful dissecting and exposure is imperative in ensuring that the facial nerve is not damaged during surgery. If the entire

PA capsule is excised along with a surrounding cuff of normal tissue, recurrence rates are as low as 4%. Common complications of parotidectomy are permanent anaesthesia of the ipsilateral ear (due to damage to the auricular nerve – occurs almost invariably), Frey's syndrome (unilateral facial sweating on eating, occurs after many months or years in 25%) and temporary facial nerve palsy (rarely permanent).

Hint: Always examine the mouth and oropharynx. Tumours in the deep lobe of the parotid gland often displace the tonsil.

Hint: Always fully inform patients undergoing salivary gland surgery of the risk of permanent facial weakness or paralysis.

3. **D – Mucoepidermoid carcinoma (high grade)** is the most common tumour of the salivary gland in childhood. Most mucoepidermoid carcinomas occur in the parotid gland (~90%). It occurs most frequently in the fifth decade of life, with the female-to male ratio being 4:1. Differentiation between low-, middle- and high-grade tumours is based on the ratio of mucous cells to epidermoid cells seen in histology. Low-grade tumours tend to have more mucous cells whereas epidermoid cells predominate in high-grade tumours. There is a greater risk of local invasion and lymph node metastasis in high-grade tumours. Malignancy is suspected in salivary gland tumours when there is rapid growth, associated pain and involvement of the facial nerve. Definitive diagnosis requires a biopsy in the form of FNA. A high-grade mucoepidermoid carcinoma is differentiated from squamous cell carcinoma by the presence of intracellular mucin. CT and MRI scanning are used for evaluation of tumour infiltration and involvement of local structures. Surgical excision is the treatment of choice. The grade of the tumour dictates the extent of surgery. If a tumour is low grade, usually a superficial partotidectomy is carried out and the facial nerve is preserved. For high-grade tumours a total parotidectomy with or without neck dissection and post-operative radiotherapy is indicated. The facial nerve is assessed and excised if there is tumour involvement. Definitive histological assessment is performed post-parotidectomy. The 5-year survival rate for high-grade mucoepidermoid carcinoma is about 50%.

Hint: Salivary gland malignancies are strongly suspected if there is rapid growth, facial pain or weakness of muscles supplied by the facial nerve.

4. **J – Warthin's tumour** (WT). Also known as an adenolymphoma, WT is the second most common benign tumour of the salivary glands, occurring in an older age group (60–80 years) as compared with pleomorphic adenomas. It has a male predominance, possibly because of its strong association with cigarette smoking. It almost exclusively affects the parotid gland, and it is the only benign salivary tumour that frequently occurs bilaterally. It usually affects individuals aged between 50 and 70 years. Of clinical importance, WT usually affects the tail of the parotid gland. There are no reports of malignant change in WT. Treatment is with superficial partotidectomy (including unaffected margins), preserving the facial nerve.

5. **B – Adenoid cystic carcinoma** (ACC). ACCs are the second most common malignant tumour of the salivary glands, and confusingly, they are not a carcinoma of the adenoids. They are the most common malignant tumours of the submandibular, sublingual and minor salivary glands. Males and females are equally affected. An ACC usually presents as a lump that has been growing for several months, and is often painful. It spreads via intraneural infiltration (i.e. along nerves), with the facial nerve being almost always affected. Another distinguishing factor from other types of carcinomas is that distant metastasis can occur up to 20 years after treatment, usually affecting the lung. Histologically, ACCs are divided into three subtypes: solid, cribiform and tubular. The solid tumour has the worst prognosis and the tubular type the best prognosis. Treatment is identical to mucoepidermoid carcinoma; however, there is a role for adjuvant post-operative radiotherapy for treatment of local infilteration.

    Hint: Malignant salivary tumours are most likely to occur in the submandibular and minor salivary glands.

    Acinic cell carcinoma occurs most commonly in the parotid glands, accounting for 15% of malignant parotid gland tumours. They are very slow growing, and the diagnosis is confirmed histologically. Surgical excision is the mainstay of treatment. The survival rate at 5 years is about 80%.

A   ENT A21 – Congenital neck swellings

1. **D – Infected thryoglossal cyst**. Embryologically, a thyroglossal cyst is the remnant of the migration of the thyroid gland from the foramen caecum at the base of the tongue along the thyroglossal duct to the root of the neck. It is the most common congenital anomaly of the neck, usually

presenting before 10 years of age. Thyroglossal cysts usually present as midline (or just off midline) lumps in the infrahyoid region, but can occur anywhere from the base of the tongue to the thyroid isthmus. Clinically, a thyroglossal cyst is characterised by moving on tongue protrusion and on swallowing, two essential steps in a complete thyroid examination. This is because it is connected to the larynx. Although thyroglossal cysts are benign, local manifestations such as dysphagia and difficulty in breathing may occur due to local compression. Another important complication is infection. A thyroglossal cyst is normally non-painful and not tender to palpation. The atypical presentation in this scenario suggests an infection of the cyst. The ultrasound scan findings are further suggestive of this, as a non-infected thyroglossal cyst is typically thin-walled and anechoic. Patients with thyroglossal abscesses may additionally have a discharging cyst and signs of systemic infection. An abscess must be treated promptly because of the risk of fistula formation with adjacent structures. The surgical treatment of choice is the Sistrunk's procedure, in which an en bloc resection of the sinus tract and the midportion of the hyoid bone is performed. There is usually an 8% rate of recurrence.

2. **H – Second branchial cleft cyst**. Branchial cysts usually present from late adolescence to the third decade of life. They can be characterised according to origin:
   - First branchial cleft cyst – originating in the angle of the mandible and extending posteriorly to the retroauricular scalp.
   - Second branchial cleft cyst – found along the anterior surface of the sternocleidomastoid muscle.
   - Third branchial cleft cyst – located in the lateral aspect of the neck.

Branchial cysts are asymptomatic but can become painful and swollen if a secondary infection develops, most typically following an upper respiratory tract infection. Various theories regarding the origin of branchial cysts have been postulated, which are beyond the scope of this book. Diagnosis of the lump is clinical. The lump is usually soft and cystic but it may feel solid to palpation. Diagnosis may be aided by FNA and cytological examination of the fluid to rule out other sinister differentials such as a lymphoma. Treatment is conservative after ruling out sinister differentials. Surgical excision may be considered to prevent secondary infections, for histological examination or for cosmetic purposes. Surgery to excise branchial cysts can be complicated by the involvement of local structures such as the facial nerve, and recurrence can occur in up to 20% of cases.

3. **B – Dermoid cyst**. The term dermoid cyst is used in different subspecialties referring to cysts in various locations in the body. Dermoid cysts contain mature and well-differentiated tissue. They may contain hair, teeth, cartilage, blood, fat and other tissue. In the context of neck swellings, dermoid cysts are congenital in origin and may present later in life. They are invariably midline as they occur at lines of fusion in embryological development whereby epithelial tissue becomes trapped beneath the lines of fusion. Clinically, dermoid cysts are painless and do not move on tongue protrusion and swallowing. This may aid the clinician in differentiating between a dermoid and thryoglossal cyst. Complications include abscess formation, local compression and cosmetic concerns. Malignant change is rare. Complete surgical excision is the treatment of choice.

4. **A – Cystic hygroma**. Cystic hygromas, otherwise known as lymphangiomas, arise due to abnormalities of the lymphatic system, including failure of appropriate drainage of the lymphatic system into the venous system. They are smooth, soft and non-tender. In 75% of cases, cystic hygromas affect the head and neck region. Of note, the majority of hygromas affect the left side of the neck and are mainly located in the posterior triangle. The incidence of cystic hygromas is about 1 per 15 000 live births, with an equal sex distribution. Sixty per cent are present at birth and up to 90% by 2 years of age. They can be visualised in antenatal imaging. They are also associated with an increase in alpha-fetoprotein levels in the amniotic fluid. Various manifestations occur depending on the anatomical location of the hygroma. They may be large at birth, necessitating a tracheostomy. Sudden increase in the size of the lesion is an emergency as this may represent a large haemorrhage that may be fatal. Management of the lesion on an elective basis consists of either surgical excision or injection with a sclerosing agent, OK-432 (strains of attenuated *Streptococcus pyogenes*).

5. **E – Laryngocele**. A layrngocele is a benign neck swelling that forms because of the herniation of the laryngeal mucosa through the thyrohyoid membranes. Although rare, it is found mostly in glass-blowers and patients with chronic obstructive pulmonary disease. Patients may present with a change in voice, dysphagia, dyspnoea or a feeling of a 'lump' in the throat. On examination the lump is tense, resonant and translucent. It would be easily compressible and enlarges when asking the patient to blow against a closed nose. A secondary infection may develop, known as a laryngopyocele.

A ENT A22 – Acquired neck swellings

1. **E – Infectious mononucleosis** is caused by the Epstein–Barr virus (EBV). It is commonly referred to as glandular fever or the 'kissing' disease. EBV is a DNA herpesvirus that is mainly transmitted via saliva, hence why it is known as the kissing disease in colloquial terms. Infected B-cells spread EBV throughout the body and mainly affect the reticular-endothelial system and deposit in the spleen, liver and lymph nodes. Patients can range from being asymptomatic to being severely unwell. Serious complications consist of haematological abnormalities (haemolytic anaemia and thrombocytopenia), hepatitis, encephalitis, cranial nerve pathologies, petechial haemorrhage, hepatosplenomegaly and splenic rupture. Most patients present with a fever, sore throat, headache and lymphadenopathy. Most patients report feeling lethargic and this may persist for months after the infection. A full blood count shows raised white cell count with a lymphocytosis. Heterophil antibody tests (e.g. Monospot and Paul–Bunnell test) are more specific investigations to confirm one's suspicion of infectious mononucleosis; the tests involve using horse and sheep red blood cells respectively to investigate if the cells agglutinate in the presence of the EBV antibodies. Ninety per cent of patients develop heterophil antibodies by week 3. False positives can occur in certain conditions (e.g. hepatitis). Other tests include immunoglobulin assays for IgG and IgM, where elevated IgG levels reflect past infection and raised IgM levels reflect a recent infection.

   Patients are advised to avoid contact sports for up to 6 weeks from the onset of symptoms to reduce the risk of splenic rupture. Infectious mononucleosis usually resolves without active treatment. NSAIDs may be used for symptomatic relief. There is some evidence for the use of oral steroids when the symptoms are severe. Of note, antibiotics such as amoxicillin and ampicillin are contraindicated when infectious mononucleosis is suspected, as they lead to the development of a severe, widespread macular rash. Penicillin V can be used for the treatment of bacterial tonsillitis, and does not cause the described macular rash in patients with glandular fever, unless the patient has an allergy to penicillins.

2. **F – Ludwig's angina** is an ENT emergency when respiratory compromise is suspected. It is a cellulitis of the submandibular space. It is commonly preceded by a recent dental infection or abscess. Ludwig's angina is very rare, especially after the development of antibiotics. It is more common in patients who are immunocompromised. Patients usually present with a

recent history of a dental infection and neck swelling. Neck pain, tongue protrusion and dysphagia may develop if not treated early (due to laryngeal oedema). Abiding by the ABCDE approach to acutely unwell patients, confirming a patent airway is the most important step in management. If the patient's airway is not secure they will require immediate intubation. After the immediate step of securing the airway and breathing, intravenous broad-spectrum antibiotics is the immediate mainstay of management. There is some evidence for the use of intravenous steroids. After the acute phase in management some patients experience suppurative complications (accumulation of pus in the submandibular spaces) that require surgical drainage. CT images of the neck are needed to guide a surgeon in locating the site of accumulation.

3. **D – Hyperplastic carotid body tumour**. The carotid body is present at the bifurcation of the common carotid artery. It is formed by a group of chemoreceptors that sense a drop in the partial pressure of oxygen or carbon dioxide. The cells also sense changes to temperature and pH. Type I cells also known as chief cells sense a drop in pO_2 or rise in pCO_2 and trigger an action potential and in turn regulate the respiratory rate and blood pressure accordingly. Carotid body tumours (chemodectomas) are categorised as (a) familial, (b) hyperplastic and (c) sporadic.

   The familial type mainly affects young adults; there are four genes identified that are responsible in its inheritance. The hyperplastic type is seen in patients experiencing states of chronic hypoxia such as inhabitants of high altitude countries, patients with chronic obstructive pulmonary disease and patients with cyanotic heart disease (such as the patient with Eisenmenger's in this scenario). The cells in the carotid body undergo hyperplasia because of constant exposure to low partial pressures of oxygen and triggering of action potentials. Patients usually present with a painless lump that only moves in the horizontal plane when palpated. Enlargement of the tumour may lead to local compression of surrounding nerves leading to hoarseness of voice, dysphagia and Horner's syndrome. Surgical excision is the treatment of choice, however imaging in the form of CT, MRI and angiography should precede any surgical treatment to assess the degree of local involvement.

4. **C – Hodgkin's lymphoma** (HL) is a malignant lymphoma that was first described by Thomas Hodgkin in the early nineteenth century. It has a bimodal presentation typically affecting individuals between the ages of 15 and 35 years and patients above the age of 55 years. There are five

subtypes of HL that are distinguished histologically. Microscopic evaluation of a biopsy sample from an affected lymph node characteristically shows evidence of Reed–Sternberg cells. Those are neoplastic cells of B-cell origin. The five types of HL are: (a) nodular sclerosing, (b) mixed-cellularity, (c) lymphocyte rich, (d) lymphocyte depleted, and (e) nodular lymphocyte predominant HL. Patients with HL present with generalised lymphadenopathy mainly affecting the cervical chains and the lymph nodes in the axillae. The lymphadenopathy is painless and characteristically described as being rubbery. Furthermore, they present with what is termed as the B symptoms, which refers to the fevers, night sweats and unexplained weight loss. The fever may be intermittent, it may wax and wane – this is described as the Pel–Ebstein fever. Patients may present with other symptoms secondary to lymph node enlargement in the mediastinum, which may lead to shortness of breath, chest pain and a cough. Apart from the rubbery lymph nodes, examination of a patient may reveal hepatosplenomegaly. Histological diagnosis is the most important investigation in order to ascertain the exact subtype of HL. However, initially anyone suspected to have HL will need a full blood count; this may reveal anaemia of chronic disease, generalised increase in white cell count with associated lymphopenia. Other blood investigations such as lactate hydrogenase and erythrocyte sedimentation rate are non-specific; however, elevated erythrocyte sedimentation rate levels have been associated with a worse prognosis. Anteroposterior and lateral chest X-rays are requested to assess for any mediastinal masses. The investigation of choice to aid in the staging of HL is a positron emission tomography scan to assess for extranodal involvement. The Ann Arbor Classification for staging is used for HL: stage I, single affected LN region; stage II, two or more affected LN regions on the same side of the diaphragm; stage III, affected LN on both sides of the diaphragm; stage IV, multiple involvement of extranodal organs (e.g. liver and bone marrow). A further 'B' can be added to the staging system – this indicates the presence of the B symptoms mentioned; an 'A' refers to the absence of such symptoms. HL is a potentially curable malignancy. The treatment options depend on the individual's age, stage of disease at presentation, subtype and co-morbidities. In essence, early stages (i.e. stages I–II) are treated with a combination of radiotherapy to affected regions and chemotherapy. More advanced stages are treated with chemotherapy alone. Treatment response to the aforementioned agents is monitored using regular positron emission tomography scans that are conducted 6–8 weeks after a chemotherapy cycle.

5. **G – Non-Hodgkin's lymphoma** (NHL) is an umbrella term for a diverse group of malignancies. NHL has a poorer prognosis than HL and mainly affects the elderly. NHL comprises around 85% of lymphoma malignancies. Subtypes include anaplastic large cell lymphoma, B-cell lymphoma, mantle cell lymphoma, lymphoblastic lymphoma, cutaneous T-cell lymphoma and other subtypes. The type of affected cells (e.g. B-cell, T-cell or natural killer cells) can be used to classify the type of NHL. Patients with NHL have a similar presentation to individuals with HL. The presenting symptoms depend on the time or presentation and the grade of lymphoma (i.e. low, intermediate or high grade). B symptoms and extranodal involvement occur at intermediate- to high-grade lymphomas and vary rarely in low-grade ones. Intermediate- or high-grade lymphomas can also present secondary to local manifestations of large lymph nodes; compression of soft tissue may lead to superior vena cava obstruction, cranial nerve palsies and bowel obstruction. In addition to the aforementioned investigations related to HL, bone marrow aspirate and serum β_2-microglobulin levels (elevate levels correlate to a poor prognosis) are important. Staging is similar to that for HL; however, letters may be added to reflect organ involvement (B, bone; D, skin; E, extranodal; H, liver; L, lung; P, pleura). Treatment depends on many factors such as the age at presentation, stage of disease and co-morbidities. Treatment is usually with the CHOP regimen (cyclophosphamide, hydroxydaunorubicin, Oncovin (vincristine) and prednisolone). Rituximab, a monocloncal antibody, has been shown to be effective in combination with chemotherapy in improving remission rates.

A   **ENT A23 – Sleep apnoea**

Breathing disorders related to sleep can cause severe mortality and morbidity and should therefore be thoroughly investigated. The questions here tackle snoring and apnoeas. Either or both can cause episodes of oxygen deprivation. The long-term effects will therefore include pulmonary hypertension and dysrhythmias. Interrupted sleep can lead to hypersomnolence, lethargy during the day and reduced concentration. Sudden infant death has also been associated with apnoea. Snoring is essentially stridor and may be indicative of airway obstruction. Note that 20% of people snore, but only 1%–2% of women and 2%–4% of men suffer from apnoeas.

1. **A – 10-second cessation of breathing**. The definition of apnoea varies between professional bodies. However, commonalities are a 10-second pause in breathing. Reduction of ventilation by at least 50% for 10 seconds defines hypopnea. Sleep apnoea is defined as at least five episodes per hour of cessation of breathing lasting 10 seconds over a 7-hour sleep period. One is more likely to find apnoeas during the rapid eye movement phase of sleep. This is because this phase has a higher tolerance for lower saturations of oxygen. Also, during sleep, there is a reduced tone of the airway muscles. There are three types of apnoeas: obstructive, central and complex. These will be discussed further shortly.

2. **D – Advise to stop work**. Carlos is a bus driver and therefore poses a risk in terms of public safety with his symptoms of daytime lethargy, somnolence and reduced alertness. The key to identifying this risk is a thorough history. The first step in managing Carlos is to advise him against working until he is investigated and treated. Investigations into apnoeas include flexible laryngoscopies to assess the upper airway, imaging with CT and lateral X-rays of the post-nasal space, and sleep studies.

3. **H – Obstructive sleep apnoea** (OSA) is the most common apnoea and occurs as a result of intermittent airway collapse during sleep. Patients at risk are usually obese males with short, wide necks and a history of smoking, as described in the patient in the example. Excessive alcohol intake and sedative drugs may also exacerbate sleep disturbance. Patients often present with daytime lethargy, somnolence, reduced alertness, irritability and reduced libido. Clinical examinations are non-specific; however, patients who have a raised body mass index and a neck circumference of >48 cm are at risk. Acromegaly and hypothyroidism also increase the risk of OSA. Anatomically, there are three main sites that can cause snoring and OSA:
   - nasopharynx – polyps; defects in nasal septum
   - oropharynx – macroglossia; tonsillar hypertrophy (more common in children); jaw abnormalities, e.g. micrognathia
   - larynx/trachea – lesions, e.g. tumours.

For all of these sites, the main principle is that the upper airway is drawn close when a patient breathes in. As with the patient described in the example, patients tend to snore and thrash in an attempt to shift air. This patient underwent sleep studies or polysomnography. The parameters measured are oxygen saturations, electro-encephalogram, two electro-oculograms to measure eye movements, electro-myelogram to measure muscle movement (placed on the chin) and ECG to check for arrhythmias. Polysomnographies are expensive and often pulse oximeters are used in the first instance to monitor oxygen saturation levels during sleep. Specialists also observe chest and abdominal wall movements, and body position during sleep.

4. **F – Continuous positive airway pressure** (CPAP). The scenario given describes an extreme complication of poorly managed sleep apnoea. Such patients are also at risk of hypertension, myocardial infarction, dysrhythmias and stroke. CPAP is used to keep airways patent using compressed air at a titrated pressure in inspiration. On expiration, the bronchi and alveoli are prevented from collapsing. CPAP has the added advantage of minimising snoring. However, some patients find CPAP difficult to tolerate and it may also have social implications for patients and their partners. Non-compliance is therefore common. Management of sleep apnoea is multifaceted. It can be conservative with advice on weight loss, not sleeping on one's back, smoking cessation and avoiding alcohol in the evenings. Sedatives are relatively contraindicated in patients with known apnoea. Other interventions include intra-oral devices or mandibular positioning splints. These act by displacing the jaw anteriorly. This increases the diameter of the upper airway. Respiratory stimulants have also been suggested. In the case of polyps or a deflected septum, surgery may be required. Laser-assisted palatoplasty or uvulopharyngopalatoplasty with or without a tonsillectomy may be used to correct any upper airway narrowing. Maxillomandibular advancement surgery has become the surgical treatment of choice; studies have shown cure rates of up to 95% in treating sleep apnoea. In extreme cases a tracheostomy may be required to essentially bypass the upper airway.

5. **E – Central sleep apnoea** (CSA). The other types of apnoea are CSA and mixed sleep apnoea. The former is thought to occur as a result of cerebral assaults causing poor signals to the body's respiratory system. The respiratory system therefore does not respond appropriately to episodes of desaturation. The causes range from alcohol, opiates or sedation to cerebrovascular accidents, Parkinson's disease and high altitudes. However, many cases are also idiopathic. CSA is rare and occurs in less than 5% of patients with apnoea. Symptoms are similar to that of OSA (described earlier). A key difference is that in sleep studies of patients with CSA, there is no obvious chest wall movements or struggles for breath. Cheyne–Stokes breathing (progressively faster and deeper breathing that subsequently

becomes slower and more shallow until it temporarily stops – this pattern is cyclical) is a type of CSA. CPAP is recommended in managing these patients, as the cause of apnoea is usually irreversible or unknown. Acetazolamid (carbonic anhydrase inhibitor) has been used in treating CSA by reducing the pH of blood and hence encouraging respiration. Mixed sleep apnoea is a combination of OSA and CSA.

A ENT A24 – ENT disorders

1. **B – Glottic laryngeal carcinoma**. The cardinal symptoms such as dysphagia, malaise and weight loss should trigger your mind to think of some type of carcinoma. In this case, the involvement of the vocal cords should make a glottic laryngeal carcinoma the most likely diagnosis. Laryngeal carcinoma (LC) is the most common head and neck tumour, affecting 3.6 per 100 000 individuals in the United Kingdom. Patients usually present in their sixties. Males and females are affected at a ratio of 4:1. There are many risk factors attributed to LC; however, smoking and alcohol are the most implicated. Other risk factors include human papilloma virus infection, laryngopharyngeal reflux and exposure to radiation, fuel fumes and asbestos. Tumours are classified according to the affected region: (a) supraglottic, (b) glottis, and (c) subglottic. Individuals with LC present with symptoms of dysphagia, dysphonia (mainly glottic LC), dyspnoea (mainly supraglottic LC), lethargy, weight loss, neck lump and other non-specific symptoms. Haemoptysis, aspiration and otalgia are signs of more advanced LC. Although the history may be characteristic of LC, further testing in the form of flexible laryngoscopy enables a clinician to visualise the larynx. Biopsies can be taken via the same route under general anaesthetic. CT scanning and MRI can be used to assess the extent of the tumour and local tissue involvement. Positron emission tomography and CT scanning is useful in identifying the presence of metastasis. The investigations mentioned will aid in accurate staging of the tumour using the tumour, node and metastasis staging system. Staging allows the clinician to provide the largest amount of information to the patient concerning prognosis and treatment options. Treatment is tailored to every individual according to patient choice, staging and co-morbidities. In general, radical radiotherapy is the treatment of choice for T1 and T2 tumours. T4 tumours are treated by total laryngectomy and post-operative radiotherapy. The treatment of T3 tumours is debatable, as some advocate partial or total laryngectomy and others advocate radiotherapy. If nodal involvement is present a modified radical neck dissection is indicated with the addition of post-operative

radiotherapy. The exact surgical choice depends on the site, size and grade of tumour, which is beyond the realms of this book.

2. **F – Oral squamous cell carcinoma**. The vast majority of oral cancers (OCs) are squamous cell carcinomas. The diagnosis of OC in this particular case should be the top of your differential diagnosis because of the chronic nature of the lesion, the heterogenous colour (red and white), the exophytic (outward growing) margins and the pain experienced by the patient. Early oral squamous cell carcinoma appears as an indurated nodule or shallow ulcer, and often results in otalgia. Mouth ulcers that do not heal within 2 weeks should be biopsied to exclude neoplasia. Other signs that may suggest malignancy include bleeding from the ulcer, difficulty chewing and swallowing and palpable neck lumps. Risk factors for developing OC include smoking, drinking alcohol, poor dentition and chewing betel nuts. The latter is common among people in the Far East. Pipe smokers have an increased risk of lower lip cancer. As the mentioned risk factors are more associated with the male gender, OC affects males to females at a 2:1 ratio, with a peak incidence between the fifth and sixth decades. Individuals with OC usually present with a chronic lump/ulcer in the base of the mouth. The typical appearance of a malignant ulcer is a raised, exophytic lesion with a granular surface. The red regions of the ulcer represent malignant tissue with more dysplasia than the white region. Assessment of such lesions would require a full history and examination of the oral cavity and regional lymph nodes. Involvement of surrounding structures can be grossly assessed by palpating the size of tumour. Any palpable lymph nodes warrant further investigations with an ultrasound-guided FNA. Flexible nasoendoscopy should be done to visualise the oropharynx, larynx and oesophagus to investigate for other primary tumours. Imaging in the form of an orthopantogram should be done to assess for mandibular invasion. An MRI or spiral CT scan is useful in investigation for local invasion and to accurately measure the tumour. A chest X-ray is mandatory in all cases to exclude lung metastases. The information gathered from the investigations along with a biopsy of the lesion enables the clinician to stage the tumour. Surgery is indicated for all tumour stages and adjuvant radiotherapy is indicated post-operatively for T3/T4 tumours. Nodal involvement warrants a functional or radical neck dissection.

3. **D – Lichen planus** (LP) is a chronic inflammatory condition of the skin. Oral lesions may be found in about half of patients. LP may also affect the genitals. Oral LP occurs most commonly on the inside of the cheek

(buccal mucosa), appearing as white lines in a lace-like pattern. They may be asymptomatic, or may cause a stinging sensation in the mouth on eating/drinking. Unlike oral candidiasis, both oral LP and leukoplakia cannot be scraped off. Oral LP is a benign lesion of the oral mucosa. This has the appearance of a white plaque, with a characteristic smooth and shiny white surface. The aetiology of oral LP is not known, but there is an association with tobacco chewing, heavy alcohol drinking, chronic irritation of the mucosa (ill-fitted dentures, cheek biting) and oral candidiasis. Of importance, oral LP is pre-malignant and monitoring of the lesion with repeated biopsies is therefore essential. Treatment is decided by the size of the lesion; smaller lesions can be surgically excised or treated using laser therapy. Obtaining a biopsy is important, as different subtypes have different malignant potentials (verrucous oral LP has a larger potential for malignant change than homogenous oral LP).

4. **H – Pharyngeal diverticulum** (PD). The terms pharyngeal pouch and pharyngeal diverticulum are used interchangeably. You may even come across the term Zenker's diverticulum, which refers to a German physician, Friedrich von Zenker, who first described the pathology in 1877. A PD usually originates from the posterior aspect of the oesophagus. It is postulated that such pathology arises from an overactive upper-oesophageal sphincter. The herniation occurs through Killian's triangle, also called Killian's dehiscence (superior to the cricopharyngeus muscle, between the two heads of the inferior constrictor muscle). The condition most commonly occurs in elderly males. Symptoms of dysphagia, cachexia and aspiration pneumonia should always add PD to your differential diagnosis. Patients may also present with difficulty coughing, gurgling sounds in the neck, halitosis and regurgitation of undigested food. These symptoms may not be elicited if they are not asked about directly. A barium swallow is diagnostic of this condition and gives more information regarding the exact location and size of the diverticulum. Once the immediate illness is managed (i.e. treating the aspiration pneumonia, keeping the patient nil by mouth and inserting a nasogastric tube for feeding) and the patient is stable, definitive treatment for the PD can be considered. Open surgical repairs have been superseded by endoscopic procedures. The current treatment of choice is endoscopic stapling of pharyngeal pouch – namely, Dolman's procedure. It is imperative to investigate a patient fully for any upper gastrointestinal malignancies first, and the diverticulum is visualised clearly with a diverticuloscope to biopsy any suspicious lesions.

5. **J – Tracheo-oesophageal fistula** (TOF). As the name implies, a TOF is an abnormal connection between the trachea and the oesophagus. It is a common congenital anomaly, but may be acquired later in life. The most common cause of acquired TOFs is mediastinal malignancy (~75% oesophageal), followed by endotracheal cuff-related trauma. Ono's sign is characteristic, referring to uncontrolled coughing after swallowing solids or liquids. Other symptoms include coughing, chest pain, dyspnoea, hoarseness and recurrent pneumonias. The diagnosis can be confirmed by barium swallow, flexible oesophagoscopy or flexible bronchoscopy. It is important to exclude underlying malignancies, such as oesophageal cancer, which may be present in this patient. The mainstay of treatment is surgical repair. Oesophageal stenting is used as a palliative measure in inoperable malignancy-related TOF.

An **aphthous ulcer** or canker sore (more accurately termed 'recurrent aphthous stomatitis') can be minor or major. Most (~80%) are classified as minor aphthous ulcers, and are experienced by most people at some point in their lives. They are characterised by recurrent, painful, small, punched-out mucosal lesions that are surrounded by an erythematous halo. These do not normally last for more than 2 weeks. They typically start in childhood and resolve by the third decade. A positive family history is common. The aetiology is unknown, and no treatment is usually required. The two other less common types of recurrent aphthous stomatitis are major aphthous ulcers and herpitoform ulcers. Systemic conditions (e.g. coeliac disease, Crohn's disease, Behçet's disease) can also be associated with aphthous-like mouth ulcers.

The incidence of laryngeal cancer is about five folds that of **oropharyngeal cancer** (OPC). Moreover, the mortality rate from OPC has decreased by around 35% over the last 3 decades. OPC has a male predominance of 3:1 and usually affects men in their sixth to seventh decades. Patients characteristically present late when symptoms of local compression of adjacent structures have developed. Symptoms include dysphagia, the feeling of a lump in the throat, sore throat and otalgia. The latter is secondary to compression to divisions of the vagus nerve that cause referred pain in the ear. Moreover, symptoms reflecting advanced disease such as haemoptysis, weight loss, hoarse voice and laryngeal stridor can manifest as the disease progresses. Investigations and treatment options are very similar to laryngeal carcinoma, as described earlier.

Index

CPD with Radcliffe

You can now use a selection of our books to achieve CPD (Continuing Professional Development) points through directed reading.

We provide a free online form and downloadable certificate for your appraisal portfolio. Look for the CPD logo and register with us at: www.radcliffehealth.com/cpd

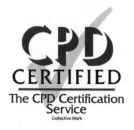

CERTIFIED
The CPD Certification
Service
Collective Mark